Maternity Nursing

Shannon E. Perry
RN, CNS, PhD, FAAN
Professor Emerita, School of Nursing
San Francisco State University
San Francisco, California

Deitra Leonard Lowdermilk
RNC, PhD, FAAN
Clinical Professor Emerita, School of Nursing
University of North Carolina at Chapel Hill
Chapel Hill, North Carolina

CONSULTANT
Kitty Cashion, RN, BC, MSN
Clinical Nurse Specialist
University of Tennessee Health Science Center
Department of Obstetrics and Gynecology
Division of Maternal-Fetal Medicine
Memphis, Tennessee

MOSBY

ELSEVIER

MOSBY
ELSEVIER

11830 Westline Industrial Drive
St. Louis, Missouri 63146

CLINICAL COMPANION FOR MATERNITY NURSING, SEVENTH EDITION

ISBN-10: 0-323-03163-3
ISBN-13: 978-0-323-03163-9

Notice

Knowledge and best practice in this field are constantly changing. As new research and experience broaden our knowledge, changes in practice, treatment, and drug therapy may become necessary or appropriate. Readers are advised to check the most current product information provided (i) on procedures featured or (ii) by the manufacturer of each product to be administered to verify the recommended dose or formula, the method and duration of administration, and contraindications. It is the responsibility of the practitioner, relying on his or her own experience and knowledge of the patient, to make diagnoses, to determine dosages and the best treatment for each individual patient, and to take all appropriate safety precautions. To the fullest extent of the law, neither the Publisher nor the Authors assume any liability for any injury and/or damage to persons or property arising from or related to any use of the material contained in this book.

ISBN-10: 0-323-03163-3
ISBN-13: 978-0-323-03163-9

Acquisitions Editor: Catherine Jackson
Senior Developmental Editor: Laurie K. Gower
Publishing Services Manager: Jeff Patterson
Project Manager: Anne Konopka
Cover Design: Amy Buxton
Design Direction: Paula Ruckenbrod

Printed in the United States of America.

Last digit is the print number: 9 8 7 6 5 4 3 2 1

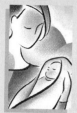

Preface

Purpose

This Clinical Companion was written for nursing students and practicing nurses. Its handy size makes it a portable reference book that can easily be carried to the clinical area where information that relates to hands-on practice is most useful. Although the authors briefly explain essential background information and describe expected medical interventions, the focus is on nursing assessments and interventions. This Clinical Companion complements the seventh edition of *Maternity Nursing* by Lowdermilk and Perry, but it can be used alone by nurses who need only a review or a quick reference.

Content and Organization

The companion book is divided into six units. Unit 1 provides an overview community and home care. Unit 2 addresses women's health with a focus on risk identification and anticipatory guidance. Common reproductive system concerns are considered, including problems of the breast and common neoplasms. Contraception is reviewed.

Unit 3, Pregnancy, includes antepartum assessment, maternal and fetal nutrition, and nursing care during pregnancy. In addition, this section addresses therapeutic management and nursing considerations of complications of pregnancy.

Unit 4, Childbirth, describes management of discomfort, fetal assessment, and nursing care during labor. This section also addresses therapeutic management and nursing considerations of complications of labor and birth.

Unit 5, Postpartum, describes nursing care required during normal and complicated postpartum periods.

Unit 6, Newborn, describes assessment and care of the newborn and nutrition and feeding. Problems of the newborn related to gestational age and acquired and congenital problems are addressed. Nursing considerations related to grieving the loss of a newborn are included.

Guides for some of the most common procedures in maternal-newborn nursing are included. Tools for assessment are included where relevant.

Appendices include English-Spanish translations, as well as useful words and phrases, and medication guides. Also included are Standard Precautions guidelines, temperature equivalents, conversion of pounds to grams, NANDA-Approved nursing diagnoses, the most current JCAHO Do Not Use list, and a table on traditional cultural beliefs and practices of childbearing and parenting. A bibliography is included for reference.

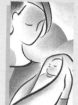

Contents

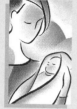

Community and Home Care

Most health care for women occurs outside the acute care setting. The movement to reduce health care costs has shortened hospitalization time and led to an increase of home- and community-based options for the provision of care. Hospital stays after childbirth may be abbreviated. By minimizing inpatient length of stay, much of acute care nursing has been transferred to home-based nursing services in local communities.

HEALTH AND WELLNESS IN THE COMMUNITY

Public Health Services

Public health services are essential to provide for the needs of the community, especially for those who do not have the resources to access needed health care (Box 1-1). Communities must do assessments to determine the needs of the populations they serve.

ASSESSING THE COMMUNITIES IN WHICH FAMILIES LIVE

Mothers assume much of the health-related decision making for their families, with up to 83% of them having sole or shared responsibility for financial decisions affecting family health. A significant link exists between the maternal roles of health care provider and decision maker and family health behavior. The health and well-being of women and children will be in jeopardy as long as the communities in which they live are ill prepared to provide the quantity and quality of services they need.

BOX 1-1

Essential Public Health Services

1. Monitor health status to identify community health problems.
2. Diagnose and investigate health problems and health hazards in the community.
3. Enforce laws and regulations that protect health and ensure safety.
4. Inform, educate, and empower people about health issues.
5. Mobilize community partnerships to identify and solve health problems.
6. (a) Link people to needed personal health services. (b) Ensure the provision of health care when otherwise unavailable.
7. Evaluate effectiveness, accessibility, and quality of personal and population-based health services.
8. Ensure a competent public health and personal health care workforce.
9. Develop policies and plans that support individual and community health efforts.
10. Research for new insights and innovative solutions to health problems.

Source: Essential Public Health Services Work Group of the Public Health Functions Steering Committee. Internet document available from www.phf.org/essential.htm (accessed July 9, 2005).

Methods of Community Assessment

With the community as the focus of perinatal health care, the nurse must become familiar with the neighborhoods and resources that influence patients. Community assessment is a complex although well-defined process through which the unique characteristics of the populations and their special needs are identified to plan and evaluate health services for the community as a whole.

The most critical indicators of perinatal health in a community are related to access to health care; maternal mortality; infant mortality; low birth weight; first-trimester prenatal care;

and rates for mammography, Papanicolaou smears, and other similar screening tests. Nurses may use these indicators as a reflection of access, quality, and continuity of health care in a community. They may use a variety of sources of data to assess the community.

Data collection methods may include visual surveys that can be completed by walking through a community (Box 1-2); participant observation, interviews, and analysis of existing data; focus groups or community forums; and formal surveys, conducted by mail, by telephone, or by face-to-face interviews.

COMMUNITY HEALTH PROMOTION

Health promotion efforts for childbearing families are primarily focused on early intervention through prenatal care and prevention of complications during the perinatal period. Often this early exposure to health information sets the stage for a successful birth and positive outcomes for mother and baby. Involving expectant mothers and fathers in identification of their learning needs is an essential first step to securing their participation in the health promotion process.

PERINATAL CONTINUUM OF CARE

Within the community, perinatal care is provided on a continuum. A continuum of care is defined as a range of clinical services provided for an individual or group that reflects care given during a single hospitalization or care for multiple conditions over a lifetime. Home care is one delivery component available along the perinatal continuum of care.

HOME CARE PERINATAL SERVICES

Patient Selection and Referral

The office- or hospital-based nurse is often the key person in making effective referrals to home care. When a referral to home care is considered, the following factors are evaluated:

- Health status of mother and fetus or infant: Is the condition serious enough to warrant home care? Is it stable enough for intermittent observation to be sufficient?

BOX 1-2

Community Walk-Through

Physical environment—Older neighborhood or newer addition? Sidewalks, streets, and buildings in good or poor repair? Billboards and signs, and what are they advertising? Lawns kept up? Trash in the streets? Parks or playgrounds? Parking lots? Empty lots?

People in the area—Old, young, homeless, children, predominant ethnicity, language?

Services available—Restaurants—chain, local, ethnic? Grocery stores—neighborhood or chain? Department stores, gas stations, real estate or insurance offices, travel agencies, pawn shops, liquor stores, discount or thrift stores, newspaper stands?

Social and religious—Clubs, bars, fraternal organizations (e.g., Elks, American Legion), museums, churches, synagogues, mosques?

Health services—Drug stores, physicians' offices, clinics, dentists' offices, mental health services, veterinarians' offices, urgent care facilities, hospital, shelters?

Transportation—Cars, buses, taxis, light rail, sidewalks, bicycle paths, access for disabled persons?

Education—Schools, before- and after-school programs, child care, libraries, book stores? Reputation of the schools?

Government—What is the governance structure? Is there a mayor? City council? Meetings open to the public?

Safety—How safe is the community? Crime rate? Types of crimes committed? Police visible? Is there a fire station?

Evaluation of the community based on your observations—Your impression of the community? Pleasing environment? Adequate services and transportation? How difficult is it for residents to obtain needed services; that is, how far do they have to travel? Would you want to live in this community? Why or why not?

- Availability of professionals to provide the needed services within the patient's community
- Family resources, including psychosocial, social, and economic resources: Will the family be able to provide care between nursing visits? Are relationships supportive? Is third-party reimbursement available, or can it be negotiated with the insurer? Could a voluntary or tax-supported community agency provide needed care without payment?
- Cost-effectiveness: Is it more reasonable for the patient to receive these services at home or to go to a local outpatient facility to receive them?

Preparing for the Home Visit

The home care nurse reviews the available clinical data, demographic information, and completed plan of care form and consults with the home care pharmacist or other health care team members who have previously contacted the woman to determine the goals of the visit. At this point the nurse uses the medical diagnosis and place on the perinatal continuum as a starting point to organize the woman's care. The nurse reviews agency policies and procedures, professional literature about diagnosis, and community resources as part of the previsit preparation work (Box 1-3).

First Home Care Visit

Assessment

The major areas of the assessment are demographics, medical history, general health history, medication history, sociocultural assessment, home and community environment, and physical assessment. Some of this information can be obtained from patient records sent to the home care agency at the time of referral or from the previsit interview. These data will be used to develop the nursing care plan and complete the plan of care, which is required for many licensed home health care agencies.

Social assessment includes information regarding the number of people in the family, the roles of each household member, which family members or individuals have taken on the roles

Text continued on p. 9.

BOX 1-3

Protocol for Perinatal Home Visits

PREVISIT INTERVENTIONS

1. Contact family to arrange details for home visit.
   a. Identify self, credentials, and agency role.
   b. Review purpose of home visit follow-up.
   c. Schedule convenient time for visit.
   d. Confirm address and route to family home.
2. Review and clarify appropriate data.
   a. Review all available assessment data for mother and fetus or infant (e.g., referral forms, hospital discharge summaries, family-identified learning needs).
   b. Review records of any previous nursing contacts.
   c. Contact other professional caregivers as necessary to clarify data (e.g., obstetrician, nurse-midwife, pediatrician, referring nurse).
3. Identify community resources and teaching materials appropriate to meet needs already identified.
4. Plan the visit; and prepare bag with equipment, supplies, and materials necessary for assessments of mother and fetus or infant, actual care anticipated, and teaching.

IN-HOME INTERVENTIONS: ESTABLISHING A RELATIONSHIP

1. Reintroduce self and establish purpose of visit for mother, infant, and family; offer family opportunity to clarify their expectations of contact.
2. Spend brief time socially interacting with family to become acquainted and establish trusting relationship.

IN-HOME INTERVENTIONS: WORKING WITH FAMILY

1. Conduct systematic assessment of mother and fetus or newborn to determine physiologic adjustment and any existing complications.
2. Throughout visit, collect data to assess the emotional adjustment of individual family members to pregnancy or birth and lifestyle changes. Note evidence of family-newborn bonding and sibling

BOX 1-3

Protocol for Perinatal Home Visits—cont'd

rivalry; note relationships among mother, father, children, and grandparents.

3. Determine adequacy of support system.
   a. To what extent does someone help with cooking, cleaning, and other home management tasks?
   b. To what extent is help being provided in caring for the newborn and any other children?
   c. Are support persons encouraging the new mother to care for herself and get adequate rest?
   d. Who is providing helpful information? Emotional support?
4. Throughout the visit, observe home environment for adequacy of resources.
   a. Space: privacy, safe play of children, sleeping
   b. Overall cleanliness and state of repair
   c. Number of steps pregnant woman/new mother must climb
   d. Adequacy of cooking arrangements
   e. Adequacy of refrigeration and other food storage areas
   f. Adequacy of bathing, toilet, and laundry facilities
   g. Arrangements in home for newborn: sleeping, bathing, formula preparation (if needed), layette items, and diapers
5. Throughout the visit, observe home environment for overall state of repair and existence of safety hazards.
   a. Storage of medications, household cleaners, and other substances hazardous to children
   b. Presence of peeling paint on furniture, walls, or pipes
   c. Factors that contribute to falls, such as dim lighting, broken steps, scatter rugs
   d. Presence of vermin
   e. Use of crib or playpen that fails to meet safety guidelines
   f. Existence of emergency plan in case of fire; fire alarm or extinguisher

Continued

BOX 1-3

Protocol for Perinatal Home Visits—cont'd

6. Provide care to mother, newborn, or both as prescribed by their respective primary care provider or in accord with agency protocol.
7. Provide teaching on basis of previously identified needs.
8. Refer family to appropriate community agencies or resources, such as warm lines and support groups.
9. Ascertain that woman knows potential problems to watch for and whom to call if they occur.
10. Ensure that used disposable items have been handled appropriately and that reusable items are cleaned and repacked appropriately in the nurse's bag.

IN-HOME INTERVENTIONS: ENDING THE VISIT

1. Summarize the activities and main points of the visit. ·
2. Clarify future expectations, including schedule of next visit.
3. Review teaching plan, and provide major points in writing.
4. Provide information about reaching the nurse or agency if needed before the next scheduled visit.

POSTVISIT INTERVENTIONS

1. Document the visit thoroughly, using the necessary agency forms to serve as a legal record of the visit and to allow third-party reimbursement, as possible.
2. Initiate the plan of care on which the next encounter with the woman and family will be based.
3. Communicate appropriately (by telephone, letter, progress notes, or referral form) with primary care provider, other health professionals, or referral agencies on behalf of woman and family.

of caregivers, and the woman's social support network (Box 1-4). Identifying the roles of each member is helpful for developing the plan of care.

Physical assessment of the home environment is an essential element of the home care assessment. The major areas of the home environment assessment include physical features of the home, access to the home, sanitary conditions, the presence of utilities (e.g., indoor plumbing, telephone, and electricity), safety features, and access to transportation and emergency support. During the physical inspection, careful consideration should be taken to avoid moving personal belongings that are not affected by the care.

Safety issues for the home care nurse

- Be aware of the home environment and neighborhood in which the home care is being provided.
- Take necessary safety precautions, and avoid dangerous areas.
- Conduct a violence potential assessment by telephone before the visit, and enlist the patient's cooperation in minimizing risk.
- If necessary, have hired full-time security personnel accompany nurses on their visits.
- Personal strategies recommended for nurses visiting families with a history of violence or substance abuse
  - Self-awareness
  - Environmental assessment
  - Use of listening and observation skills with patients to be aware of behavioral changes indicating aggression or lack of impulse control
  - Available plan for dealing with aggressive behavior (e.g., allowing personal space and taking a nonaggressive stance)
  - Making visits in pairs
  - Access to a cellular phone at all times
- Personal safety considerations
  - Dress should be casual but professional in appearance.
  - Wear a name identification tag.
  - Limited jewelry should be worn.
  - Valuable personal items, such as an expensive purse or coat, should not be worn on a visit.

BOX 1-4

Psychosocial Assessment

LANGUAGE

Identify the primary language spoken in the home.
Assess whether there are any language barriers to
receiving support.

COMMUNITY RESOURCES AND ACCESS TO CARE

Identify primary and secondary means of
transportation.
Identify community agencies the family currently uses
for health care and support.
Assess cultural and psychosocial barriers to receiving
care.

SOCIAL SUPPORT

Determine the people living with the pregnant woman.
Identify who assists with household chores.
Identify who assists with child care and parenting
activities.
Identify to whom the pregnant woman turns when
problems occur or during a crisis.

INTERPERSONAL RELATIONSHIPS

Identify the way decisions are made in the family.
Identify the family's perception of the need for home
care.
Identify roles of adults in caring for family members.

CAREGIVERS

Identify the primary caregiver for home care treatments.
Identify other caregivers and their roles.
Assess the caregiver's knowledge of treatments and
care process.
Identify potential strain from the caregiver role.
Identify the level of satisfaction with the caregiver role.

STRESS AND COPING

Identify what the woman perceives as lifestyle changes
and their impact on her and her family.
Identify the changes she and her family have made to
adjust to her health condition and home health care
treatments.

—Carrying an extra set of car keys in the nursing home care bag saves time and frustration if the nurse becomes locked out of the automobile. Automobile keys spread between the fingers with sharp ends outward can be used as a weapon if necessary.

—The same commonsense behaviors and precautions that guide a person's behavior when alone in any setting should be followed by home care nurses.

- Agency considerations

  —The agency is responsible for safety of home care staff. All home care agencies should have policies to follow in unsafe situations.

- Transportation for home care visits

  —The automobile used for the home care visits should have regular preventive maintenance checks, an adequate fuel level, and road safety items stored in the trunk.

  —Items to carry in the vehicle include change for telephone calls and tolls, maps, emergency telephone numbers, a flashlight, a first aid kit, flares, a blanket, and equipment for inclement weather conditions.

  —When a visit is made to a patient in a more remote rural setting, other travel considerations may be needed, as well as additional supplies or medication to be taken to the patient.

  —Home care nurses should park and lock their cars in a safe place that is visible from the street and the patient's home and away from hidden alleys.

  —While driving to the patient's home, the nurse should assess the neighborhood for safety, especially if the neighborhood is unfamiliar.

  —All valuable items should be stored out of sight before the nurse leaves the office.

  —While walking to the patient's home, nurses should not walk near groups of strangers hanging out in doorways or alleys, enter vacant buildings, or enter a yard that has an unrestrained dog.

  —The home or building should not be entered if the nurse has any safety concerns.

- Unsafe situations in the patient's home

—The nurse may encounter unsafe situations such as the presence of weapons, abusive behavior, or health hazards.

—Each potentially hazardous situation must be dealt with according to agency policies and procedures.

—If abuse or neglect is reasonably suspected, the home care nurse should follow home care agency and state and federal regulations for reporting and documenting the situation.

—Nurses should maintain their own safety first and act accordingly throughout the visit.

Infection control

The nurse carries the necessary supplies and equipment to provide nursing care to the woman. Standard Precautions should be used whenever a treatment is performed.

Handwashing remains the single most important infection-control procedure. Hands should be washed thoroughly for 15 to 20 seconds before and after each patient contact. Wearing gloves does not eliminate the necessity for handwashing. If running water or clean facilities are unavailable, the hands can be cleaned with a self-drying antibacterial solution.

Medication administration

A careful medication history should be obtained to see if the woman is taking her medications correctly and understands the desired action and potential side effects. Sometimes when orders are changed, women continue to take both the old and new prescriptions, which can lead to dangerous overdoses or medication interactions. Over-the-counter drugs or herbal supplements may not be considered medications by the woman and not mentioned unless such information is specifically requested.

Documentation

Clear documentation of assessments, problems identified, treatments and interventions performed, and the patient's responses is essential. Third-party payers base reimbursement on the nurse's written record of providing skilled nursing care and assessments that support the woman's continuing need for those services. The nurse must promptly inform the health care provider by telephone or facsimile (fax) of any significant changes. When new orders are transmitted by telephone, a written copy must be sent for the physician's signature.

Nursing documentation should reflect an objective description of the nursing assessment data collected at each visit. Once the home care outcomes are achieved and the patient is discharged from the home care agency, documentation should include information about the patient's status at the time of discharge, progress toward attaining health care goals, and plans for follow-up care. Appropriate care should be taken to complete the necessary home health care records accurately and in a timely manner. Documentation guidelines include writing or dictating notes or using a laptop computer at the patient's home or shortly after the visit.

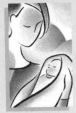

CHAPTER 2

Assessment and Health Promotion

HEALTH ASSESSMENT

Interview

- Communication may be hindered by different beliefs even when the nurse and patient speak the same language. The Cultural Considerations box lists examples of communication variations.

- Women with emotional or physical disorders have special needs. Women who are visually, aurally, emotionally, or physically disabled should be respected and involved in the assessment and physical examination to the full extent of their abilities. The assessment and physical examination can be adapted to each woman's individual needs.

- All women entering the health care system should be screened for potential abuse. An abuse assessment screen can be used as part of the interview or written history (Fig. 2-1). If a male partner is present, he should be asked to leave the room, because the woman may not disclose experiences of abuse in his presence or he may try to answer questions for her to protect himself.

- The areas most commonly injured in women are the head, neck, chest, abdomen, breasts, and upper extremities. Burns and bruises in patterns resembling hands, belts, cords, or other weapons and multiple traumatic injuries may be seen.

- An interview with a teenager should assess for hints about risky behaviors, eating disorders, and depression. Do not assume that a teenager is not sexually active. After rapport has been established, it is best to talk to a teen with the parent (or partner or friend) out of the room. Questions should be

Cultural Considerations

Communication Variations

- *Conversational style and pacing:* Silence may show respect or acknowledgment that the listener has heard. In cultures in which a direct "no" is considered rude, silence may mean no. Repetition or loudness may mean emphasis or anger.
- *Personal space:* Conceptions of personal space differ, based on one's culture. Someone may be perceived as distant for backing off when approached or aggressive for standing too close.
- *Eye contact:* Eye contact varies among cultures from intense to fleeting. In an effort to refrain from invading personal space, avoiding direct eye contact may be a sign of respect.
- *Touch:* The norms about how people should touch each other vary among cultures. In some cultures, physical contact with the same gender (embracing, walking hand in hand) is more appropriate than that with an unrelated person of the opposite gender.
- *Time orientation:* In some cultures, involvement with people is more valued than being "on time." In other cultures, life is scheduled and paced according to clock time, which is valued over personal time.

Reference: Mattson, S. (2000). Striving for cultural competence: Providing care for the changing face of the U.S. *AWHONN Lifelines, 4*(3), 48-52.

asked with sensitivity and in a gentle and nonjudgmental manner.

History

A medical history usually includes the following:

1. *Identifying data.* Name, age, sex, race, and occupation are obtained.
2. *Chief complaint(s).* A verbatim response to the question, "What problem or symptom brought you here today?"
3. *History of present illness.* A chronologic narrative that includes onset of the problem, the setting in which it developed, its manifestations, and any treatments received is noted. The woman's state of health before the onset of the present

ABUSE ASSESSMENT SCREEN

1. Have you ever been emotionally or physically abused by your partner or someone important to you?

   YES ☐ NO ☐

2. Within the last year, have you been hit, slapped, kicked, or otherwise physically hurt by someone?

   YES ☐ NO ☐

   If YES, by whom ______________________

   Number of times ______________________

   Mark the area of injury on body map.

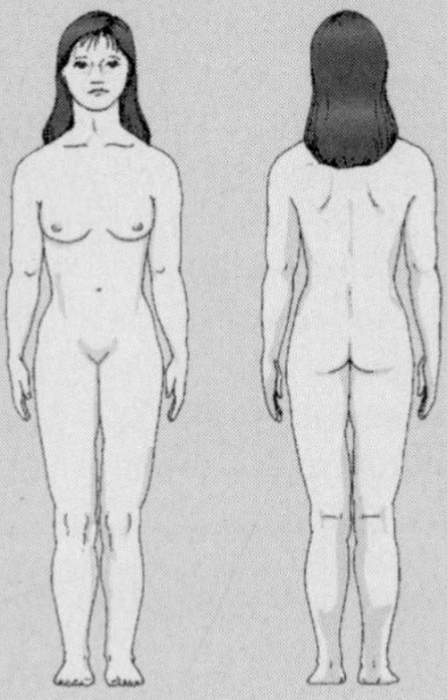

3. Within the last year, has anyone forced you to have sexual activities?

   YES ☐ NO ☐

   If YES, by whom ______________________

   Number of times ______________________

4. Are you afraid of your partner or anyone you listed above?

   YES ☐ NO ☐

Fig. 2-1 Abuse assessment screen. (Modified from the Nursing Research Consortium on Violence and Abuse.)

problem is determined. If the problem is long-standing, the reason for seeking attention at this time is elicited. The principal symptoms should be described with regard to the following:

- Location
- Quality
- Quantity or severity
- Timing (onset, duration, frequency)
- Setting
- Factors that aggravate or relieve
- Associated manifestations

4. *Past medical history.* Determine general state of health and strength:
   - Infectious diseases: measles, mumps, rubella, whooping cough, chicken pox, rheumatic fever, scarlet fever, diphtheria, polio, tuberculosis (TB), or hepatitis
   - Chronic diseases and system disorders: arthritis, cancer, diabetes, heart, lung, kidney, seizures, stroke, or ulcers
   - Adult injuries, accidents, illnesses, disabilities, hospitalizations, or blood transfusions

5. *Present health status.*
   - Allergies: medications, previous transfusion reactions, or environmental allergies
   - Immunizations: diphtheria, pertussis, tetanus; polio; measles, mumps, rubella (MMR); hepatitis B, varicella, influenza, and pneumococcal vaccine; last TB skin test
   - Screening tests: Pap test, mammogram, stool for occult blood, sigmoidoscopy or colonoscopy, chest x-ray study, hematocrit, hemoglobin, rubella titer, urinalysis, and cholesterol test; blood type and Rh; last eye examination; last dental examination
   - Environmental and chemical hazards: home, school, work, and leisure setting; exposure to extreme heat or cold, noise, industrial toxins such as asbestos or lead, pesticides, diethylstilbestrol (DES), radiation, cat feces, or cigarette smoke
   - Use of safety measures: seat belts, bicycle helmets, designated driver
   - Exercise and leisure activities: regular
   - Sleep patterns: length and quality

- Sexuality: Is she sexually active? With men, women, or both? Safer sex practices?
- Diet, including beverages: 24-hour dietary recall
- Medications: name, dose, frequency, duration, reason for taking, and compliance with prescription medications; home remedies, over-the-counter drugs, vitamin and mineral supplements used over a 24-hour period; herbal therapies
- Nicotine, alcohol, illicit or recreational drugs: type, amount, frequency, duration, and reactions
- Caffeine: coffee, tea, cola, or chocolate intake

6. *Past surgical history.* Type, date, reason, outcome, and any complications should be noted.

7. *Family history.* Information about age and health of family members may be presented in narrative or genogram: age, health status, or death of parents, siblings, spouse, and children. Check for history of diabetes, heart disease, hypertension, stroke, respiratory disorders, renal disorders, thyroid disorders, cancer, bleeding disorders, hepatitis, allergies, asthma, arthritis, TB, epilepsy, mental illness, HIV, and other conditions.

8. *Social history.* Note birthplace, education, employment, marital status, living accommodations, children, persons at home, and hobbies. Does she enjoy what she is doing?
   - Screen for abuse: Has she ever been hit, kicked, slapped, or forced to have sex against her wishes? Has she been verbally or emotionally abused? Does she have a history of childhood sexual abuse? If yes, has she received counseling or does she need referral?

9. *Review of systems.* It is probable that all questions in each system will not be included every time a history is taken. Some questions regarding each system should be included in every history. The essential areas to be explored are listed in the following head-to-toe sequence. If a woman gives a positive response to a question about an essential area, more detailed questions should be asked.
   - General: weight change, fatigue, weakness, fever, chills, or night sweats
   - Skin: skin, hair, and nail changes; itching; bruising; bleeding; rashes; sores; lumps; or moles

- Lymph nodes: enlargement, inflammation, pain, suppuration (pus), or drainage
- Head, eyes, ears, nose, and throat (HEENT): head–trauma, vertigo (dizziness), convulsive disorder, syncope (fainting), headache location, frequency, pain type, nausea or vomiting, or visual symptoms; eyes–glasses, contact lenses, blurriness, tearing, itching, photophobia, diplopia, inflammation, trauma, cataracts, glaucoma, or acute visual loss; ears–hearing loss, tinnitus (ringing), vertigo, discharge, pain, fullness, recurrent infections, or mastoiditis; nose and sinuses–trauma, rhinitis, nasal discharge, epistaxis, obstruction, sneezing, itching, allergy, or smelling impairment; mouth, throat, and neck–hoarseness, voice changes, soreness, ulcers, bleeding gums, goiter, swelling, or enlarged nodes
- Breasts: masses, pain, lumps, dimpling, nipple discharge, fibrocystic changes, or implants; BSE practice (see Patient Instructions for Self-Care box, p. 24)
- Respiratory: shortness of breath, wheezing, cough, sputum, hemoptysis, pneumonia, pleurisy, asthma, bronchitis, emphysema, or TB; date and result of last chest x-ray examination
- Cardiac: hypertension, rheumatic fever, murmurs, angina, palpitations, dyspnea, tachycardia, orthopnea, edema, chest pain, cough, cyanosis, cold extremities, ascites, intermittent claudication (calf pain), phlebitis, or skin color changes
- GI: appetite, nausea, vomiting, indigestion, dysphagia, abdominal pain, ulcers, hematochezia (bleeding with stools), melena (black, tarry stools), bowel habit changes, diarrhea, constipation, bowel movement frequency, food intolerance, hemorrhoids, jaundice, or hepatitis; sigmoidoscopy, colonoscopy, barium enema, or ultrasound
- Genitourinary (GU): frequency, hesitancy, urgency, polyuria, dysuria, hematuria, nocturia, incontinence, stones, infection, or urethral discharge; dysmenorrhea, intermenstrual bleeding, dyspareunia, discharge, sores, itching, STIs, gravidity (G), parity (P), problems in pregnancy, contraception, menopause, hot flashes, or sweats (may be included here or as part of endocrine assessment)

- Vascular: leg edema, claudication, varicose veins, thromboses, or emboli
- Endocrine: heat or cold intolerance, dry skin, excessive sweating, polyuria, polydipsia, polyphagia, thyroid problems, diabetes, or secondary sex characteristic changes; age at menarche, length and flow of menses, last menstrual period (LMP), age at menopause; libido or sexual concerns
- Hematologic: anemia, easy bruising, bleeding, petechiae, purpura, or transfusions
- Musculoskeletal: muscle weakness, pain, joint stiffness, scoliosis, lordosis, kyphosis, range-of-motion instability, redness, swelling, arthritis, or gout
- Neurologic: loss of sensation, numbness, tingling, tremors, weakness, vertigo, paralysis, fainting, twitching, blackouts, seizures, convulsions, loss of consciousness or memory
- Psychiatric: moodiness, depression, anxiety, obsessions, delusions, illusions, or hallucinations

Physical Examination

Objective data are recorded by system or location. A general statement of overall health status is a good way to start. Findings are described in detail.

- General appearance: age, race, gender, state of health, stature, development, dress, hygiene, affect, alertness, orientation, cooperativeness, communication skills
- Vital signs: temperature, pulse, respiration, blood pressure
- Height and weight
- Skin: color; integrity; texture; hydration; temperature; edema; excessive perspiration; unusual odor; presence and description of lesions; hair texture and distribution; nail configuration; color, texture, condition of nails or presence of nail clubbing
- Head: size, shape, trauma, masses, scars, rashes, or scaling; facial symmetry; presence of edema or puffiness
- Eyes: pupil size, shape, reactivity; conjunctival injection; scleral icterus; fundal papilledema; hemorrhage; lids; extraocular movements; visual fields and acuity

- Ears: shape and symmetry, tenderness, discharge, external canal, and tympanic membranes; hearing: Weber test should be midline (loudness of sound equal in both ears) and Rinne test negative (no conductive or sensorineural hearing loss); should be able to hear whisper at 3 feet
- Nose: symmetry, tenderness, discharge, mucosa, turbinate inflammation, frontal and maxillary sinus tenderness; discrimination of odors
- Mouth, throat: hygiene, condition of teeth, dentures, appearance of lips, tongue, buccal and oral mucosa, erythema, edema, exudate, tonsillar enlargement, palate, uvula, gag reflex, ulcers
- Neck: mobility, masses, range of motion, trachea deviation, thyroid size, carotid bruits
- Lymphatic: cervical, intraclavicular, axillary, trochlear, or inguinal adenopathy; size, shape, tenderness, consistency
- Breasts: skin changes, dimpling, symmetry, scars, tenderness, discharge or masses; characteristics of nipples and areolae
- Heart: rate, rhythm, murmurs, rubs, gallops, clicks, heaves, or precordial movements
- Peripheral vascular: jugular vein distention, bruits, edema, swelling, vein distention, Homans sign, or tenderness of extremities
- Lungs: chest symmetry with respirations, wheezes, crackles, rhonchi, vocal fremitus, whispered pectoriloquy, percussion, and diaphragmatic excursion; breath sounds equal and clear bilaterally
- Abdomen: shape, scars, bowel sounds, consistency, tenderness, rebound, masses, guarding, organomegaly, liver span, percussion (tympany, shifting, dullness), costovertebral angle tenderness
- Extremities: edema, ulceration, tenderness, varicosities, erythema, tremor, or deformity
- GU: external genitalia, perineum, vaginal mucosa, cervix, inflammation, tenderness, discharge, bleeding, ulcers, nodules, masses, internal vaginal support, bimanual and rectovaginal examination; palpation of cervix, uterus, and adnexa

- Rectal: sphincter tone, masses, hemorrhoids, rectal wall contour, tenderness, and stool for occult blood
- Musculoskeletal: posture, symmetry of muscle mass, muscle atrophy, weakness, appearance of joints, tenderness or crepitus, joint range of motion, instability, redness, swelling, or spine deviation
- Neurologic: mental status, orientation, memory, mood, speech clarity and comprehension, cranial nerves II through XII, sensation, strength, deep tendon and superficial reflexes, gait, balance, and coordination with rapid alternating motions

Pelvic Examination

- The woman is assisted into the lithotomy position for the pelvic examination. External inspection and palpation are done before the internal examination. A speculum is inserted to view the vaginal vault and cervix (see Procedure box, Assisting with Pelvic Examination).
- The collection of specimens for cytologic examination is an important part of the gynecologic examination. Infection and cancer (potential or actual) can be diagnosed through examination of specimens collected during the pelvic examination (see Procedure box, Papanicolaou [Pap] Test).
- After the specimens are obtained, the speculum is removed and bimanual palpation is performed. The vagina and cervix are palpated with one hand. The other hand is placed on the abdomen halfway between the umbilicus and symphysis pubis and exerts pressure downward toward the pelvic hand to trap reproductive structures for assessment by palpation.
- The rectovaginal examination permits assessment of the rectovaginal septum, the posterior surface of the uterus, and the region behind the cervix and the adnexa. The vaginal finger is removed and folded into the palm, leaving the middle finger free to rotate 360 degrees. The rectum is palpated for rectal tenderness and masses.

Procedure

Assisting with Pelvic Examination

Wash hands. Assemble equipment.

Ask woman to empty her bladder before the examination (obtain clean-catch urine specimen as needed).

Assist with relaxation techniques. Have the woman place her hands on her chest at about the level of the diaphragm, breathe deeply and slowly (in through her nose and out through an O-shaped mouth), concentrate on the rhythm of breathing, and relax all body muscles with each exhalation.

Encourage the woman to become involved with the examination if she shows interest. For example, a mirror can be placed so that she can see the area being examined.

Assess for and treat signs of problems such as supine hypotension.

Warm the speculum in warm water if a prewarmed one is not available.

Instruct the woman to bear down when the speculum is being inserted.

Apply gloves and assist the examiner with collection of specimens for cytologic examination, such as a Pap test. After handling specimens, remove gloves and wash hands.

Lubricate the examiner's fingers with water or water-soluble lubricant before bimanual examination.

Assist the woman at completion of the examination to a sitting position and then a standing position.

Provide tissues to wipe lubricant from perineum.

Provide privacy for the woman while she is dressing.

Laboratory and Diagnostic Procedures

The following laboratory and diagnostic procedures are ordered at the discretion of the clinician: complete blood count or hemoglobin and hematocrit, total blood cholesterol, fasting plasma glucose, urinalysis for bacteria, syphilis serology (Venereal Disease Research Laboratory [VDRL] test or rapid plasma reagin test [RPR]) and other screening tests for

Text continued on p. 27.

PATIENT INSTRUCTIONS FOR SELF-CARE

Breast Self-Examination

1. The best time to do breast self-examination is about 1 week after your period, when breasts are not tender or swollen. If you do not have regular periods or sometimes skip a month, do it on the same day every month. If you are breastfeeding or no longer menstruating, choose a date and examine your breasts at the same time each month.
2. Lie down and put a pillow under your right shoulder. Place your right arm behind your head (Fig. 1).

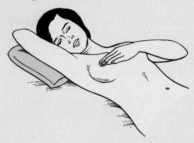

Fig. 1

3. Use the finger pads of your three middle fingers on your left hand to feel for lumps or thickening. Your finger pads are the top third of each finger.
4. Press firmly enough to know how your breast feels. If you're not sure how hard to press, ask your health care provider or try to copy the way your health care provider uses the finger pads during a breast examination. Learn what your breast feels like most of the time. A firm ridge in the lower curve of each breast is normal.
5. Move around the breast in a set way. You can choose either circles (Fig. 2, *A*), vertical lines (Fig. 2, *B*), or wedges (Fig. 2, *C*). Do it the same way every time. It will help you to make sure that you've gone over the entire breast area and to remember how your breast feels.

Continued

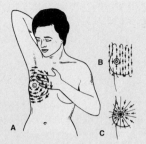

Fig. 2

6. Gently compress the nipple between your thumb and forefinger, and look for discharge.
7. Now examine your left breast using the finger pads of your right hand.
8. If you find any changes, see your health care provider right away.
9. You may want to check your breasts while standing in front of a mirror right after you do your breast self-examination each month. See if there are any changes in the way your breasts look: dimpling of the skin, changes in the nipple, or redness or swelling.
10. You may also want to do an extra breast self-examination while you're in the shower (Fig. 3). Your soapy hands will glide over the wet skin, making it easy to check how your breasts feel.
11. It is important to check the area between the breast and the underarm and the underarm itself. Also examine the area above the breast to the collarbone and to the shoulder.

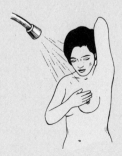

Fig. 3

Procedure

Papanicolaou (Pap) Test

In preparation, make sure the woman has not douched, used vaginal medications, or had sexual intercourse for 24 to 48 hours before the procedure. Reschedule the test if the woman is menstruating. Midcycle is the best time for the test.

Explain to the woman the purpose of the test and what sensations she will feel as the specimen is obtained (e.g., pressure but not pain).

The woman is assisted into a lithotomy position. A speculum is inserted into the vagina.

The cytologic specimen is obtained before any digital examination of the vagina is made or endocervical bacteriologic specimens are taken. A cotton swab may be used to remove excess cervical discharge before the specimen is collected.

The specimen is obtained by using an endocervical sampling device (Cytobrush, Cervex-Brush, papette, or broom). If the two-sample method of obtaining cells is used, the Cytobrush is inserted into the canal and rotated 90 to 180 degrees, followed by a gentle smear of the entire transformation zone by using a spatula. Broom devices are inserted and rotated 360 degrees five times. They obtain endocervical and ectocervical samples at the same time. If the patient has had a hysterectomy, the vaginal cuff is sampled. Areas that appear abnormal on visualization will require colposcopy and biopsy. If using a one-slide technique, the spatula sample is smeared first. This is followed by applying the Cytobrush sample (rolling the brush in the opposite direction from which it was obtained), which is less subject to drying artifact; then the slide is sprayed with preservative within 5 seconds.

The ThinPrep Pap Test is a liquid-based method of preserving cells that reduces blood, mucus, and inflammation. The Pap specimen is obtained in the manner described above except that the cervix is not swabbed before collection of the sample. The collection device (brush, spatula, or broom) is rinsed in a vial of preserving

Procedure—cont'd

solution that is provided by the laboratory. The sealed vial with solution is sent off to the appropriate laboratory. A special processing device filters the contents, and a thin layer of cervical cells is deposited on a slide, which is then examined microscopically. The AutoPap and Papnet tests are similar to the ThinPrep test. If cytology is abnormal, liquid-based methods allow follow-up testing for human papillomavirus (HPV) DNA with the same sample.

Label the slides or vial with the woman's name and site. Include on the form to accompany the specimens the woman's name, age, parity, and chief complaint or reason for taking the cytologic specimens.

Send specimens to the pathology laboratory promptly for staining, evaluation, and a written report, with special reference to abnormal elements, including cancer cells.

Advise the woman that repeated tests may be necessary if the specimen is not adequate.

Instruct the woman concerning routine checkups for cervical and vaginal cancer.

Record the examination date on the woman's record.

STIs, mammogram, tuberculin skin test, hearing test, electrocardiogram, chest x-ray film, fecal occult blood, and bone mineral density. HIV and drug screening may be offered or encouraged with informed consent, especially in high risk populations.

ANTICIPATORY GUIDANCE FOR HEALTH PROMOTION AND PREVENTION

- **Nutrition.** Foods low in saturated fat and cholesterol, moderate sodium and sugar intake, whole grain products, and a variety of fruits and vegetables should be selected. At least four to six glasses of water in addition to other fluids such as juices should be included in the diet daily. Coffee, tea, soft drinks, and alcoholic beverages should be used in moderation. Red meats and processed meats as well as refined grains should be limited. Women who are unlikely to get enough calcium in the diet may need calcium supplements.

- **Exercise.** Stress the importance of daily exercise throughout life for weight management and health promotion, suggesting exercises that are enjoyable to the individual.
- **Kegel exercises,** or pelvic muscle exercises, were developed to strengthen the supportive pelvic floor muscles to control or reduce incontinent urine loss. Educational strategies for teaching women how to perform Kegel exercises that were compiled by nurse researchers involved in the project are described in the Teaching Guidelines box.

Text continued on p. 33.

TEACHING GUIDELINES
Kegel Exercises

DESCRIPTION AND RATIONALE

Kegel exercise, or pelvic muscle exercise, is a technique used to strengthen the muscles that support the pelvic floor. This exercise involves regularly tightening (contracting) and relaxing the muscles that support the bladder and urethra. By strengthening these pelvic muscles, a woman can prevent or reduce accidental urine loss.

TECHNIQUE

The woman needs to learn how to target the muscles for training and how to contract them correctly. One suggestion for teaching is to have the woman pretend she is trying to prevent the passage of intestinal gas. Have her use this tightening motion on the muscles around her vagina and the upper pelvis. She should feel these muscles drawing inward and upward. Other suggested techniques are to have the woman pretend she is trying to stop the flow of urine in midstream or to have her think about how her vagina is able to contract around and move up the length of the penis during intercourse.

The woman should avoid straining or bearing-down motions while performing the exercise. She should be taught how bearing down feels by having her take a breath, hold it, and push down with her abdominal muscles as though she were trying to have a bowel movement. Then the woman can be taught how to avoid straining down by exhaling gently and keeping her mouth open each time she contracts her pelvic muscles.

SPECIFIC INSTRUCTIONS

1. Each contraction should be as intense as possible without contracting the abdomen, thighs, or buttocks.
2. Contractions should be held for at least 10 seconds. The woman may have to start with as little as 2 seconds per contraction until her muscles get stronger.
3. The woman should rest for 10 seconds or more between contractions, so that the muscles have time to recover and each contraction can be as strong as the woman can make it.
4. The woman should feel the pulling up over the three muscle layers so that the contraction reaches the highest level of her pelvis.

OTHER SUGGESTIONS FOR IMPLEMENTATION

1. At first the woman should set aside about 15 minutes each day to do the Kegel exercises.
2. The woman may want to put up reminders, such as notes on her bathroom mirror, her refrigerator, her television, or her calendar, to do the exercises.
3. Guidelines for practicing Kegel exercises suggest performing between 24 and 100 contractions per day; however, positive results can be achieved with only 24 to 45 per day.
4. The best position for learning how to do Kegel exercises is to lie supine with the knees bent. Another position to use is on the hands and knees. Once the woman learns the proper technique, she can perform the exercises in other positions such as standing or sitting.

From Sampselle, C. (2000). Behavioral interventions for urinary incontinence in women: Evidence for practice. *Journal of Midwifery & Women's Health, 45*(2), 94-103; Sampselle, C. (2003). Behavior interventions in young and middle-aged women: Simple interventions to combat a complex problem. *American Journal of Nursing, 103*(suppl), 9-19; Sampselle, C. et al. (2000). Continence for women: A test of AWHONN's evidence-based protocol. *Journal of Obstetric, Gynecologic, and Neonatal Nursing, 29*(1), 312-317.

TABLE 2-1

Health Screening Recommendations for Women Aged 18 Years and Older

INTERVENTION	RECOMMENDATION*
PHYSICAL EXAMINATION	
Blood pressure	Every visit, but at least every 2 yr
Height and weight	Every visit, but at least every 2 yr
Pelvic examination	Annually until age 70 yr; recommended for any woman who has ever been sexually active
Breast examination	
Self-examination	Initiated or taught at time of first pelvic examination; done monthly at end of menses
Clinical examination[†]	Every 3 yr, ages 20-39; annually after age 40 Annually after age 18 with history of premenopausal breast cancer in first-degree relative
Risk groups	At least annually:
Skin examination	Family history of skin cancer or increased exposure to sunlight after age 40; every 3 yr between ages 20 and 40; monthly self-examinations also recommended

*Unless otherwise noted, the recommended intervention should be performed routinely every 1 to 3 years.
[†]American Cancer Society (ACS) (2005).
Sources: American Cancer Society (ACS). (2005). *Cancer facts and figures 2005*. New York: ACS; Centers for Disease Control and Prevention (CDC). (2002). Sexually transmitted diseases treatment guidelines 2002. *Morbidity and Mortality Weekly Report, 51*(RR-6), 1-80; Expert Panel on Detection, Evaluation, and Treatment of High Blood Cholesterol in Adults. (2001). Executive summary of the third report of the national education program (NCEP) expert panel on detection, evaluation, and treatment of high blood cholesterol in adults (Adult Treatment Panel III). *Journal of the American Medical Association, 285*(19), 2486-2497; National Women's Health Resource Center. (2001). Screening tests and women's health. *National Women's Health Report, 23*(6), 1-7; U.S. Preventive Services Task Force. (2005). *Guide to clinical preventive services, 2005*. AHRQ Publication no. 05-0570, June 2005. Rockville, MD: Agency for Healthcare Research and Quality.

TABLE 2-1

Health Screening Recommendations for Women Aged 18 Years and Older—cont'd

INTERVENTION	RECOMMENDATION*
Oral cavity examination	Mouth lesion or exposure to tobacco or excessive alcohol
LABORATORY AND DIAGNOSTIC TESTS	
Blood cholesterol (fasting lipoprotein analysis)	Every 5 yr
	More often per clinical judgment with potential for cardiac or lipid abnormalities
Papanicolaou test[†]	Initially, 3 yr after becoming sexually active but no later than age 21; yearly with conventional Pap test or every 2 yr with liquid-based Pap tests; after age 30 and after three normal test results in a row, every 2-3 yr; after age 70 and no abnormal test results in 10 yr, screening may be stopped
Mammography[‡]	Annually over age 50 Annually over age 40 Every 1-2 yr between ages 40 and 49 and annually thereafter
Colon cancer screening	Fecal occult blood test annually and flexible sigmoidoscopy every 5 yr after age 50; more often if family history of colon cancer or polyps

[‡]Note: There is no consensus regarding mammograms for women between 40 and 49 years of age; therefore various recommendations are listed. Women are urged to discuss circumstances with their health care providers.

Continued

TABLE 2-1

Health Screening Recommendations for Women Aged 18 Years and Older—cont'd

INTERVENTION	RECOMMENDATION*
Risk groups	
Fasting blood sugar	Annually with family history of diabetes or gestational diabetes or if significantly obese; every 3-5 yr for all women older than 45 yr
Hearing screen	Annually with exposure to excessive noise or when loss is suspected
Sexually transmitted infection screen	As needed with multiple sexual partners
Tuberculin skin test	Annually with exposure to persons with tuberculosis or in risk categories for close contact with the disease
Endometrial biopsy	At menopause for women at risk for endometrial cancer
Vision	Every 2 yr between ages 40 and 64; annually after age 65
Bone mineral density testing	All women age 65 and older; younger women with risk for osteoporosis may need periodic screenings
IMMUNIZATIONS	
Tetanus-diphtheria	Booster given every 10 yr after primary series
Measles, mumps, rubella	Once if born after 1956 and no evidence of immunity
Hepatitis B	Primary series of three for all who are in risk categories
Influenza	Annually after age 65 or in risk categories, such as chronic diseases, immunosuppression, renal dysfunction

- **Stress management.** Role playing, relaxation techniques, biofeedback, meditation, desensitization, imagery, assertiveness training, yoga, diet, exercise, and weight control are techniques nurses can include in their repertoire of helping skills.
- **Substance use cessation.** Counseling women who appear to be smoking or drinking excessively or using drugs may include strategies to increase self-esteem and teaching new coping skills to resist and maintain resistance to alcohol abuse and drug use. General referral to sources of support should also be provided.
- **Safer sexual practices.** Specific self-care measures for "safer sex" are described in Chapter 3.
- **Health screening schedule.** Periodic health screening includes history, physical examination, education, counseling, and selected diagnostic and laboratory tests. Table 2-1 gives an overview of health screening recommendations for women older than 18 years of age.
- **Health risk prevention.** Reinforce commonsense concepts that will protect the individual, such as wearing seat belts at all times in a moving vehicle and protecting the skin from ultraviolet light by use of sunscreen and clothing.

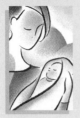

CHAPTER 3

Common Reproductive Concerns

MENSTRUAL PROBLEMS

Amenorrhea

The absence or cessation of menstrual flow is a clinical sign of a variety of disorders:

- Primary—failure of menses to occur by age 16 years
- Secondary—menses has not occurred for 3 months; common reasons—pregnancy; lactation; menopause; anorexia; stress; strenuous exercise; medications, such as phenytoin (dilantin); endocrine disorders, such as hypothyroidism or hyperthyroidism

Care management

- Confirm that the woman is not pregnant.
- Treatment varies, depending on cause. Counseling and education are primary interventions because many of the causes are potentially reversible (e.g., stress, weight loss for nonorganic reasons). Hormonal therapy may be needed if these interventions do not correct amenorrhea.

Primary Dysmenorrhea

- Painful menstruation that begins within 1 to 2 years after menarche
- Occurs only with ovulatory cycles
- Excessive prostaglandin secretion released with menses: causes ischemia and abdominal cramping

Clinical manifestations

- Lower abdominal pain, bloating, nausea, headaches, backache

- Usually begin with menstrual flow and last for several hours to several days

Care management
- Pharmacologic—nonsteroidal antiinflammatory drugs (NSAIDs) (e.g., ibuprofen, naproxen), oral contraceptive pills (OCPs), aspirin (see Medications Used to Treat Dysmenorrhea in Appendix B)
- Nonpharmacologic—exercise, heat to abdomen, relaxation techniques, massage, orgasm; decrease sodium, sugar, red meat; increase natural diuretic intake
- Herbal preparations—have long been used for management of menstrual problems, including dysmenorrhea (e.g., dong quai, black haw, black cohosh); however, it is essential that women understand that these therapies are not without potential toxicity and may cause drug interactions and that research is inconclusive about the effectiveness of use.

NURSE ALERT   *If one NSAID is ineffective often a different one may be effective. If the second drug is unsuccessful after a 6-month trial, combined OCPs may be used. Women with a history of aspirin sensitivity or allergy should avoid all NSAIDs.*

Secondary Dysmenorrhea
- Associated with pathologic conditions—endometriosis, pelvic inflammatory disease (PID), polyps, and so on
- Usually develops after age 25 years

Clinical manifestations
- Symptoms vary—pain can begin at ovulation, begin a few days before menses, or begin after menses starts
- Pain—usually dull lower abdominal aching and can radiate to back and thighs

Care management
- The underlying cause is identified and treated.
- Interventions for primary dysmenorrhea may also provide relief.

Premenstrual Syndrome

- Premenstrual syndrome (PMS) is a group of physical and psychologic symptoms for which there is no known cause.
- Theories of etiology include progesterone deficiency, prolactin and prostaglandin excesses, and dietary deficiencies.
- Premenstrual dysphoric disorder (PDD) is a more severe variant of PMS in which women have marked irritability, dysphoria, mood lability, anxiety, fatigue, appetite changes, and a sense of feeling overwhelmed.

Clinical manifestations

- Begin in the luteal phase of the menstrual cycle; symptoms do not occur in the follicular phase
- Fluid retention (bloating, edema of lower extremities, breast tenderness, weight gain, pelvic fullness)
- Emotional changes (depression, crying, irritability, panic attacks, inability to concentrate)
- Premenstrual cravings (sweets, salt, increased appetite, food binges)
- Headaches, fatigue, backache

Care management

- There is little agreement on management; a daily log of symptoms and mood changes for several cycles may be useful.
- Nonpharmacologic management includes diet changes: limit salt, sugar, red meats, alcohol, caffeine; natural diuretics, vitamin E, magnesium, calcium; exercise; stress reduction techniques; and counseling/support groups.
- Pharmacologic management includes diuretics, prostaglandin inhibitors (NSAIDs), progesterone, and OCPs. Fluoxetine (Sarafem or Prozac, 20 mg/day), a selective serotonin reuptake inhibitor (SSRI), is the only U.S. Food and Drug Administration (FDA)–approved agent for PMS.
- Herbal therapies such as black cohosh, dong quai, and chaste tree fruit have long been used to treat PMS.

Endometriosis

- Endometriosis is a benign disease.
- Implantation of endometrial tissue occurs outside the uterine cavity. The tissue responds to hormonal stimulation and bleeds into tissues, causing an inflammatory response.
- The cause is not well understood. Theories include retrograde menstruation, lymphatic spread, hematogenous spread (spread through blood), surgical implantation, and spontaneous formation.
- It usually develops in women older than 30 years; and it may be familial.

Clinical manifestations

- Peak of pain—usually just before the menstrual flow
- Located in the lower abdomen; sacral backache, painful defecation, infertility, hypermenorrhea, dyspareunia
- May worsen over time or be asymptomatic; disappears with menopause unless the woman is taking hormonal therapy

Care management

- Management is based on symptoms and goals of the woman (e.g., mild or severe symptoms; desires pregnancy or not).
- Nonpharmacologic management, which includes application of heat, relaxation techniques, yoga, biofeedback, and other nursing care measures discussed in the section on dysmenorrhea, is appropriate for managing chronic pelvic pain.
- Pharmacologic management includes analgesics, low-dose OCPs, and hormonal antagonists to suppress ovulation (gonadotropin-releasing hormone [GnRH] therapy to suppress pituitary gonadotropin secretion); or danazol (androgenic synthetic steroid) to suppress follicle-stimulating hormone (FSH) and luteinizing hormone (LH) secretion to produce anovulation (see Appendix B).
- Surgical intervention involves removal of endometrial tissue (laser therapy) or hysterectomy and bilateral salpingo-oophorectomy.

- Counseling and education are critical components of nursing care. Women need an honest discussion of treatment options with potential risks and benefits of each option reviewed.
- Sexual dysfunction resulting from painful intercourse (dyspareunia) may be present and may necessitate referral for counseling.
- Referral to support groups for women with endometriosis may be appropriate.

Dysfunctional Uterine Bleeding

Abnormal uterine bleeding (AUB) is any form of uterine bleeding that is irregular in amount, duration, or timing and not related to regular menstrual bleeding. Box 3-1 lists possible causes of AUB. Although often used interchangeably, the terms *AUB* and *dysfunctional uterine bleeding (DUB)* are not synonymous. Dysfunctional uterine bleeding is a subset of AUB defined as "excessive uterine bleeding with no demonstrable organic cause, genital or extragenital." A diagnosis of DUB is made only after all other causes of abnormal menstrual bleeding have been ruled out.

Care management
- The most effective medical treatment of acute bleeding episodes of DUB is administration of oral or intravenous estrogen. A dilation and curettage may be done if the bleeding has not stopped in 12 to 24 hours. An oral conjugated estrogen and progestin regimen is usually given for at least 3 months.
- If the recurrent, heavy bleeding is not controlled by hormonal therapy, ablation of the endometrium through laser treatment may be performed.
- Nursing roles include informing women of their options, counseling and education as indicated, and referring to the appropriate specialists and health care services.

Sexually Transmitted Infections

Sexually transmitted infections (STIs) are infections or infectious disease syndromes primarily transmitted by sexual contact. Table 3-1 summarizes the most common STIs in women. *Text continued on p. 46.*

BOX 3-1

Possible Causes of Abnormal Uterine Bleeding

ANOVULATION
- Hypothalamic dysfunction
- Polycystic ovary syndrome

PREGNANCY-RELATED CONDITIONS
- Threatened or spontaneous miscarriage
- Retained products of conception after elective abortion
- Ectopic pregnancy

LOWER REPRODUCTIVE TRACT INFECTIONS
- Chlamydial cervicitis
- Pelvic inflammatory disease

NEOPLASMS
- Endometrial hyperplasia
- Cancer of cervix and endometrium
- Endometrial polyps
- Hormonally active tumors (rare)
- Leiomyomata
- Vaginal tumors (rare)

TRAUMA
- Genital injury (accidental, coital trauma, sexual abuse)
- Foreign body
- Primary coagulation disorders

SYSTEMIC DISEASES
- Diabetes mellitus
- Thyroid dysfunction (hypothyroidism, hyperthyroidism)
- Severe organ disease (renal or liver failure)

IATROGENIC CAUSES
- Exogenous hormone use (oral contraceptives, menopausal hormone therapy)
- Medications with estrogenic activity
- Herbal preparation (ginseng)

Sources: American College of Nurse-Midwives (ACNM). (2002). Abnormal and dysfunctional uterine bleeding. ACNM Clinical Bulletin no. 6. *Journal of Midwifery and Women's Health, 47*(3), 207-213; Stenchever, M. et al. (2001). *Comprehensive gynecology* (4th ed.). St. Louis: Mosby.

TABLE 3-1

Infections

STI		SCREENING/ DIAGNOSIS	LESION	DIS- CHARGE	DYSURIA	DYS- PAREUNIA	TREATMENT	COMMENTS
Chlamydia	Yes	Culture	No	Muco- purulent	Yes	No—may cause postcoital bleeding	Doxycycline, 100 mg orally 2 times daily for 7 days, or azithromycin, 1 g orally 1 time	Most common bacterial STI in United States; risk of pelvic inflammatory disease (PID), ectopic pregnancy, and tubal factor infertility
Gonorrhea	Yes	Culture	No	Green- yellow	Yes	Yes	One dose of ceftriaxone, 125 mg IM; cefixime, 400 mg orally; ciprofloxacin, 500 mg orally; ofloxacin, 400 mg orally;	Gonorrhea is a reportable disease; infection can cause PID

Syphilis	Yes	Non-treponemal antibody test (VDRL or RPR) for screening; treponemal test for confirming diagnosis (FTA-ABS)	Yes, chancre	No	Yes	Yes	or levofloxacin 250 mg orally. CDC also suggests treatment for chlamydia because coinfection is common Penicillin G benzathine, 2.4 million units IM once	Primary stage—chancre; secondary—rash, fever; tertiary—systemic; syphilis is a reportable disease
Human papilloma virus (HPV)	Yes	Pap test; HPV DNA test for screening; biopsy for diagnosis	Yes, wartlike growths	No	No	Yes	Untreated warts may resolve on their own; podofilox, 0.5% solution or gel applied topically; cryosurgery, electrocautery, and laser therapy	Most common viral STI; primary cause of cervical neoplasia

Continued

TABLE 3-1

Infections—cont'd

STI	SCREENING/ DIAGNOSIS	LESION	DIS- CHARGE	DYSURIA	DYS- PAREUNIA	TREATMENT	COMMENTS
						are used but no treatment eradicates HPV	
Genital herpes simplex virus (HSV)	Yes	Viral tissue culture; serologic tests for HSV-2 antibodies	Ulcerative lesions "Blisters"	Yes	Yes	Yes	First episode: acyclovir, 400 mg orally 3 times daily for 7-10 days, or acyclovir, 200 mg orally 5 times daily for 7-10 days or famciclovir, 250 mg orally 3 times daily for 7-10 days, or valacyclovir, 1 g orally twice daily for 7-10 days	No known cure; management includes comfort measures, support, and counseling

Human immunodeficiency virus (HIV)	Yes	HIV-1 and HIV-3 antibody tests for screening; Western blot or immunofluorescence assay for diagnosis after reactive screening	No	No	No	No	Complex management that includes behavioral, psychologic, and medical services—discussion beyond the scope of this chapter	Informed consent is needed before testing; no cure at this time
Hepatitis B (HBV)	Yes	HBsAg screening test	Possible skin eruptions	No	No	No	No specific treatment	A disease of the liver and often a silent infection; hepatitis B vaccine recommended for women at high risk (e.g., IV drug user, sex workers, heath care providers who are exposed to blood and needlesticks)

Continued

43

TABLE 3-1

Infections—cont'd

	STI	SCREENING/ DIAGNOSIS	LESION	DIS- CHARGE	DYSURIA	DYS- PAREUNIA	TREATMENT	COMMENTS
Bacterial vaginosis (BV)	Not usually	Wet prep—normal saline smear for presence of clue cells or whiff test (10% potassium hydroxide [KOH] and vaginal secretions)—releases fishy odor	No	Yes—white, thin discharge	No	No	Metronidazole, 500 mg orally twice daily for 7 days, or gel 0.75%, 1 full applicator (5 g) intravaginally once for 5 days	Most common vaginitis—at least 50% of women are asymptomatic
Vulvovaginal candidiasis (VVC)	Not usually	Wet prep—normal saline or 10% KOH or Gram stain of vaginal discharge—shows yeast cells	No	Yes—white, thick, cottage cheese like	Yes	Yes	Intravaginal agents—butoconazole 2% cream, 5 g for 5 days, or clotrimazole 1% cream, 5 g for 7-14 days	Many of the intravaginal preparations are available over the counter but should be used by

Trichomoniasis	Yes	Saline wet smear; culture	No	Yes—profuse, frothy, yellow-green, malodorous	Yes	Yes	or miconazole 2% cream, 5 g for 7 days, or terconazole 0.4% cream, 5 g for 7 days; Oral—fluconazole, 150 mg once	women only if they have been previously diagnosed with VVC
							Metronidazole, 2 g orally once	Sex partners should be treated

Source: Centers for Disease Control and Prevention (CDC). (2002). Sexually transmitted diseases treatment guidelines 2002. *Morbidity and Mortality Weekly Report, 51*(RR-6), 1-82.

STI, Sexually transmitted infection; *VDRL*, Venereal Disease Research Laboratory; *RPR*, rapid plasma reagin; *FTA-ABS*, fluorescent treponemal antibody absorption; *DNA*, deoxyribonucleic acid; *IM*, intramuscular; *CDC*, Centers for Disease Control and Prevention.

Prevention

- Preventing infection (primary prevention) is the most effective way of reducing the adverse consequences of STIs for women.
- Preventing the spread of STIs requires that women at risk for transmitting or acquiring infections change their behavior. A critical first step is to include questions about a woman's sexual history, sexual risk behaviors, and drug-related risky behaviors as a part of her assessment.
- Techniques that are effective in providing prevention counseling include using open-ended questions, using understandable language, and reassuring the woman that treatment will be provided regardless of consideration such as ability to pay, language spoken, or lifestyle.
- Prevention messages should include descriptions of specific actions to be taken to prevent contracting or transmitting STIs (e.g., refraining from sexual activity when STI-related symptoms are present) and should be tailored to the individual woman, with attention given to her specific risk factors.
- An essential component of primary prevention is counseling women regarding safer sex practices, including knowledge of partners, reduction of number of partners, low risk sex, and avoiding the exchange of body fluids.
- Currently, the sole physical barrier promoted for the prevention of sexual transmission of STIs is the condom.
- Evidence has shown that vaginal spermicides do not protect against certain STIs (e.g., chlamydia, cervical gonorrhea) and that frequent use of spermicides containing nonoxynol-9 has been associated with genital lesions and may increase human immunodeficiency virus (HIV) transmission. Condoms lubricated with nonoxynol-9 are not recommended.

Pelvic Inflammatory Disease

Pelvic inflammatory disease (PID) is an infectious process that most commonly involves the uterine tubes (salpingitis), uterus (endometritis), and, more rarely, the ovaries and peritoneal surfaces. In addition to gonorrhea and chlamydia, a wide variety of anaerobic and aerobic bacteria are recognized to cause PID. Because PID may be caused by many different infectious agents and encompasses a wide variety of pathologic processes, the infection can be acute, subacute, or chronic and has a wide range of symptoms. Women are at increased risk for ectopic pregnancy, infertility, and chronic pelvic pain.

Clinical manifestations

The symptoms of PID vary, depending on whether the infection is acute, subacute, or chronic; however, pain is common to all types of infection. It may be dull, cramping, and intermittent (subacute) or severe, persistent, and incapacitating (acute). Women may also report one or more of the following: fever, chills, nausea and vomiting, increased vaginal discharge, symptoms of a urinary tract infection, and irregular bleeding. Abdominal pain is usually present; upper abdominal pain may result from liver capsule inflammation (Fitz-Hugh–Curtis syndrome).

Care management

- Primary prevention includes education in preventing the acquisition of STIs, and secondary prevention involves preventing a lower genital tract infection from ascending to the upper genital tract. Instructing women in self-protective behaviors, such as practicing safer sex and using barrier methods, is critical. A woman with a history of PID should not choose an intrauterine device (IUD) as her contraceptive method.

- Although treatment regimens vary with the infecting organism, a broad-spectrum antibiotic generally is used. Treatment may be oral (ofloxacin plus metronidazole) or parenteral (e.g., cefotetan [intravenous] plus doxycycline [oral]), and regimens can be administered in in-patient or out-patient settings. The woman with acute PID should be on bed rest in a semi-Fowler position. Comfort measures include analgesics for pain and all other nursing measures applicable to a patient confined to bed.

PROBLEMS OF THE BREASTS

Benign Problems

Table 3-2 compares the common manifestations of benign breast masses.

Cancer of the Breast

Although the exact cause of breast cancer continues to elude investigators, certain risk factors that increase a woman's risk for developing a malignancy have been identified (Box 3-2). The most important predictor for breast cancer is age; the risk increases as the woman ages.

Clinical manifestations

- It is estimated that 90% of all breast lumps are detected by the woman. More than one half of all lumps are discovered in the upper outer quadrant of the breast. The most common presenting symptom is a lump or thickening of the breast. The lump may feel hard and fixed or soft

---

BOX 3-2

Risk Factors for Breast Cancer*

Age
Previous history of breast cancer
Family history of breast cancer, especially a mother or sister (particularly significant if premenopausal)
Previous history of ovarian, endometrial, colon, or thyroid cancer
Early menarche (before age 12 years)
Late menopause (after age 55 years)
Nulliparity or first pregnancy after age 30 years
Use of estrogen replacement therapy
Obesity after menopause
Previous history of benign breast disease with epithelial hyperplasia
Race (Caucasian women have highest incidence)
High socioeconomic status
Sedentary lifestyle

*Risk factors are cumulative—the more risk factors present, the greater the likelihood of breast cancer occurring.

TABLE 3-2

Comparison of Common Manifestations of Benign Breast Masses

FIBROCYSTIC CHANGES	FIBROADENOMA	LIPOMA	INTRADUCTAL PAPILLOMA	MAMMARY DUCT ECTASIA
Multiple lumps	Single lump	Single lump	Single or multiple	Mass behind nipple
Nodular	Well delineated	Well delineated	Not well delineated	Not well delineated
Palpable	Palpable	Palpable	Nonpalpable	Palpable
Movable	Movable	Movable	Nonmobile	Nonmobile
Round, smooth	Round, smooth	Round, lobular	Small, ball-like	Irregular
Firm or soft	Firm	Soft	Firm or soft	Firm
Tenderness influenced by menstrual cycle	Usually asymptomatic	Nontender	Usually nontender	Painful, burning, itching
Bilateral	Unilateral	Unilateral	Unilateral	Unilateral
May or may not have nipple discharge	No nipple discharge	No nipple discharge	Serous or bloody nipple discharge	Thick, sticky nipple discharge

and spongy. It may have well-defined or irregular borders. It may be fixed to the skin, thereby causing dimpling to occur. A nipple discharge that is bloody or clear also may be present.

- When a suspicious finding on a mammogram is noted or a lump is detected, diagnosis is confirmed by needle aspiration, a core needle biopsy, or surgical excision. Ultrasound may also be used to assess a specific area of abnormality found during a mammogram procedure.

- Laboratory diagnosis of breast cancer and possible metastases includes complete blood count, liver enzyme levels, serum calcium, and alkaline phosphatase level. Elevated liver enzyme levels indicate possible liver metastases, and increased serum calcium and alkaline phosphatase levels suggest bone metastases. HER2 testing may be done on the biopsied breast tissue; elevated levels with unfavorable prognosis.

- Other tests to determine the spread of the cancer include chest x-ray examination, bone scan, computed tomography (CT), magnetic resonance imaging (MRI), and positron emission tomography (PET scan). Once the stage or spread of cancer is determined, treatment options can be identified.

- Nodal involvement and tumor size are the most significant prognostic criteria for long-term survival. One factor that has been helpful in predicting response to therapy and survival is whether the tumor is estrogen or progesterone-receptor positive or hormone-receptor (HR) positive. Women with HR-positive tumors tend to respond better to treatment and have higher survival rates.

Care management

- Controversy continues regarding the best treatment of breast cancer. Most health care providers recommend that the malignant mass be removed, as well as the axillary nodes for staging purposes.

- The most frequently recommended surgical approaches for the treatment of breast cancer are lumpectomy and modified radical mastectomy.

- Breast-conserving surgery, such as a lumpectomy or quadrantectomy, removes the tumor. Sampling of axillary lymph nodes is usually done through a separate incision at the time of these procedures, and surgery is usually followed by radiation therapy to the remaining breast tissue. Lumpectomy offers survival equivalent to that with modified radical mastectomy.

- A simple mastectomy is the removal of the breast containing the tumor. A modified radical mastectomy is the removal of the breast tissue, skin, and fascia of the pectoralis muscle and dissection of the axillary nodes. A radical mastectomy, although rarely performed, is the removal of the breast and underlying pectoralis muscles and complete axillary node dissection. After surgery, follow-up treatment may include radiation, chemotherapy, or hormonal therapy.

- The decision to include follow-up therapy is based on the stage of disease, age and menopausal status of the woman, the woman's preference, and her hormonal receptor status. Follow-up treatment is usually used to decrease the risk of recurrence in women who have no evidence of metastasis.

- Radiation is generally recommended as follow-up therapy for women who have stage I or II cancer.

- Hormone therapy with tamoxifen, an estrogen agonist, is recommended for women over the age of 50 for at least 5 years (see Medication Guide: Tamoxifen in Appendix B). Tamoxifen therapy may be followed with letrozole (Femara) tablets as extended adjuvant therapy to reduce the risk of cancer return in women who had estrogen receptor positive breast cancer.

- Chemotherapy is often given to premenopausal women who have positive nodes.

- Surgery may be performed in an out-patient surgical setting or as an in-patient procedure, depending on what type of surgery is being done. Preoperatively, women need to be assessed for psychologic preparation and specific teaching needs related to the procedure to be performed and what to expect after surgery. A visit from a woman who has had a similar experience may be beneficial preoperatively as well as postoperatively.

- Postoperative nursing care focuses on recovery. Women who had surgery in an out-patient setting generally go home within a few hours after surgery. A 24- to 48-hour stay is usual after modified radical mastectomy. Precautions should be taken to avoid taking the blood pressure, giving injections, or taking blood from the arm on the affected side. The woman is usually discharged to home after being given self-care instructions (see Patient Instructions for Self-Care box).

PATIENT INSTRUCTIONS FOR SELF-CARE

Mastectomy

- Wash hands well before and after touching incision area or drains.
- Empty surgical drains twice each day and as needed, recording the date, time, drain site (if more than one drain is present), and amount of drainage in milliliters in diary you will take to each surgical checkup until your drains are removed. (Before discharge, you may receive a graduated container for emptying drains and measuring drainage.)
- Avoid driving, lifting more than 10 pounds, or reaching above your head until given permission by surgeon.
- Take medications for pain as soon as pain begins.
- Perform arm exercises as directed.
- Call physician if inflammation of incision or swelling of the incision or the arm occurs.
- Avoid tight clothing, tight jewelry, and other causes of decreased circulation in the affected arm.
- Until drains are removed, wear loose-fitting underwear (camisole or half-slip) and clothes, pinning surgical drains inside clothing. (You will be taught how to do this safely.)
- After drains are removed and surgical sites are healing and still tender, wear a mastectomy bra or camisole with a cotton-filled, muslin temporary prosthesis. Temporary prostheses of this type are often available from Reach to Recovery.
- Avoid depilatory creams, strong deodorants, and shaving of affected chest area, axilla, and arm.
- Sponge bathe until drains are removed.
- Return to the surgeon's office for incision check, drain inspection, and possible drain removal as directed.

- Contact Reach to Recovery for assistance in obtaining external prosthesis and lingerie when dressings, drains, and staples are removed and wound is healing and nontender.
- Contact insurance company for information about coverage of prosthesis and wig if needed. Obtain prescriptions for prosthesis and wig to submit with receipts of purchase for these items to the insurance company. If insurance does not pay for these items, contact hospital or agency social worker or local American Cancer Society for assistance.
- Continue with monthly breast self-examination (BSE) of unaffected side and affected surgical site and axilla.
- Encourage mother, sisters, and daughters (if applicable) to learn and practice monthly BSE and to have annual professional breast examinations and mammography (if appropriate).
- Keep follow-up visits for professional examination, mammography, and testing to detect recurrent breast cancer.
- Expect decreased sensation and tingling at incision sites and in the affected arm for weeks to months after surgery.
- Resume sexual activities as desired.

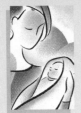

Contraception

CONTRACEPTION

Methods of Contraception

Coitus interruptus

- Coitus interruptus (withdrawal or "pulling out") involves the male partner withdrawing the entire penis from the woman's vagina and moving away from her external genitalia before he ejaculates.
- Adolescents and men with premature ejaculation may find this method difficult to use.
- This method is immediately available, costs nothing, and involves no hormonal alterations or chemicals; the effectiveness of this birth control technique is similar to that of barrier methods.
- Some religions and cultures prohibit this technique.
- Coitus interruptus does not adequately protect against sexually transmitted infections (STIs) or human immunodeficiency virus (HIV) infection.

Fertility awareness methods
Periodic Abstinence

- Periodic abstinence, or natural family planning (NFP), provides contraception by using methods that rely on avoidance of intercourse during fertile periods. NFP methods are the only contraceptive practices acceptable to the Roman Catholic Church. Fertility awareness is the combination of charting signs and symptoms of the menstrual cycle with the use of abstinence during fertile periods.
- Pregnancy is unlikely to occur if a couple abstains from intercourse for 4 days before and for 3 or 4 days after

ovulation (fertile period). Unprotected intercourse on the other days of the cycle (safe period) should not result in pregnancy.
- Women with irregular menstrual periods have the greatest risk of failure with this form of contraception.

Calendar Rhythm Method

- Practice of the calendar rhythm method is based on the number of days in each cycle counting from the first day of menses. The beginning of the fertile period is estimated by subtracting 18 days from the length of the shortest cycle. The end of the fertile period is determined by subtracting 11 days from the length of the longest cycle. If the shortest cycle is 24 days and the longest is 30 days, application of the formula is as follows:

Shortest cycle: 24 − 18 = sixth day

Longest cycle: 30 − 11 = nineteenth day

- To avoid conception the couple would abstain during the fertile period—days 6 through 19. If the woman has very regular cycles of 28 days each, the formula indicates the fertile days to be as follows:

Shortest cycle: 28 − 18 = tenth day

Longest cycle: 28 − 11 = seventeenth day

- To avoid pregnancy, the couple abstains from days 10 through 17 because ovulation occurs on day 14 plus or minus 2 days.

Ovulation Method

- The cervical mucus ovulation-detection method (also called the Billings method and the Creighton model ovulation method) requires that the woman recognize and interpret the cyclic changes in the amount and consistency of cervical mucus that characterize her own unique pattern of changes (see Patient Instructions for Self-Care box).

Basal Body Temperature Method

- The basal body temperature (BBT) is the lowest body temperature of a healthy person, taken immediately after

PATIENT INSTRUCTIONS FOR SELF-CARE

Cervical Mucus Characteristics

SETTING THE STAGE

- Show charts of menstrual cycle along with changes in the cervical mucus.
- Have woman practice with raw egg white.
- Supply her with a basal body temperature (BBT) log and graph if she does not already have one.
- Explain that assessment of cervical mucus characteristics is best when mucus is not mixed with semen, contraceptive jellies or foams, or discharge from infections. Douching should not be done before assessment.

CONTENT RELATED TO CERVICAL MUCUS

- Explain to woman (couple) how cervical mucus changes throughout the menstrual cycle.
  - a. Postmenstrual mucus: scant
  - b. Preovulation mucus: cloudy, yellow or white, sticky
  - c. Ovulation mucus: clear, wet, sticky, slippery
  - d. Postovulation fertile mucus: thick, cloudy, sticky
  - e. Postovulation, postfertile mucus: scant
- Right before ovulation, the watery, thin, clear mucus becomes more abundant and thick. It feels like a lubricant and can be stretched 5+ cm between the thumb and forefinger; this is called *spinnbarkeit*. This indicates the period of maximal fertility. Sperm deposited in this type of mucus can survive until ovulation occurs.

ASSESSMENT TECHNIQUE

- Stress that good handwashing is imperative to begin and end all self-assessment.
- Start observation from last day of menstrual flow.
- Assess cervical mucus several times each day for several cycles. Mucus can be obtained from vaginal introitus; no need to reach into vagina to cervix.
- Record findings on the same record on which BBT is entered.

waking and before getting out of bed. The BBT usually varies from 36.2° C to 36.3° C during menses and for about 5 to 7 days afterward. At about the time of ovulation, a slight decrease in temperature (approximately 0.05° C) may occur in some women, but others may have no decrease at all. After ovulation, in concert with the increasing progesterone levels of the early luteal phase of the cycle, the BBT increases slightly (approximately 0.4° C to 0.8° C). The temperature remains on an elevated plateau until 2 to 4 days before menstruation, and then it decreases to the low levels recorded during the previous cycle, unless pregnancy has occurred, and the temperature remains elevated. If ovulation fails to occur, the pattern of lower body temperature continues throughout the cycle.

- To use this method, the fertile period is defined as the day of first temperature drop, or first elevation through 3 consecutive days of elevated temperature. Abstinence begins on the first day of menstrual bleeding and lasts through 3 consecutive days of sustained temperature rise (at least 0.2° C).
- Infection, fatigue, less than 3 hours of sleep per night, awakening late, and anxiety may cause temperature fluctuations, altering the expected pattern. Jet lag, alcohol, and antipyretic medications taken the evening before or sleeping in a heated waterbed also must be noted on the chart because each affects the BBT.

Symptothermal Method

- The symptothermal method combines at least two methods, usually cervical mucus changes with BBT, in addition to heightened awareness of secondary, cycle phase-related symptoms (e.g., increased libido, mid-cycle spotting, mittelschmerz, pelvic fullness or tenderness, and vulvar fullness). The woman notes days on which coitus, changes in routine, illness, and so on have occurred. Calendar calculations and cervical mucus changes are used to estimate the onset of the fertile period; changes in cervical mucus or the BBT are used to estimate its end.

Barrier methods
Spermicides

- Spermicides, such as nonoxynol-9, work by reducing the sperm's mobility, because the chemicals attack the sperm flagella and body, thereby preventing the sperm from reaching the cervical os. Spermicides provide little to no protection against STIs.
- Nonoxynol-9, the chemical used in spermicidal products in the United States, is a surfactant that destroys the sperm cell membrane; however, recent data suggest that frequent use (more than two times per day) of nonoxynol-9, or use as a lubricant during anal intercourse, may increase the transmission of HIV and can cause lesions.
- Women with high risk behaviors that increase their likelihood of contracting HIV and other STIs are advised to avoid the use of spermicidal products containing nonoxynol-9, including those lubricated condoms, diaphragms, and cervical caps to which nonoxynol-9 is added.
- Intravaginal spermicides are marketed and sold without a prescription as foams, tablets, suppositories, creams, films, and gels. Preloaded, single-dose applicators small enough to be carried in a small purse are available. The spermicide should be inserted high into the vagina so that it makes contact with the cervix. Some spermicide should be inserted at least 15 minutes before, and no longer than 1 hour before, sexual intercourse. Spermicide needs to be reapplied for each additional act of intercourse, even if a barrier method is used.

Condoms

- The male condom is a thin, stretchable sheath that covers the penis before genital, oral, or anal contact and is removed when the penis is withdrawn from the partner's orifice after ejaculation.
- In addition to providing a physical barrier for sperm, non-spermicidal latex condoms also provide a barrier for STIs (particularly gonorrhea, chlamydia, and *Trichomonas*) and HIV transmission. Condoms lubricated with nonoxynol-9 are not recommended for preventing STIs or HIV.
- Latex condoms will break down with oil-based lubricants and should be used only with water-based or silicone lubricants.

- Condoms need to be discarded after each single use. They are available without a prescription.
- A small percentage of condoms are made from the lamb cecum (natural skin). Natural skin condoms do not provide the same protection against STIs and HIV infection as latex condoms.
- Instructions, such as those listed in Box 4-1, can be used for patient teaching.
- The female condom is a lubricated vaginal sheath made of polyurethane and has flexible rings at both ends. The closed end of the pouch is inserted into the vagina and is anchored around the cervix, and the open ring covers the labia.
- The female condom is available in one size, is intended for single use only, and is sold over the counter.
- Male condoms should not be used concurrently, because the friction from both sheaths can increase the likelihood of either or both tearing.

Diaphragms and Cervical Caps

- Diaphragms and cervical caps are soft latex or silicone barriers that cover the cervix and prevent the sperm from migrating to fertilize the ovum. They are washable and reusable and need inspection for holes, tears, or other problems before each use. Each needs to be filled with spermicidal jelly or cream before vaginal insertion. These mechanical barriers are nonhormonal but still require a prescription from a licensed health care provider. It is essential the patient undergo proper fitting of the device. Women who choose to use these methods need to be willing to touch their genitalia and be capable of providing accurate return demonstrations of proper insertion and removal techniques.
- Instruct the woman about ways to reduce her risk for toxic shock syndrome (TSS). These measures include prompt removal 6 to 8 hours after intercourse, not using the diaphragm or cervical cap during menses, and learning and watching for danger signs of TSS. The most common signs include a sunburn-type rash, diarrhea, dizziness, faintness, weakness, sore throat, aching muscles and joints, sudden high fever, and vomiting.
- Because various types of diaphragms are on the market, the nurse uses the package insert for teaching the woman

how to use and care for the diaphragm and cervical cap
(see Patient Instructions for Self-Care box).

Contraceptive Sponges

- The vaginal sponge is a small, round, polyurethane sponge
  that contains nonoxynol-9 spermicide. It is designed to fit
  over the cervix (one size fits all). The side that is placed

Text continued on p. 67.

BOX 4-1

Male Condoms

MECHANISM OF ACTION

Sheath is applied over the erect penis before insertion
or loss of preejaculatory drops of semen. Used
correctly, condoms prevent sperm from entering the
cervix. Spermicide-coated condoms cause ejaculated
sperm to be immobilized rapidly, thus increasing
contraceptive effectiveness.

FAILURE RATE

Typical users, 15%
Correct and consistent users, 2%

ADVANTAGES

- Safe.
- No side effects.
- Readily available.
- Premalignant changes in cervix can be prevented or
  ameliorated in women whose partners use condoms.
- Method of male nonsurgical contraception.

DISADVANTAGES

- Must interrupt lovemaking to apply sheath.
- Sensation may be altered.
- If condom is used improperly, spillage of sperm can
  result in pregnancy.
- Condoms occasionally may tear during intercourse.

**PROTECTION AGAINST SEXUALLY TRANSMITTED
INFECTIONS (STIs)**

If a condom is used throughout the act of intercourse
and there is no unprotected contact with female
genitalia, a latex rubber condom, which is impermeable
to viruses, can act as a protective measure against STIs.

Continued

BOX 4-1

Male Condoms—cont'd

NURSING CONSIDERATIONS

Teach man to do the following:

- Use a new condom (check expiration date) for each act of sexual intercourse or other acts between partners that involve contact with the penis.
- Place condom after penis is erect and before intimate contact.
- Place condom on head of penis (Fig. A) and unroll it all the way to the base (Fig. B).
- Leave an empty space at the tip (see Fig. A); remove any air remaining in the tip by gently pressing air out toward the base of the penis.
- If a lubricant is desired, use water-based products, such as K-Y lubricating jelly. Do not use petroleum-based products because they can cause the condom to break.
- After ejaculation, carefully withdraw the still-erect penis from the vagina, holding onto condom rim; remove and discard the condom.
- Store unused condoms in cool, dry place.
- Do not use condoms that are sticky, brittle, or obviously damaged.

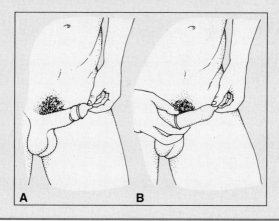

A   B

PATIENT INSTRUCTIONS FOR SELF-CARE

Use and Care of the Diaphragm

POSITIONS FOR INSERTION OF DIAPHRAGM

Squatting
Squatting is the most commonly used position, and most women find it satisfactory.

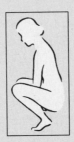

Leg-up Method
Another position is to raise the left foot (if right hand is used for insertion) on a low stool and, while in a bending position, insert the diaphragm.

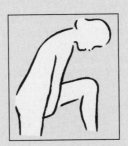

Chair Method

Another practical method for diaphragm insertion is to sit far forward on the edge of a chair.

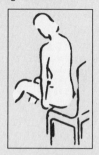

Reclining

You may prefer to insert the diaphragm while in a semireclining position in bed.

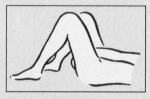

INSPECTION OF DIAPHRAGM

Your diaphragm must be inspected carefully before each use. The best way to do this is as follows:

- Hold the diaphragm up to a light source. Carefully stretch the diaphragm at the area of the rim, on all sides, to make sure there are no holes. Remember, it is possible to puncture the diaphragm with sharp fingernails.
- Another way to check for pinholes is carefully to fill the diaphragm with water. If there is any problem, it will be seen immediately.
- If your diaphragm is puckered, especially near the rim, this could mean thin spots.
- The diaphragm should not be used if you see any of these; consult your health care provider.

PREPARATION OF DIAPHRAGM

Rinse off cornstarch. Your diaphragm must always be used with a spermicidal lubricant to be effective. Pregnancy cannot be prevented effectively by the diaphragm alone.

Continued

Always empty your bladder before inserting the diaphragm. Place about 2 teaspoonfuls of contraceptive jelly or contraceptive cream on the side of the diaphragm that will rest against the cervix (or whichever way you have been instructed). Spread it around to coat the surface and the rim. This aids in insertion and offers a more complete seal. Many women also spread some jelly or cream on the other side of the diaphragm (Fig. A).

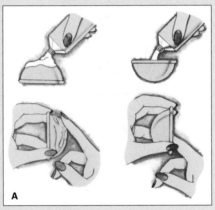

A

INSERTION OF DIAPHRAGM
The diaphragm can be inserted as long as 6 hours before intercourse. Hold the diaphragm between your thumb and fingers. The dome can be either up or down, as directed by your health care provider. Place your index finger on the outer rim of the compressed diaphragm (Fig. B).

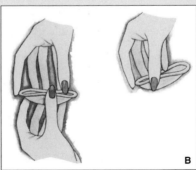

B

Use the fingers of the other hand to spread the labia (lips of the vagina). This will assist in guiding the diaphragm into place.

Insert the diaphragm into the vagina. Direct it inward and downward as far as it will go to the space behind and below the cervix (Fig. C).

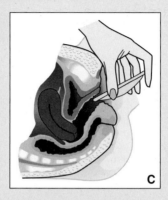

C

Tuck the front of the rim of the diaphragm behind the pubic bone so that the rubber hugs the front wall of the vagina (Fig. D).

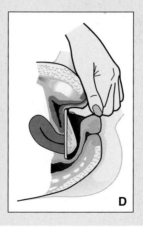

D

Continued

Feel for your cervix through the diaphragm to be certain it is properly placed and securely covered by the rubber dome (Fig. E).

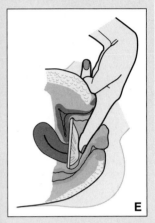

GENERAL INFORMATION

Regardless of the time of the month, you must use your diaphragm every time intercourse takes place. Your diaphragm must be left in place for at least 6 hours after the last intercourse. If you remove your diaphragm before the 6-hour period, your chance of becoming pregnant could be greatly increased. If you have repeated acts of intercourse, you must add more spermicide for each act of intercourse.

REMOVAL OF DIAPHRAGM

The only proper way to remove the diaphragm is to insert your forefinger up and over the top side of the diaphragm and slightly to the side.

Next, turn the palm of your hand downward and backward, hooking the forefinger firmly on top of the inside of the upper rim of the diaphragm, breaking the suction (Fig. F).

Pull the diaphragm down and out. This avoids the possibility of tearing the diaphragm with the fingernails. You should not remove the diaphragm by trying to catch the rim from below the dome.

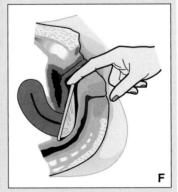

CARE OF DIAPHRAGM

When using a vaginal diaphragm, avoid using oil-based products, such as certain body lubricants, mineral oil, baby

Continued

oil, vaginal lubricants, or vaginitis preparations. These products can weaken the rubber.

A little care means longer wear for your diaphragm. After each use, wash the diaphragm in warm water and mild soap. Do not use detergent soaps, cold-cream soaps, deodorant soaps, and soaps containing oil products, because they can weaken the rubber.

After washing, dry the diaphragm thoroughly. All water and moisture should be removed with a towel. Then dust the diaphragm with cornstarch. Scented talc, body powder, baby powder, and the like should not be used because they can weaken the rubber.

To clean the introducer (if one is used), wash with mild soap and warm water, rinse, and dry thoroughly.

Place the diaphragm back in the plastic case for storage. Do not store it near a radiator or heat source or exposed to light for an extended period.

next to the cervix is concave for better fit. The opposite side has a woven polyester loop to be used for removal of the sponge.

- The sponge must be moistened with water before it is inserted. It provides protection for up to 24 hours and for repeated instances of sexual intercourse. The sponge should be left in place for at least 6 hours after the last act of intercourse. Wearing it longer than 24 to 30 hours may put the woman at risk for TSS.

Hormonal methods

More than 30 different contraceptive formulations are available in the United States today. Because of the wide variety of preparations available, the woman and nurse must read the package insert for information about specific products prescribed. Formulations include combined estrogen-progestin medications and progestational agents. The formulations are administered orally, transdermally, vaginally, by implantation, by injection, or by the intrauterine route.

Combined Estrogen-Progestin Contraceptives
Oral contraceptives

- Regular ingestion of combined oral contraceptive pills (COCs) suppresses the action of the hypothalamus and anterior pituitary, leading to inappropriate secretion of follicle-stimulating hormone (FSH) and luteinizing hormone (LH); therefore follicles do not mature, and ovulation is inhibited.
- Maturation of the endometrium is altered, making it a less favorable site for implantation. COCs also have a direct effect on the endometrium, so that from 1 to 4 days after the last COC is taken, the endometrium sloughs and bleeds as a result of hormone withdrawal. The withdrawal bleeding usually is less profuse than that of normal menstruation and may last only 2 to 3 days.
- Monophasic pills provide fixed dosages of estrogen and progestin. Multiphasic pills (e.g., biphasic and triphasic oral contraceptives) alter the amount of progestin and sometimes the amount of estrogen within each cycle. These preparations reduce the total dosage of hormones in a single cycle without sacrificing contraceptive efficacy.
- To maintain adequate hormonal levels for contraception and enhance compliance, COCs should be taken at the same time each day.
- If a pill is missed, it is suggested to take it as soon as it is remembered and to take the next pill at the regular time. No backup method usually is needed. If more then 1 pill is missed recommendations for taking pills vary, and a backup method of contraception usually is recommended.
- Use of oral hormonal contraceptives is initiated on one of the first days of the menstrual cycle (day 1 of the cycle is the first day of menses). With a "Sunday start," women begin taking pills on the first Sunday after the start of their menstrual period.

DISADVANTAGES AND SIDE EFFECTS

- Contraindications for COC use include a history of thromboembolic disorders, cerebrovascular or coronary artery disease, breast cancer or other estrogen-dependent tumors, impaired liver function, liver tumor, smoking if the woman is older than 35 years of age (more than 15 cigarettes per day), headaches with focal neurologic symptoms, surgery with prolonged immobilization or any surgery on the legs, hypertension (160/100), and diabetes mellitus (of more than 20 years' duration) with vascular disease.

- Serious adverse effects documented with high doses of estrogen and progesterone include stroke, myocardial infarction, thromboembolism, hypertension, gallbladder disease, and liver tumors.

- Common side effects of estrogen excess include nausea, breast tenderness, fluid retention, and chloasma.

- Side effects of estrogen deficiency include early spotting (days 1 to 14), hypomenorrhea, nervousness, and atrophic vaginitis leading to painful intercourse (dyspareunia).

- Side effects of progestin excess include increased appetite, tiredness, depression, breast tenderness, vaginal yeast infection, oily skin and scalp, hirsutism, and postpill amenorrhea. Side effects of progestin deficiency include late spotting and breakthrough bleeding (days 15 to 21), heavy flow with clots, and decreased breast size.

- One of the most common side effects of combined COCs is bleeding irregularities.

- The effectiveness of oral contraceptives can be negatively influenced when the following medications are taken simultaneously.
  - Anticonvulsants: barbiturates, oxcarbazepine, phenytoin, phenobarbital, felbamate, carbamazepine, primidone, and topiramate
  - Systemic antifungals: griseofulvin
  - Antituberculosis drugs: rifampicin and rifabutin
  - Anti-HIV protease inhibitors

- Over-the-counter medications, as well as some herbal supplements (e.g., St. John's wort) can alter the effectiveness of COCs. Women should be asked about their use when COCs are being considered for contraception.

- Oral contraceptives do not protect a woman against STIs or HIV. A barrier method such as condoms and spermicide should be used for protection.

Oral contraceptives 91-day regimen

- Levonorgestrel–ethinyl estradiol (Seasonale) contains both estrogen and progestin, taken in 3-month cycles of 12 weeks of active pills followed by 1 week of inactive pills. Menstrual periods occur during the thirteenth week of the cycle. There is no protection from STIs, and risks are similar to those of COCs. Seasonale is available only by prescription and must be taken on a daily schedule, regardless of the frequency of intercourse. Because users will have fewer menstrual flows, they should consider the possibility of pregnancy if they do not experience their thirteenth-week flow.

Transdermal contraceptive system

- The contraceptive transdermal patch, which is available by prescription only, delivers continuous levels of norelgestromin (progesterone) and ethinyl estradiol. The patch can be applied to intact skin of the upper outer arm, upper torso (front and back, excluding the breasts), lower abdomen, or buttocks. Application is on the same day once each week for 3 weeks, followed by 1 week without the patch. Withdrawal bleeding occurs during the "no patch" week. Mechanism of action, efficacy, contraindications, skin reactions, and side effects are similar to those of COCs. This method is not recommended for use in women who weigh more than 198 pounds.

Vaginal contraceptive ring

- The vaginal contraceptive ring, which is available only with a prescription, is a flexible ring worn in the vagina to deliver continuous levels of etonorgestrel (progesterone) and ethinyl estradiol. One vaginal ring is worn for 3 weeks, followed by 1 week without the ring. Withdrawal bleeding occurs during the "no ring" week. The ring is inserted by the woman and does not have to be fitted. Some wearers may experience vaginitis, leukorrhea, and vaginal discomfort. Mechanism of action, efficacy, contraindications, and side effects are similar to those of COCs.

Progestin-Only Contraceptives. Progestin-only methods impair fertility by inhibiting ovulation, thickening and decreasing the amount of cervical mucus, thinning the endometrium, and altering cilia in the uterine tubes.

- **Oral progestins (minipill).** Failure rate of progestin-only pills for typical users is about 8% in the first year of use. Effectiveness is increased if minipills are taken correctly. Because minipills contain such a low dose of progestin, the minipill must be taken at the same time every day. Users often complain of irregular vaginal bleeding.

- **Injectable progestins**. Depot medroxyprogesterone acetate (DMPA or Depo-Provera), 150 mg, is given intramuscularly in the deltoid or gluteus maximus muscle. A 21- to 23-gauge needle, 2.5 to 4 cm long, should be used. DMPA should be initiated during the first 5 days of the menstrual cycle and administered every 11 to 13 weeks.

> **NURSE ALERT** *When administering an intramuscular injection of progestin (e.g., Depo-Provera), do not massage the site after the injection, because this action can hasten the absorption and shorten the period of effectiveness.*

Advantages of DMPA include a contraceptive effectiveness comparable with that of combined oral contraceptives, long-lasting effects, requirement of injections only four times per year, and unlikelihood that lactation will be impaired.

Side effects at the end of 1 year include decreased bone mineral density, weight gain, lipid changes, increased risk of venous thrombosis and thromboembolism, irregular vaginal spotting, decreased libido, and breast changes. Other disadvantages include a lack of protection against STIs (including HIV). A delay in return to fertility may be as long as 18 months after discontinuing DMPA.

> **NURSE ALERT** *Women who use DMPA may lose significant bone mineral density with increasing duration of use. Women who receive DMPA should be counseled about calcium intake and exercise.*

Emergency contraception

- Emergency contraception should be taken by a woman as soon as possible but within 120 hours of unprotected intercourse or birth control mishap (e.g., broken condom, dislodged ring or cervical cap, missed oral contraceptive pills [OCPs], late for injection) to prevent unintended pregnancy. If taken before ovulation, emergency contraception prevents ovulation by inhibiting follicular development. If

TABLE 4-1

Emergency Contraceptive Pill Dosages

BRAND NAMES	FIRST DOSE (WITHIN 120 HR)	SECOND DOSE (12 HR LATER)
COMBINED ORAL CONTRACEPTIVES*		
Ovral	2 white tablets	2 white tablets
Orgestrel	2 white tablets	2 white tablets
Lo/Ovral	4 white tablets	4 white tablets
Low-Orgestrel	4 white tablets	4 white tablets
Nordette tablets	4 light orange tablets	4 light orange tablets
Levlen tablets	4 light orange tablets	4 light orange tablets
Trivora	4 yellow tablets	4 yellow tablets
Levora	4 white tablets	4 white tablets
Triphasil	4 yellow tablets	4 yellow tablets
Tri-Levlen	4 yellow tablets	4 yellow tablets
Alesse	5 pink tablets	5 pink tablets
Levlite	5 pink tablets	5 pink tablets
Aviane	5 orange tablets	5 orange tablets
PROGESTIN ONLY		
Ovrette	20 yellow tablets	20 yellow tablets
Plan B[†]	1 white tablet	1 white tablet

*Antinausea medications needed for any of the combined oral contraceptives.
[†]May take both pills at same time.
Sources: American College of Obstetricians and Gynecologists (ACOG). (2001). *Emergency oral contraception: ACOG Practice Bulletin no. 25.* Washington, DC: ACOG; Stewart, F., Trussell, J., & Van Look, P. (2004). Emergency contraception. In R. Hatcher et al. (Eds.), *Contraceptive technology* (18th ed.). New York: Ardent Media.

    taken after ovulation occurs, there is little effect on ovarian hormone production or the endometrium.
- Table 4-1 presents recommended oral medication regimens with progestin only and estrogen-progestin pills for emergency contraception.
- To minimize the side effect of nausea that occurs with high doses of estrogen and progestin, the woman can be advised to take an over-the-counter antiemetic 1 hour before each dose.

- If the woman does not begin menstruation within 21 days after taking the pills, she should be evaluated for pregnancy.
- Emergency contraception is ineffective if the woman is pregnant, because the pills do not disturb an implanted pregnancy.
- IUDs containing copper (see later discussion) provide another emergency contraception option. The IUD should be inserted within 8 days of unprotected intercourse.

Intrauterine devices

- An intrauterine device (IUD) is a small, T-shaped device with bendable arms for insertion through the cervix. Advantages to choosing this method of contraception include long-term protection from pregnancy and immediate return to fertility when removed. Disadvantages include increased risk of pelvic inflammatory disease (PID) shortly after placement, unintentional expulsion of the device, infection, and possible uterine perforation. IUDs offer no protection against HIV or other STIs. Therefore women who are in mutually monogamous relationships are the best candidates for these devices.
- There are two U.S. Food and Drug Administration (FDA)–approved IUDs. The ParaGard T-380A (copper IUD) is made of radiopaque polyethylene and fine solid copper and is approved for 10 years of use. Mirena is a hormonal intrauterine system that releases levonorgestrel and is effective for up to 5 years.
- The woman should be taught to check for the presence of the IUD strings after menstruation to rule out expulsion of the device. Signs of potential complications to be taught to the woman include abnormal spotting or bleeding, abdominal pain, infection, and abnormal vaginal discharge.

Sterilization

Sterilization refers to surgical procedures intended to render a person infertile. Most procedures involve the occlusion of the passageways for the ova and sperm. For the woman, the uterine tubes are occluded; for the man, the vasa deferentia are occluded.

PATIENT INSTRUCTIONS FOR SELF-CARE

What to Expect after Bilateral Tubal Ligation

- You should expect no change in hormones and their influence.
- Your menstrual period will be about the same as before the sterilization.
- You may feel pain at ovulation.
- The ovum disintegrates within the abdominal cavity.
- It is highly unlikely that you will become pregnant.
- You should not have a change in sexual functioning; you may enjoy sexual relations more because you will not be concerned about becoming pregnant.
- Sterilization offers no protection against sexually transmitted infections (STIs); therefore you may need to use condoms.

Female Sterilization

- A laparoscopic approach or a minilaparotomy may be used for tubal ligation (salpingectomy), tubal electrocoagulation (bipolar cautery), or the application of bands (Silastic: Fallope ring or Yoon Band) or clips (Hulka-Clemens spring clip or Filshie clip). Electrocoagulation and ligation are considered to be permanent methods. Use of the bands or clips has the theoretic advantage of possible removal and return of tubal patency.
- For the mini-laparotomy, the woman is admitted the morning of surgery, having taken nothing by mouth since midnight. Preoperative sedation is given. The procedure may be carried out with the patient under local anesthesia, but general anesthesia also may be used. A small incision is made in the abdominal wall below the umbilicus (see Patient Instructions for Self-Care box).

Male Sterilization

- Vasectomy can be carried out with the patient under local anesthesia on an outpatient basis. Pain, bleeding, infection, and other postsurgical complications are considered the disadvantages to the surgical procedure.

- The man is instructed in self-care to promote a safe return to routine activities. To reduce swelling and relieve discomfort, ice packs are applied to the scrotum intermittently for a few hours after surgery. A scrotal support may be applied to decrease discomfort. Moderate inactivity for about 2 days is advisable because of local scrotal tenderness. Sexual intercourse may be resumed as desired; however, sterility is not immediate. Some sperm will remain in the proximal portions of the sperm ducts after vasectomy. One week to several months are required to clear the ducts of sperm (i.e., after approximately 20 ejaculations); therefore some form of contraception is needed until the sperm count in the ejaculate on two consecutive tests is down to zero.

Laws and Regulations

- All states have strict regulations for informed consent.
- If federal funds are used for sterilization, the person must be age 21 years or older.
- Informed consent must include an explanation of the risks, benefits, and alternatives; a statement that describes sterilization as a permanent, irreversible method of birth control; and a statement that mandates a 30-day waiting period between giving consent and the sterilization.
- Informed consent must be in the person's native language, or a translator must be provided to read the consent form to the person.

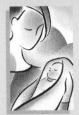

CHAPTER 5

Antepartum Assessment

BIOPHYSICAL ASSESSMENT

The major expected outcome of all antepartum testing is the detection of potential fetal compromise. No single test can provide this information. Assessment tests should be selected based on their effectiveness, and the results must be interpreted in light of the complete clinical picture.

Daily Fetal Movement Count

Indications
- Daily fetal movement count (DFMC, also called "kick counts") is frequently used to monitor the fetus in pregnancies complicated by conditions that may affect fetal oxygenation.

Procedure and interpretation
- Can be done at home, is noninvasive, is simple to understand, and usually does not interfere with a daily routine.
- Several protocols are used for counting. One protocol is to instruct the pregnant woman to lie down on her side and count every fetal movement for 60 minutes.
- The clinical value of the absolute number of fetal movements has not been established, except in the situation in which fetal movements cease entirely for 12 hours. A count of fewer than three fetal movements within 1 hour usually warrants further evaluation.
- The presence of movements is generally a reassuring sign of fetal health.
- In assessing fetal movements, it is important to remember that they are usually not present during the fetal sleep cycle; also, they may be temporarily reduced if the woman is taking depressant medications, drinking alcohol, or smoking a cigarette.

- Women should be taught the significance of the presence or absence of fetal movements, the procedure for counting that is to be used, how to record findings on a DFMC record, and when to notify their health care provider.

Ultrasonography

Indications

- Diagnostic ultrasonography is an important, safe technique in antepartum fetal surveillance. It provides critical information to health care providers regarding fetal activity and gestational age, normal versus abnormal fetal growth curves, visual assistance with which invasive tests may be performed more safely, fetal and placental anatomy, and fetal well-being. Major indications for obstetric sonography appear by trimester in Table 5-1.

Procedure and interpretation

- For abdominal scans, the woman usually should have a full bladder to get a better image of the fetus. Transmission gel or paste is applied to the woman's abdomen before a transducer is moved over the skin to enhance transmission and reception of the sound waves.
- For transvaginal ultrasonography, in which the probe is inserted into the vagina, a full bladder is not necessary. A protective cover such as a condom or the finger of a clean rubber surgical glove is used to cover the transducer probe. The probe is lubricated with a water-soluble gel and placed in the vagina either by the examiner or by the woman herself.
- Interpretation depends on why the scan was done.

Doppler Blood Flow Analysis

Indications

- Doppler ultrasound is used to study the uteroplacental blood flow in umbilical arteries in the management of pregnancies at risk because of hypertension, intrauterine growth restriction (IUGR), diabetes mellitus, multiple fetuses, preterm labor, or other causes of uteroplacental insufficiency.

TABLE 5-1

Major Uses of Ultrasonography During Pregnancy

FIRST TRIMESTER	SECOND TRIMESTER	THIRD TRIMESTER
Confirm pregnancy	Establish or confirm dates	Confirm gestational age
Confirm viability	Confirm viability	Confirm viability
Determine gestational age	Detect polyhydramnios, oligohydramnios	Detect macrosomia
Rule out ectopic pregnancy	Detect congenital anomalies	Detect congenital anomalies
Detect multiple gestation	Detect intrauterine growth restriction (IUGR)	Detect IUGR
Visualize during chorionic villus sampling	Confirm placenta placement	Determine fetal position
Detect maternal abnormalities, such as bicornuate uterus, ovarian cysts, fibroids	Visualize fetus during amniocentesis	Detect placenta previa or abruptio placentae
		Visualize fetus during amniocentesis, external version
		Do biophysical profile
		Do amniotic fluid volume assessment
		Do Doppler flow studies
		Detect placental maturity

Procedure and interpretation

- A pulsed Doppler device is positioned over the fetus, and umbilical artery blood flow is measured. A plot of velocity versus time and the shape of these waveforms can be analyzed to give information about blood flow and resistance in a given circulation.
- Velocity waveforms reported as systolic/diastolic (S/D) ratios can be first detected at 15 weeks of pregnancy. Because of the progressive decline in resistance in both the umbilical and uterine arteries, this ratio decreases as pregnancy advances. Most fetuses will achieve an S/D ratio of 3 or less by 30 weeks.
- Persistent elevation of S/D ratios after 30 weeks is considered abnormal.

Amniotic Fluid Volume Index

Indications

- The amniotic fluid index (AFI) evaluates the quantity of amniotic fluid to determine adequate uteroplacental function. Decreased (oligohydramnios) or increased (polyhydramnios) amniotic fluid volume is frequently associated with fetal disorders. Oligohydramnios is associated with congenital anomalies (e.g., renal agenesis), growth restriction, and fetal distress during labor. Polyhydramnios is associated with neural tube defects, obstruction of the fetal gastrointestinal tract, multiple fetuses, and fetal hydrops.

Procedure and interpretation

- The total amniotic fluid volume (AFV) can be evaluated by using ultrasound to measure the depths (in centimeters) of the amniotic fluid in all four quadrants surrounding the maternal umbilicus. The measurements are totaled.
- An AFI less than 5 cm indicates oligohydramnios; 5 to 19 cm is considered a normal measurement; and a measurement greater than 20 cm reflects polyhydramnios.

Biophysical Profile

Indications

- The biophysical profile (BPP) is a noninvasive dynamic assessment of fetal well-being. The presence of normal fetal biophysical activities indicates that the central nervous system (CNS) is functional, and the fetus therefore is not hypoxemic.

Procedure and interpretation

- An abdominal ultrasound scan is done to evaluate fetal breathing movements (FBMs), fetal movements, fetal tone, and AFV; fetal heart rate (FHR) patterns are assessed by means of a nonstress test.
- When the BPP score is normal and the risk of fetal death low, intervention is indicated only for obstetric or maternal factors. BPP variables and scoring are detailed in Table 5-2.

BIOCHEMICAL ASSESSMENT

Biochemical assessment involves biologic examination (e.g., as chromosomes in exfoliated cells) and chemical determinations (e.g., lecithin/sphingomyelin [L/S] ratio and bilirubin level) (Table 5-3). Procedures used to obtain the needed specimens include amniocentesis, percutaneous umbilical blood sampling, chorionic villus sampling, and maternal sampling.

Amniocentesis

Indications

- Amniocentesis is performed to obtain amniotic fluid, which contains fetal cells. Indications for the procedure include prenatal diagnosis of genetic disorders or congenital anomalies (neural tube defects in particular), assessment of pulmonary maturity, and diagnosis of fetal hemolytic disease.

Procedure and interpretation

- The examiner uses direct ultrasonographic visualization to insert a needle transabdominally into the uterus, withdraw amniotic fluid into a syringe, and perform various assessments. Amniocentesis is possible after week 14 of pregnancy, when the uterus becomes an abdominal organ, and sufficient amniotic fluid is available for testing.
- Complications in the mother and fetus occur in fewer than 1% of the cases and include the following:

TABLE 5-2

Biophysical Profile

VARIABLES	NORMAL (SCORE = 2)	ABNORMAL (SCORE = 0)
Fetal breathing movements	One or more episodes in 30 min, each lasting ≥30 sec	Episodes absent or no episode ≥30 sec in 30 min
Gross body movements	Three or more discrete body or limb movements in 30 min (episodes of active continuous movement being considered as a single movement)	Less than three episodes of body or limb movements in 30 min
Fetal tone	One or more episodes of active extension with return to flexion of fetal limb(s) or trunk, opening and closing of hand being considered normal tone	Slow extension with return to flexion, movement of limb in full extension, or fetal movement absent
Reactive fetal heart rate	Two or more episodes of acceleration (≥15 beats/min) in 20 min, each lasting ≥15 sec and associated with fetal movement	Less than two episodes of acceleration or acceleration of <15 beats/min in 20 min
Amniotic fluid volume	One or more pockets of fluid measuring ≥1 cm in two perpendicular planes	Pockets absent or pocket <1 cm in two perpendicular planes

SCORE

Normal 8-10 (if amniotic fluid index is adequate)

Equivocal 6

Abnormal <4

Reference: Harman, C. (2004). Assessment of fetal health. In R. Creasy, R. Resnik, & J. Iams (Eds.), *Maternal-fetal medicine: Principles and practice* (5th ed.). Philadelphia: Saunders.

- —Maternal: hemorrhage, fetomaternal hemorrhage with possible maternal Rh isoimmunization, infection, labor, abruptio placentae, inadvertent damage to the intestines or bladder, and amniotic fluid embolism.
- —Because of the possibility of fetomaternal hemorrhage, it is standard practice after an amniocentesis to administer Rh_oD immune globulin (e.g., RhoGAM) to the woman who is Rh negative.
- —Fetal: death, hemorrhage, infection (amnionitis), direct injury from the needle, miscarriage or preterm labor, and leakage of amniotic fluid.
- Table 5-3 lists possible findings and clinical significance of amniotic fluid analysis.

Chorionic Villus Sampling

Indications

- Chorionic villus sampling (CVS) is done for genetic studies. Although indications for CVS are similar to those for amniocentesis, the benefits of earlier diagnosis must be weighed against the increased risk of pregnancy loss and risk of anomalies.

Procedure and interpretation

- The procedure is performed between 10 and 12 weeks of gestation and involves the removal of a small tissue specimen from the fetal portion of the placenta.
- In transcervical sampling, the examiner uses continuous ultrasonographic guidance to introduce a sterile catheter into the cervix and aspirate a small portion of the chorionic villi with a syringe. The aspiration cannula and obturator must be placed at a suitable site, and rupture of the amniotic sac must be avoided.
- If the abdominal approach is used, the examiner uses sterile conditions and ultrasound guidance to insert an 18-gauge spinal needle with stylet through the abdominal wall into the chorion frondosum. The stylet is then withdrawn, and the chorionic tissue is aspirated into a syringe.
- Complications of the procedure include vaginal spotting or bleeding immediately afterward and, uncommonly, miscarriage, rupture of membranes, and chorioamnionitis.

TABLE 5-3

Summary of Biochemical Monitoring Techniques

TEST	POSSIBLE FINDINGS	CLINICAL SIGNIFICANCE
MATERNAL BLOOD		
Coombs' test	Titer of 1:8 and rising	Significant Rh incompatibility
Alpha fetoprotein (AFP)	See below	
AMNIOTIC FLUID ANALYSIS		
Color	Meconium	Possible hypoxia or asphyxia
Lung profile		Fetal lung maturity
Lecithin-sphingomyelin (L/S ratio)	>2:1	
Phosphatidylglycerol	Present	
Creatinine	>2 mg/dl	Gestational age >36 wk
Bilirubin delta optical density (ΔOD 450/nm)	<0.015	Gestational age >36 wk, normal pregnancy
		Fetal hemolytic disease in Rh-isoimmunized pregnancies
Lipid cells	>10%	Gestational age >35 wk
AFP	High levels after 15-wk gestation	Open neural tube or other defect
Osmolality	Decline after 20-wk gestation	Advancing gestational age
Genetic disorders	Dependent on cultured cells for karyotype and enzymatic activity	Counseling possibly required
Sex linked		
Chromosomal		
Metabolic		

- Because of the possibility of fetomaternal hemorrhage, women who are Rh negative should receive Rh_oD immune globulin to avoid isoimmunization.
- An increased risk of limb anomalies (transverse digital anomalies) has been noted when CVS is done before 10 weeks of gestation.
- Interpretation is based on what is being evaluated.

Percutaneous Umbilical Blood Sampling

Indications

- Percutaneous umbilical blood sampling (PUBS), or cordocentesis, is used for fetal blood sampling and transfusion. Indications for use of PUBS include prenatal diagnosis of inherited blood disorders, karyotyping of malformed fetuses, detection of fetal infection, determination of the acid-base status of fetuses with IUGR, and assessment and treatment of isoimmunization and thrombocytopenia in the fetus.

Procedure and interpretation

- PUBS involves the insertion of a needle directly into a fetal umbilical vessel using ultrasound guidance.
- Generally, 1 to 4 ml of blood is removed and tested immediately by the Kleihauer-Betke procedure to ensure that it is fetal in origin.
- Complications that can occur include leaking of blood from the puncture site, cord laceration, thromboembolism, preterm labor, premature rupture of membranes, and infection.
- Follow-up includes continuous FHR monitoring for several minutes to 1 hour and a repeated ultrasound examination 1 hour later to ensure that no further bleeding or hematoma formation has occurred.
- Interpretation is based on why PUBS was performed.

Maternal Assays

Alpha-Fetoprotein

Indications

- Maternal serum alpha-fetoprotein (MSAFP) levels have been used as a screening tool for neural tube defects

(NTDs) in pregnancy. Through this technique, approximately 80% to 85% of all open NTDs and open abdominal wall defects can be detected early in pregnancy. Screening is recommended for all pregnant women.

Procedure and interpretation

- MSAFP screening can be done with reasonable reliability any time between 15 and 22 weeks of gestation (16 to 18 weeks being ideal).
- A blood sample is drawn and sent for analysis.
- Once the maternal level of AFP is determined, it is compared with normal values for each week of gestation. Values also should be correlated with maternal age, weight, race, and whether the woman has insulin-dependent diabetes.
- Higher-than-normal levels are associated with NTDs.
- Down syndrome and probably other autosomal trisomies are associated with lower-than-normal levels of MSAFP.
- If findings are abnormal, follow-up procedures include genetic counseling for families with a history of NTD, repeated AFP, ultrasound examination, and possibly amniocentesis.

Triple-Marker Test
Indications

- The triple-marker test also is performed at 16 to 18 weeks of gestation and uses the levels of three maternal serum markers: MSAFP, unconjugated estriol, and human chorionic gonadotropin (hCG), in combination with maternal age to calculate the risk of a fetus with Down syndrome.

Procedure and interpretation

- A blood sample is drawn and sent for analysis.
- In the presence of a fetus with Down syndrome, the MSAFP and unconjugated estriol levels are low, whereas the hCG level is elevated.
- As with MSAFP, these tests are screening procedures only and are not diagnostic. A definitive examination of amniotic fluid for AFP and chromosomal analysis combined with ultrasound visualization of the fetus is necessary for diagnosis.

Coombs' Test

Indications

- The indirect Coombs' test is a screening for Rh incompatibility. Coombs' test also can detect other antibodies that may place the fetus at risk for incompatibility with maternal antigens.

Procedure and interpretation

- A blood sample is drawn and sent for analysis.
- If the maternal titer for Rh antibodies is greater than 1:8, amniocentesis for determination of bilirubin in amniotic fluid is indicated to establish the severity of fetal hemolytic anemia.

ANTEPARTAL ASSESSMENT USING ELECTRONIC FETAL MONITORING

Indications

- First- and second-trimester antepartal assessment is directed primarily at the diagnosis of fetal anomalies. The goal of third-trimester testing is to determine whether the intrauterine environment continues to be supportive to the fetus.
- The testing is often used to determine the timing of childbirth for women at risk for uteroplacental insufficiency (UPI). Gradual loss of placental function results first in inadequate nutrient delivery to the fetus, leading to IUGR. Subsequently, respiratory function also is compromised, resulting in fetal hypoxia.
- Box 5-1 lists common indications for both the nonstress test (NST) and the contraction stress test (CST).

Procedure and interpretation

- For the *nonstress test*, the woman is seated in a reclining chair (or in semi-Fowler position) with a slight left tilt to optimize uterine perfusion and avoid supine hypotension.
  - The FHR is recorded with a Doppler transducer, and a tocodynamometer is applied to detect uterine contractions or fetal movements.
  - The tracing is observed for signs of fetal activity and a concurrent acceleration of FHR.

BOX 5-1

Indications for Electronic Fetal Monitoring Assessment Using NST and CST

Maternal diabetes mellitus
Chronic hypertension
Hypertensive disorders in pregnancy
Intrauterine growth restriction
Sickle cell disease
Maternal cyanotic heart disease
Postmaturity
History of previous stillbirth
Decreased fetal movement
Isoimmunization
Meconium-stained amniotic fluid at third-trimester
   amniocentesis
Hyperthyroidism
Collagen disease
Older pregnant woman
Chronic renal disease

NST, Nonstress test; *CST,* contraction stress test.

—The test is usually completed within 20 to 30 minutes, but it may take longer if the fetus must be awakened from a sleep state.

—Table 5-4 lists the interpretation and clinical significance of findings.

- *Vibroacoustic stimulation* (also called fetal acoustic stimulation test) is another method of testing antepartum FHR response and is sometimes used in conjunction with the NST.

   —The test takes approximately 15 minutes to complete, with the fetus monitored for 5 to 10 minutes before stimulation to obtain a baseline FHR.

   —If the fetal baseline pattern is nonreactive, the sound source (usually a laryngeal stimulator) is then activated for 3 seconds on the maternal abdomen over the fetal head. Monitoring continues for another 5 minutes, after which the monitor tracing is assessed.

TABLE 5-4

Interpretation of the Nonstress Test

RESULT	INTERPRETATION	CLINICAL SIGNIFICANCE
Reactive	Two or more accelerations of FHR of 15 beats/min lasting ≥15 sec, associated with each fetal movement in a 20-min period	As long as twice-weekly NSTs remain reactive, most high risk pregnancies are allowed to continue
Nonreactive	Any tracing with either no FHR accelerations or accelerations <15 beats/min or lasting <15 sec throughout any fetal movement during testing period	Further indirect monitoring may be attempted with abdominal fetal electrocardiography in an effort to clarify FHR pattern and quantitate variability; external monitoring should continue, and CST or BPP should be done
Unsatisfactory	Quality of FHR recording not adequate for interpretation	Test is repeated in 24 hr or CST is done depending on clinical situation

Reference: Tucker, S. (2004). *Pocket guide to fetal monitoring and assessment* (5th ed.). St. Louis: Mosby.
FHR, Fetal heart rate; *NST,* nonstress test; *CST,* contraction stress test; *BPP,* biophysical profile.

—A test is considered reactive if there is an immediate and sustained increase in long-term variability and FHR accelerations. The accelerations produced may have a significant increase in duration. The test may be repeated at 1-minute intervals up to three times when there is no response.

—Further evaluation is needed with BPP or CST if the pattern is still nonreactive.

- For the *contraction stress* test the woman is placed in semi-Fowler position or sits in a reclining chair with a slight left tilt to optimize uterine perfusion and avoid supine hypotension.

  —She is monitored electronically with the fetal ultrasound transducer and uterine tocodynamometer.

  —The tracing is observed for 10 to 20 minutes for baseline rate, long-term variability, and the possible occurrence of spontaneous contractions. The two methods of CST are the nipple-stimulated contraction test and the oxytocin-stimulated contraction test.

  —Table 5-5 lists interpretation and clinical significance of findings.

  —*Nipple-Stimulated Contraction Test*—Several methods of nipple stimulation have been described. In one approach, the woman applies warm, moist washcloths to both breasts for several minutes. The woman is then asked to massage one nipple for 10 minutes. Massaging the nipples causes a release of oxytocin from the posterior pituitary. An alternative approach is for her to massage the nipple for 2 minutes, rest for 5 minutes, and repeat the cycles of massage and rest as necessary to achieve adequate uterine activity. When adequate contractions or hyperstimulation (defined as uterine contractions lasting more than 90 seconds or five or more contractions in 10 minutes) occurs, stimulation should be stopped.

  —*Oxytocin-Stimulated Contraction Test*—Exogenous oxytocin also can be used to stimulate uterine contractions. An intravenous (IV) infusion is begun with a scalp needle. The oxytocin is diluted in an IV solution (e.g., 10 units in 1000 ml fluid), infused into the tubing of the main IV device through a piggyback port and delivered by an

TABLE 5-5

Guide for Interpretation of the Contraction Stress Test

INTERPRETATION	CLINICAL SIGNIFICANCE
NEGATIVE No late decelerations, with minimum of three uterine contractions lasting 40-60 sec within 10-min period	Reassurance that the fetus is likely to survive labor should it occur within 1 wk; more frequent testing may be indicated by clinical situation
POSITIVE Persistent and consistent late decelerations occurring with more than one half of contractions	Management lies between use of other tools of fetal assessment, such as BPP, and termination of pregnancy (e.g., labor induction, cesarean birth); a positive test result indicates that fetus is at increased risk for perinatal morbidity and mortality; physician may perform expeditious vaginal birth after successful induction or may proceed directly to cesarean birth; decision to intervene is determined by fetal monitoring and presence of FHR reactivity

SUSPICIOUS

Late decelerations occurring in less than one half of uterine contractions once adequate contraction pattern established

NST and CST should be repeated within 24 hr; if interpretable data cannot be achieved, other methods of fetal assessment must be used*

HYPERSTIMULATION

Late decelerations occurring with excessive uterine activity (contractions more often than every 2 min or lasting longer than 90 sec) or persistent increase in uterine tone

UNSATISFACTORY

Inadequate uterine contraction pattern or tracing too poor to interpret

Reference: Tucker, S. (2004). *Pocket guide to fetal monitoring and assessment* (5th ed.). St. Louis: Mosby.
BPP, Biophysical profile; *CST,* contraction stress test; *FHR,* fetal heart rate; *NST,* nonstress test.
*Applies to results noted as suspicious, hyperstimulation, or unsatisfactory.

infusion pump to ensure accurate dosage. One method of oxytocin infusion is to begin at 0.5 milliunits/min and increase the dose by 0.5 milliunits/min at 15-minute to 30-minute intervals until three uterine contractions of good quality are observed within a 10-minute period. A rate of 10 milliunits/min is usually adequate to elicit uterine contractions.

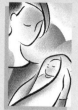

Maternal and Fetal Nutrition

Nutrition is one of many factors that influence the outcome of pregnancy. Good nutrition before and during pregnancy is an important preventive measure for a variety of problems.

NUTRIENT NEEDS BEFORE CONCEPTION

A healthful diet before conception is the best way to ensure that adequate nutrients are available for the developing fetus. Folate or folic acid intake is of particular concern in the periconceptional period.

- Folate is the form found naturally in foods.
- Folic acid is the form used in fortification of grain products and other foods and in vitamin supplements.
- All women capable of becoming pregnant are advised to consume 0.4 mg (400 mcg) of folic acid daily in fortified foods (ready-to-eat cereals and enriched grain products) or supplements, in addition to a diet rich in folate-containing foods: green leafy vegetables, whole grains, and fruits.

NUTRIENT NEEDS DURING PREGNANCY

The amount of fetal growth varies during the different stages of pregnancy. During the first trimester, the synthesis of fetal tissues places relatively few demands on maternal nutrition. In contrast, the last trimester is a period of noticeable fetal growth when most of the fetal stores of energy and minerals are deposited.

Energy Needs

Energy (kilocalories, or kcal) needs are met by carbohydrate, fat, and protein in the diet. No specific recommendations exist for the amount of carbohydrate and fat in the diet of the pregnant woman, but the intake of these nutrients should be adequate to support the recommended weight gain. The primary role of protein is to provide amino acids for the synthesis of new tissues. See Table 6-1 for nutrient intakes during pregnancy and lactation.

Weight Gain

- The optimal weight gain during pregnancy is not known precisely.
- An adequate weight gain does not necessarily indicate that the diet is nutritionally adequate, but it is associated with a reduced risk of giving birth to a small for gestational age (SGA) or preterm infant.
- The primary factor to consider in making a weight gain recommendation is the appropriateness of the prepregnancy weight for the woman's height, that is, whether the woman's weight was normal before pregnancy or whether she was underweight or overweight.
- Maternal and fetal risks in pregnancy are increased when the mother is significantly underweight or overweight before pregnancy and when weight gain during pregnancy is either too low or too high.
  - Severely underweight women are more likely to have preterm labor and to give birth to low-birth-weight (LBW) infants.
  - Both normal-weight and underweight women with inadequate weight gain have an increased risk of giving birth to an infant with intrauterine growth restriction (IUGR).
- Greater-than-expected weight gain during pregnancy may occur for many reasons, including multiple gestation, edema, gestational hypertension, and overeating.
- When obesity is preexisting or develops during pregnancy, there is an increased likelihood of macrosomia and fetopelvic disproportion; operative birth; emergency cesarean birth; postpartum hemorrhage; wound, genital tract, or urinary tract infection; birth trauma; and late fetal death.
- Obese women are more likely than normal-weight women to have gestational hypertension and gestational diabetes.

Text continued on p. 100.

TABLE 6-1

Recommendations for Daily Intakes of Selected Nutrients during Pregnancy and Lactation

NUTRIENT (UNIT)	NONPREGNANT WOMAN	PREGNANCY*	LACTATION*	ROLE IN RELATION TO PREGNANCY AND LACTATION	FOOD SOURCES
Energy (kilocalories [kcal] or kilojoules [kJ†])	Variable	First trimester, same as nonpregnant; second and third trimesters, nonpregnant + 300 kcal or 72 kJ	Nonpregnant + 500 kcal or 120 kJ	Growth of fetal and maternal tissues; milk production	Carbohydrate, fat, and protein
Protein (g)	50	60	65	Synthesis of the products of conception; growth of maternal tissue and expansion of blood volume; secretion of milk protein during lactation	Meats, eggs, cheese, yogurt, legumes (dry beans and peas, peanuts), nuts, grains

Continued

TABLE 6-1

Recommendations for Daily Intakes of Selected Nutrients during Pregnancy and Lactation—cont'd

NUTRIENT (UNIT)	NONPREGNANT WOMAN	PREGNANCY*	LACTATION*	ROLE IN RELATION TO PREGNANCY AND LACTATION	FOOD SOURCES
MINERALS					
Calcium (mg)	1300/1000	1300/1000	1300/1000	Fetal and infant skeleton and tooth formation; maintenance of maternal bone and tooth mineralization	Milk, cheese, yogurt, sardines or other fish eaten with bones left in, deep green leafy vegetables except spinach or Swiss chard, calcium-set tofu, baked beans, tortillas
Iron (mg)	15/18	30	10/9	Maternal hemoglobin formation, fetal liver iron storage	Liver, meats, whole grain or enriched breads and cereals, deep green leafy vegetables, legumes, dried fruits

Zinc (mg)	9/8	12/11	13/12	Component of numerous enzyme systems, possibly important in preventing congenital malformations	Liver, shellfish, meats, whole grains, milk
Iodine (mcg)	150	220	290	Increased maternal metabolic rate	Iodized salt, seafood, milk and milk products, commercial yeast breads, rolls, and donuts
Magnesium (mg)	360/320	400/360	350/320	Involved in energy and protein metabolism, tissue growth, muscle action	Nuts, legumes, cocoa, meats, whole grains
FAT-SOLUBLE VITAMINS					
A (mcg)	700	750/770	1200/1300	Essential for cell development, tooth bud formation, bone growth	Deep green leafy vegetables, dark yellow vegetables, and fruits, chili peppers, liver, fortified margarine and butter

Continued

TABLE 6-1

Recommendations for Daily Intakes of Selected Nutrients during Pregnancy and Lactation—cont'd

NUTRIENT (UNIT)	NONPREGNANT WOMAN	PREGNANCY*	LACTATION*	ROLE IN RELATION TO PREGNANCY AND LACTATION	FOOD SOURCES
D (mcg)	5	5	5	Involved in absorption of calcium and phosphorus, improves mineralization	Fortified milk and margarine, egg yolk, butter, liver, seafood
E (mg)	15	15	19	Antioxidant (protects cell membranes from damage), especially important for preventing breakdown of RBCs	Vegetable oils, green leafy vegetables, whole grains, liver, nuts and seeds, cheese, fish
WATER-SOLUBLE VITAMINS					
C (mg)	65/75	80/85	115/120	Tissue formation and integrity, formation of connective tissue, enhancement of iron absorption	Citrus fruits, strawberries, melons, broccoli, tomatoes, peppers, raw deep green leafy vegetables

Folate (mcg)	400	600	500	Prevention of neural tube defects, support for increased maternal RBC formation	Fortified ready-to-eat cereals and other grain products, green leafy vegetables, oranges, broccoli, asparagus, artichokes, liver
B$_6$ or pyridoxine (mg)	1.2/1.3	1.9	2.0	Involved in protein metabolism	Meat, liver, deep green vegetables, whole grains
B$_{12}$ (mcg)	2.4	2.6	2.8	Production of nucleic acids and proteins, especially important in formation of RBC and neural functioning	Milk and milk products, egg, meat, liver, fortified soy milk

*When two values appear, separated by a diagonal slash, the first is for females younger than 19 years, and the second is for those 19 to 50 years of age.

†The international metric unit of energy measurement is the joule (J).
1 kcal = 4.184 kJ.

RBCs, red blood cells.

Recommendations are the Dietary Reference Intakes (RDA or AI, see text), where available. Sources: Food and Nutrition Board, National Academy of Sciences, Institute of Medicine, 1997; *Dietary Reference Intakes for calcium, phosphorus, magnesium, vitamin D, and fluoride,* 1998; *Dietary Reference Intakes for thiamin, riboflavin, niacin, vitamin B6, folate, vitamin B12, pantothenic acid, biotin, and choline,* 2000; *Dietary Reference Intakes for vitamin C, vitamin E, selenium, and carotenoids,* 2001; *Dietary Reference Intakes for vitamin A, vitamin K, arsenic, boron, chromium, copper, iodine, iron, manganese, molybdenum, nickel, silicon, vanadium, and zinc,* Washington, DC, National Academy Press. Where DRIs are not available, the values are taken from Food and Nutrition Board, National Academy of Sciences, National Research Council: *Recommended dietary allowances,* ed 10, Washington, DC, 1989, National Academy Press.

- The risk of giving birth to a child with a major congenital defect is double that of normal-weight women.

A commonly used method of evaluating the appropriateness of weight for height is the body mass index (BMI), which is calculated by the following formula:

$$BMI = Weight/Height^2$$

where the weight is in kilograms and height is in meters. Thus for a woman who weighed 51 kg before pregnancy and is 1.57 m tall:

$$BMI = 51/(1.57)^2, \text{ or } 20.7$$

This BMI is in the normal range (Table 6-2).

Pattern of weight gain

Weight gain should take place throughout pregnancy. The woman's weight gain can be compared with standardized grids showing recommended patterns (Fig. 6-1).

- The risk of giving birth to an SGA infant is greater when the weight gain early in pregnancy has been poor.
- The likelihood of preterm birth is greater when the gains during the last half of pregnancy have been inadequate.
- The risk of mechanical complications at birth is reduced if the weight gain of short adult women (shorter than 157 cm, or 5 feet 2 inches) is near the lower end of their recommended range.

These risks exist even when the total gain for the pregnancy is in the recommended range.

Recommended weight gain during pregnancy varies with the BMI (see Table 6-2):

- Adolescents are encouraged to strive for weight gains at the upper end of the recommended range for their BMI, because it appears that the fetus and the still-growing mother compete for nutrients.
- In twin gestations, gains of approximately 16 to 20 kg appear to be associated with the best outcomes.

The recommended caloric intake corresponds to this pattern of gain:

- There is no increment for the first trimester.

TABLE 6-2

Classification of Prepregnant BMI with Recommended Weight Gain Pattern During Pregnancy

BMI	CLASSIFICATION	RECOMMENDED WEIGHT GAIN DURING PREGNANCY		
		TOTAL	FIRST TRIMESTER	WEEKLY WEIGHT GAIN IN SECOND AND THIRD TRIMESTERS
<19.8	Underweight or low	12.5-18 kg	1-2.5 kg	0.5 kg
19.8-26.0	Normal	11.5-16 kg	1-2.5 kg	0.4 kg
26.0-29.0	Overweight or high	7-11.5 kg	1-2.5 kg	0.3 kg
>29.0	Obese	At least 7 kg	1-2.5 kg	0.3 kg

BMI, Body mass index.

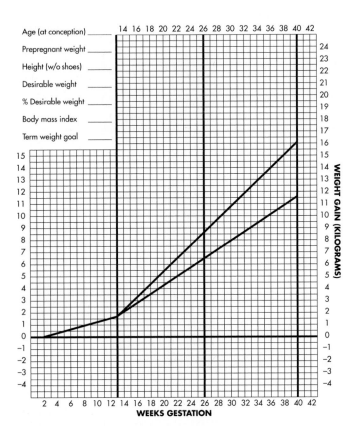

Fig. 6-1 Prenatal weight gain chart for plotting weight gain of normal weight women. NOTE: Young adolescents, African-American women, and smokers should aim for the upper end of the recommended range; short women (less than 157 cm or 5 feet 2 inches) should strive for gains at the lower end of the range.

- An additional 300 kcal/day over the prepregnant intake is recommended during the second and third trimesters.

The amount of food providing 300 kcal is not great. It can be provided by one additional serving from each of the following groups: milk, yogurt, or cheese (all skim milk products);

BOX 6-1

Calcium Sources for Women Who Do Not Drink Milk

Each of the following provides approximately the same amount of calcium as 1 cup of milk.

FISH
3-oz can of sardines
$4\frac{1}{2}$-oz can of salmon (if bones are eaten)

BEANS AND LEGUMES
3 cups cooked dried beans
$2\frac{1}{2}$ cups refried beans
2 cups baked beans with molasses
1 cup tofu (calcium is added in processing)

GREENS
1 cup collards
$1\frac{1}{2}$ cups kale or turnip greens

BAKED PRODUCTS
3 pieces cornbread
3 English muffins
4 slices French toast
2 waffles (7 inches in diameter)

FRUITS
11 dried figs
$1\frac{1}{8}$ cups orange juice with calcium added

SAUCES
3 oz pesto sauce
5 oz cheese sauce

fruits; vegetables; and bread, cereal, rice, or pasta. See Box 6-1 for calcium sources for women who do not drink milk.

The reasons for an inadequate weight gain (less than 1 kg/mo for normal-weight women or less than 0.5 kg/mo for obese women during the last two trimesters) or excessive weight gain (more than 3 kg/mo) should be thoroughly evaluated. Possible reasons for deviations from the expected rate of weight gain, besides inadequate or excessive dietary intake, include the following:

- Measurement or recording errors
- Differences in the weight of clothing

- Differences in the time of day
- The accumulation of fluids

Hazards of restricting adequate weight gain

Pregnancy is not a time for a weight reduction diet.

- Overweight or obese pregnant women need to gain at least enough weight to equal the weight of the products of conception (fetus, placenta, and amniotic fluid).
- Dietary restriction results in the catabolism of fat stores, which in turn augments the production of ketones.
- Ketonuria has been found to be correlated with the occurrence of preterm labor.
- Quality of the weight gain is important, with emphasis placed on the consumption of nutrient-dense foods and the avoidance of empty-calorie foods.

Protein

An adequate protein intake is essential to meet increasing demands in pregnancy. Milk, meat, eggs, and cheese are complete protein foods with a high biologic value. Legumes (dried beans and peas), whole grains, and nuts also are valuable sources of protein. In addition, these protein-rich foods are a source of other nutrients, such as calcium, iron, and B vitamins; plant sources of protein often provide needed dietary fiber. The recommended daily food plan (Table 6-3) is a guide to the amounts of these foods that would supply the quantities of protein needed. The recommendations provide for only a modest increase in protein intake over the prepregnant levels in adult women. Pregnant adolescents, women from impoverished backgrounds, and women adhering to unusual diets, such as a macrobiotic (highly restricted vegetarian) diet, are those whose protein intake is most likely to be inadequate. The use of high-protein supplements is not recommended because they have been associated with an increased incidence of preterm births.

Water and Other Fluids

Water is the main substance of cells, blood, lymph, amniotic fluid, and other vital body fluids.

- It aids in maintaining body temperature.

TABLE 6-3

Daily Food Guide for Pregnancy and Lactation

FOOD GROUP	SERVING SIZE	SUGGESTED NUMBER OF SERVINGS		
		NONPREGNANT, NONLACTATING WOMAN	PREGNANT WOMAN	LACTATING WOMAN
GRAIN PRODUCTS Include whole-grain and enriched breads, cereals, pasta, and rice.	1 slice bread; ½ bun, bagel, or English muffin; 1 oz ready-to-eat cereal; ½ cup cooked grains	6-11	6-11	6-11
VEGETABLES Eat dark green, leafy, and deep yellow often. Eat dried beans and peas often; count ½ cup cooked dried beans or peas as a serving of vegetables or 1 oz from meat group.	1 cup raw leafy greens; ½ cup of others	3-5	3-5	3-5

Continued

TABLE 6-3

Daily Food Guide for Pregnancy and Lactation—cont'd

FOOD GROUP	SERVING SIZE	SUGGESTED NUMBER OF SERVINGS		
		PREGNANT, LACTATING WOMAN	PREGNANT WOMAN	LACTATING WOMAN
FRUITS Include citrus fruits, strawberries, or melons frequently.	1 medium apple, orange, banana, peach, etc; ½ cup small or diced fruit; ¾ cup juice	2-4	2-4	2-4
MILK AND MILK PRODUCTS	1 cup milk or yogurt; 1½ oz cheese	2-3	3 or more	4 or more
MEAT, POULTRY, FISH, DRY BEANS, NUTS, AND EGGS Eat peanut butter or nuts rarely to avoid excessive fat intake. Limit egg intake to reduce cholesterol intake; trim fat from meat, and remove skin from poultry.	½ cup cooked dried beans, 1 egg, or 1½ T peanut butter is equivalent to 1 oz of meat	Up to 6 oz total	Up to 6 oz total	Up to 6 oz total

T, Tablespoon.

- A good fluid intake promotes good bowel function, which is sometimes a problem during pregnancy.
- The recommended daily intake is about six to eight glasses (1500 to 2000 ml) of fluid. Water, milk, and fruit juices are good sources.
- Dehydration may increase the risk of cramping, contractions, and preterm labor.
- The consumption of more than 300 mg of caffeine daily (equivalent to about 500 to 750 ml of coffee) may increase the risk of miscarriage and of giving birth to infants with IUGR. Caffeine-containing products, including caffeinated coffee, tea, soft drinks, and cocoa beverages, should be avoided or consumed only in limited quantities.
- Aspartame (Nutrasweet, Equal), acesulfame potassium (Sunett), and sucralose (Splenda), artificial sweeteners commonly used in low- or no-calorie beverages and low-calorie food products, have not been found to have adverse effects on the normal mother and fetus. Aspartame, which contains phenylalanine, should be avoided by the mother with phenylketonuria (PKU).

Minerals and Vitamins

In general, the nutrient needs of pregnant women, with perhaps the exception of folate and iron, can be met through dietary sources. Counseling about the need for a varied diet rich in vitamins and minerals should be a part of the early prenatal care of every pregnant woman and should be reinforced throughout pregnancy. Supplements of certain nutrients (see Table 6-1), however, are recommended whenever the woman's diet is very poor or whenever significant nutritional risk factors are present.

Multivitamin-multimineral supplements during pregnancy

Food can and should be the normal vehicle to meet the additional needs imposed by pregnancy, except for iron.
- A supplemental iron dose of 30 mg/day is recommended.
- The recommended folate intake may be difficult for some women to achieve.

- Some women habitually consume diets that are deficient in necessary nutrients and, for whatever reason, may be unable to change this intake.

For these women, a multivitamin-multimineral supplement should be considered to ensure that they consume the RDA for most known vitamins and minerals. The use of a vitamin-mineral supplement does not lessen the need to consume a nutritious, well-balanced diet.

Pica and Food Cravings

Pica, which is the practice of consuming nonfood substances (e.g., clay, dirt, and laundry starch) or excessive amounts of foodstuffs low in nutritional value (e.g., ice or freezer frost, baking powder or soda, and cornstarch), often is influenced by the woman's cultural background.

- In the United States, pica is most common among African-American women, women from rural areas, and women with a family history of pica.
- The regular and heavy consumption of low-nutrient products may cause more nutritious foods to be displaced from the diet, and the items consumed also may interfere with the absorption of nutrients, especially minerals.
- Women with pica have lower hemoglobin levels than do those without pica.
- These women should be counseled about the health risks associated with pica.
- It has been proposed that pica and food cravings (e.g., the urge to have ice cream, pickles, or pizza) during pregnancy are caused by an innate drive to consume nutrients missing from the diet, but research has not supported this hypothesis.

Adolescent Pregnancy Needs

Many adolescent females have diets that provide less than the recommended intakes of key nutrients, including energy, calcium, and iron.

- Pregnant adolescents and their infants are at increased risk of complications during pregnancy and parturition.
  - Growth of the pelvis is delayed in comparison with growth in stature; thus cephalopelvic disproportion and other

mechanical problems associated with labor are common among young adolescents.

–Competition between the growing adolescent and the fetus for nutrients also may contribute to some of the poor outcomes apparent in teen pregnancies.

–Pregnant adolescents are encouraged to choose a weight-gain goal at the upper end of the range for their BMI.

To improve the nutritional health of pregnant adolescents, do the following:

• Improve the nutrition knowledge, meal planning, and food preparation and selection skills of young women
• Promote access to prenatal care
• Develop nutrition interventions and educational programs that are effective with adolescents
• Strive to understand the factors that create barriers to change in the adolescent population

NUTRIENT NEEDS DURING LACTATION

Nutritional needs during lactation are similar in many ways to those during pregnancy (see Table 6-1).

• Needs for energy (calories), protein, calcium, iodine, zinc, the B vitamins (thiamin, riboflavin, niacin, pyridoxine, and vitamin B_{12}), and vitamin C remain greater than nonpregnant needs.
• The recommendations for some of these (e.g., vitamin C, zinc, and protein) are slightly to moderately higher than those during pregnancy (see Table 6-1). This allowance covers the amount of the nutrient released in the milk, as well as the needs of the mother for tissue maintenance.
• The recommendation for iron and folic acid during lactation is lower than that during pregnancy.
• The recommended energy intake is an increase of 500 kcal more than the woman's nonpregnant intake. Lactating women should consume at least 1800 kcal/day, because it is difficult to obtain adequate nutrients for the maintenance of lactation at levels less than that.
• Fluid intake must be adequate to maintain milk production, but the mother's level of thirst is the best guide to the right amount. There is no need to consume more fluids than those needed to satisfy thirst.

- Smoking, alcohol, and excessive caffeine intake should be avoided during lactation.

CARE MANAGEMENT

Assessment is based on a diet history and review of the woman's health records, physical examination, and laboratory results. Ideally a nutritional assessment is performed before conception so that any recommended changes in diet, lifestyle, and weight can be undertaken before the woman becomes pregnant.

Diet History

Box 6-2 provides a simple tool for obtaining diet history information. When potential problems are identified, they should be followed up with a careful interview.

Physical Examination

Anthropometric (body) measurements provide short- and long-term information on a woman's nutritional status and are thus essential to the assessment.

- The woman's height and weight must be determined at the time of her first prenatal visit, and her weight should be measured at every subsequent visit (see earlier discussion of BMI).
- A careful physical examination can reveal objective signs of malnutrition (Table 6-4).
  - Some of these signs are nonspecific, and the physiologic changes of pregnancy may complicate the interpretation of physical findings.
  - Lower-extremity edema often occurs when caloric and protein deficiencies are present, but it also may be a normal finding in the third trimester.

The interpretation of physical findings is made easier by a thorough health history and by laboratory testing, if indicated.

Laboratory testing

The only nutrition-related laboratory test necessary for most pregnant women is a hematocrit or hemoglobin measurement to screen for the presence of anemia.

Text continued on p. 116.

BOX 6-2

Food Intake Questionnaire

Which of the following did you eat or drink yesterday? If the way you ate yesterday wasn't the way you usually eat, choose a recent day that was typical for you.

Food or Drink	Number of Servings	Food or Drink	Number of Servings
Beer, wine, other alcoholic drinks		Orange or grapefruit juice	
Tea		Fruit juice other than orange or grapefruit	
Coffee			
Fruit drink		Soft drinks	
Water		Milk	
Cheese		Cereal with milk	
Macaroni and cheese		Yogurt	
Other foods with cheese (e.g., lasagna, enchiladas, cheeseburgers)		Pizza	
Orange or grapefruit		Melon (e.g., watermelon, cantaloupe, honeydew)	
Bananas		Berries (kind)	

Continued

BOX 6-2

Food Intake Questionnaire—cont'd

Food or Drink	Number of Servings	Food or Drink	Number of Servings
Peaches or apricots		Apples	
Green salad		Other fruit	
Spinach or greens		Broccoli	
Green peas		Green beans	
Sweet potatoes		Potatoes (other than fried)	
Carrots		Corn	
Red meat		Other vegetables	
Fish		Chicken or turkey	
Peanut butter		Egg	
Dried beans or peas		Nuts	
Bacon or sausage		Hot dog	
Bread		Cold cuts (e.g., bologna)	
Rice		Roll/bagel	

BOX 6-2

Food Intake Questionnaire—cont'd

Food or Drink	Number of Servings	Food or Drink	Number of Servings
Spaghetti or other pasta		Noodles	
Tortillas		Chips	
French fries		Cake	
Cookie		Donut or pastry	
Pie			

Are you often bothered by any of the following? (circle all that apply)
  Nausea   Vomiting   Heartburn   Constipation
Are you on a special diet? No _____ Yes _____
  If yes, what kind?_____
Do you try to limit the amount or kind of food you eat to control your weight? No _____ Yes _____
Do you avoid any foods for health or religious reasons?
  No ____ Yes ____ If yes, what foods? _____
Do you take any prescribed drugs or medications?
  No _____ Yes _____ If yes, what are they? _____
Do you take any over-the-counter medications (e.g., aspirin, cold medicines, Tylenol)?
    No ____ Yes _____ If yes, what are they?
_____
Do you take any herbal supplements? No _____
  Yes _____ If yes, what are they? _____
Do you ever have trouble affording the food you need?
  No ____ Yes _____
Do you have any help getting the food you need?
  No _____Yes _____ (circle all that apply)
  Food stamps   WIC   School lunch or breakfast
  Food from a food pantry, soup kitchen, or food bank

TABLE 6-4

Physical Assessment of Nutritional Status

SIGNS OF GOOD NUTRITION	SIGNS OF POOR NUTRITION
GENERAL APPEARANCE	
Alert, responsive, energetic, good endurance	Listless, apathetic, cachectic, easily fatigued, looks tired
MUSCLES	
Well developed, firm, good tone, some fat under skin	Flaccid, poor tone, undeveloped, tender, "wasted" appearance
NERVOUS CONTROL	
Good attention span, not irritable or restless, normal reflexes, psychologic stability	Inattentive, irritable, confused, burning and tingling of hands and feet, loss of position and vibratory sense, weakness and tenderness of muscles, decrease or loss of ankle and knee reflexes
GI FUNCTION	
Good appetite and digestion, normal regular elimination, no palpable organs or masses	Anorexia, indigestion, constipation or diarrhea, liver or spleen enlargement
CARDIO FUNCTION	
Normal heart rate and rhythm, no murmurs, normal blood pressure for age	Rapid heart rate, enlarged heart, abnormal rhythm, elevated blood pressure
HAIR	
Shiny, lustrous, firm, not easily plucked, healthy scalp	Stringy, dull, brittle, dry, thin and sparse, depigmented, can be easily plucked
SKIN (GENERAL)	
Smooth, slightly moist, good color	Rough, dry, scaly, pale, pigmented, irritated, easily bruised, petechiae
FACE AND NECK	
Skin color uniform, smooth, pink, healthy	Scaly, swollen, skin dark over cheeks and under eyes,

TABLE 6-4

Physical Assessment of Nutritional Status—cont'd

SIGNS OF GOOD NUTRITION	SIGNS OF POOR NUTRITION
appearance; no enlargement of thyroid gland; lips not chapped or swollen	lumpiness or flakiness of skin around nose and mouth; thyroid enlarged; lips swollen, angular lesions or fissures at corners of mouth

ORAL CAVITY

Reddish pink mucous membranes and gums; no swelling or bleeding of gums; tongue healthy pink or deep reddish in appearance, not swollen or smooth, surface papillae present; teeth bright and clean, no cavities, no pain, no discoloration	Gums spongy, bleed easily, inflamed or receding; tongue swollen, scarlet, and raw; magenta color, beefy, hyperemic, and hypertrophic papillae, atrophic papillae; teeth with unfilled caries, absent teeth, worn surfaces, mottled

EYES

Bright, clear, shiny, no sores at corners of eyelids, membranes moist and healthy pink color, no prominent blood vessels or mound of tissue (Bitot spots) on sclera, no fatigue circles beneath	Eye membranes pale, redness of membrane, dryness, signs of infection, Bitot spots, redness and fissuring of eyelid corners, dryness of eye membrane, dull appearance of cornea, soft cornea, blue sclerae

EXTREMITIES

No tenderness, weakness, or swelling; nails firm and pink	Edema, tender calves, tingling, weakness; nails spoon shaped, brittle

SKELETON

No malformations	Bowlegs, knock-knees, chest deformity at diaphragm, beaded ribs, prominent scapulae

- The lower limit of the normal range for hemoglobin during pregnancy is 11 g/dl in the first and third trimesters and 10.5 g/dl in the second trimester (compared with 12 g/dl in the nonpregnant state).
- The lower limit of the normal range for hematocrit is 33% during the first and third trimesters and 32% in the second trimester (compared with 36% in the nonpregnant state).
- Cutoff values for anemia are higher in women who smoke or live at high altitudes, because the decreased oxygen-carrying capacity of their RBCs causes them to produce more RBCs than other women.

A woman's history or physical findings may indicate the need for additional testing, such as a complete blood cell count with a differential to identify megaloblastic or macrocytic anemia and the measurement of levels of specific vitamins or minerals believed to be lacking in the diet.

Women may need referral to other professionals or services.

- Pregnant women with serious nutritional problems, those with intervening illnesses such as diabetes (either preexisting or gestational), and any others requiring in-depth dietary counseling should be referred to the dietitian.
- Two programs that provide nutrition services are the food stamp program and the Special Supplemental Program for Women, Infants, and Children (WIC), which provides vouchers for selected foods to pregnant and lactating women, as well as infants and children at nutritional risk. WIC foods include eggs, cheese, milk, juice, and fortified cereals; these are chosen because they provide iron, protein, vitamin C, and other vitamins.

Good nutrition practices (and the avoidance of poor practices such as smoking and alcohol or drug use) are essential content for prenatal classes designed for women in early pregnancy (see Guidelines/Guías box in Appendix A).

MyPyramid can be used as a guide to making daily food choices during pregnancy and lactation, just as it is during other stages of the life cycle (www.mypyramid.org).

Postpartum

The need for a varied diet consisting of a representation of foods from all the food groups continues throughout lactation (see Table 6-1).

Daily Food Guide and Menu Planning

The daily food plan (see Table 6-3) can be used as a guide for educating the woman about nutritional needs during pregnancy and lactation. This food plan is general enough to be used by women from a wide variety of cultures, including women following a vegetarian diet.

Medical Nutrition Therapy

During pregnancy and lactation, the food plan for women receiving special medical nutrition therapy (therapeutic diets) may have to be modified. The registered dietitian can instruct these women about their diets and assist them in meal planning. However, the nurse should understand the basic principles of the diet and be able to reinforce the diet teaching. For example, the following information is suitable for teaching pregnant women with diabetes.

- The food plan of the woman with diabetes usually includes four to six meals and snacks daily, with the daily carbohydrate intake distributed fairly evenly among the meals and snacks.
- The complex carbohydrates—fibers and starches—should be well represented in the diet.
- A diet plan with no more than approximately 40% of energy derived from carbohydrates has been used successfully in maintaining good blood glucose control during pregnancy.
- The pregnant woman with diabetes usually must monitor her own blood glucose daily.

Counseling About Iron Supplementation

- Bran, milk, egg yolks, coffee, tea, or oxalate-containing vegetables, such as spinach and Swiss chard, consumed at the same time as iron will inhibit iron absorption.
- Iron absorption is promoted by a diet rich in vitamin C (e.g., citrus fruits or melons) or "heme iron" (found in red meats, fish, and poultry).
- Iron supplements are best absorbed on an empty stomach; thus they can be taken between meals with beverages other than milk, tea, or coffee.

- Some women have gastrointestinal discomfort when they take the supplement on an empty stomach; therefore a good time for them to take the supplement is just before bedtime.
- Constipation is common with iron supplementation.
- Iron supplements should be kept away from any children in the household because their ingestion could result in acute iron poisoning and even death.

Cultural Influences and Vegetarian Diets

Women in most cultures are encouraged to eat a diet typical for them. Within each cultural group, several variations may occur. Thus careful exploration of individual preferences is needed. Many cultural food practices have some merit, or the culture would not have survived. Food cravings during pregnancy are considered normal by many cultures, but the kinds of cravings often are culturally specific. In most cultures, women crave acceptable foods, such as chicken, fish, and greens among African-Americans. Cultural influences on food intake usually lessen if the woman and her family become more integrated into the dominant culture.

Vegetarian diets represent another cultural effect on nutritional status.

- Foods basic to almost all vegetarian diets are vegetables, fruits, legumes, nuts, seeds, and grains.
- Semivegetarians, who are not truly vegetarians, include fish, poultry, eggs, and dairy products in their diets but do not eat beef or pork. Such a diet can be completely adequate for pregnant women.
- Ovolactovegetarians eat dairy products in addition to plant products. Iron and zinc intake may not be adequate in these women, but such diets can be otherwise nutritionally sound.
- Strict vegetarians, or vegans, consume only plant products. Because vitamin B_{12} is found only in foods of animal origin, this diet is deficient in vitamin B_{12}. As a result, strict vegetarians should take a supplement or consume vitamin B_{12}–fortified foods (e.g., soy milk) regularly.

—Vitamin B_{12} deficiency can result in megaloblastic anemia, glossitis (inflamed red tongue), and neurologic deficits in the mother.

—Infants born to affected mothers are likely to have megaloblastic anemia and to exhibit neurodevelopmental delays.

—Iron, calcium, zinc, and vitamin B_6 intake also may be low in women on this diet, and some strict vegetarians have excessively low caloric intakes.

—The protein intake should be assessed especially carefully, because plant proteins tend to be "incomplete" in that they lack one or more amino acids required for growth and the maintenance of body tissues.

—The daily consumption of a variety of different plant proteins—grains, dried beans and peas, nuts, and seeds—helps to provide all the essential amino acids.

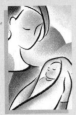

CHAPTER 7

Nursing Care during Pregnancy

PRENATAL PERIOD

- Pregnancy spans 9 months, but health care providers, in contrast to using the familiar monthly calendar to ascertain fetal age or discuss the pregnancy, use the concept of lunar months, which last 28 days, or 4 weeks. Normal pregnancy, then, lasts about 10 lunar months, which is the same as 40 weeks, or 280 days.
- Health care providers also refer to early, middle, and late pregnancy as trimesters. The first trimester lasts from weeks 1 through 13; the second, from weeks 14 through 26; and the third, from weeks 27 through 40.
- A pregnancy is considered to be at term if it advances to 38 to 40 weeks.

Estimating Date of Birth

- One formula used to calculate the estimated date of birth (EDB) is Nägele's rule, which is as follows: After determining the first day of the last menstrual period (LMP), subtract 3 calendar months and add 7 days and 1 year; or alternatively, add 7 days to the LMP and count forward 9 calendar months. Most women give birth during the period extending from 7 days before to 7 days after the EDB.

CARE MANAGEMENT

The purpose of prenatal care is to identify existing risk factors and other deviations from normal so that pregnancy outcomes may be enhanced.

Prenatal Visit Schedule

The initial visit usually occurs in the first trimester, with monthly visits through week 28 of pregnancy. Thereafter, visits are scheduled every 2 weeks until week 36 and then every week until birth. There is a growing tendency to have fewer visits with women who are at low risk for complications.

- The initial evaluation includes a comprehensive health history emphasizing the current pregnancy, previous pregnancies, the family, a psychosocial profile, a physical assessment, diagnostic testing, and an overall risk assessment. A prenatal history form is the best way to document information obtained.

- *Current pregnancy.* A review of symptoms she is experiencing and how she is coping with them helps to establish a database to develop a plan of care. Some early teaching may be provided at this time.

- *Obstetric and gynecologic history.* Data are gathered on the woman's age at menarche, menstrual history, and contraceptive history; the nature of any infertility or gynecologic conditions; her history of any sexually transmitted infections (STIs); her sexual history; and a detailed history of all her pregnancies, including the present pregnancy, and their outcomes. The date of the last Papanicolaou (Pap) test and the result are noted. The date of her LMP is obtained to establish the EDB (see Box 7-1).

- *Medical history.* The medical history includes those medical or surgical conditions that may affect the pregnancy or that may be affected by the pregnancy. The nature of previous surgical procedures, especially reproductive ones, also should be described.

- *Nutritional history.* The woman's nutritional history is an important component of the prenatal history because her nutritional status has a direct effect on the growth and development of the fetus.

- *History of drug and herbal preparations use.* A woman's past and present use of legal (over-the-counter [OTC] and prescription medications; herbal preparations; caffeine; alcohol; and nicotine) and illegal (e.g., marijuana, cocaine, and heroin) drugs must be assessed because many substances cross the placenta and may therefore harm the developing fetus. Informed consent must be obtained from a pregnant woman before she can be tested for drug use.

BOX 7-1

Gravidity and parity

Gravidity and parity information may be recorded in patient records in several ways. If gravidity and parity are described with only two digits, the first digit (gravidity) represents the number of pregnancies the woman has had including the present one, and parity is the number of pregnancies that have reached 20 weeks of gestation. For example, if a woman had twins at 36 weeks with her first pregnancy, parity would still be counted as one birth (gravida I, para I).

The five-digit GTPAL system provides more specific information about the woman's obstetric history. The first digit represents gravidity; the second digit represents the total number of term births; the third indicates the number of preterm births; the fourth identifies the number of abortions (miscarriage or elective termination of pregnancy); and the fifth is the number of children currently living. The acronym GTPAL (gravidity, term, preterm, abortions, living children) may be helpful in remembering this system of notation. For example, if a woman pregnant only once gives birth at week 34 and the infant survives, the abbreviation that represents this information is "1-0-1-0-1." With her next pregnancy, she gives birth to a single infant at 39 weeks of gestation; the abbreviation is "2-1-1-0-2."

- *Family history.* The family history provides information about familial or genetic disorders or conditions that could affect the present health status of the woman or her fetus.
- *Social, experiential, and occupational history.* Situational factors, such as the family's ethnic and cultural background and socioeconomic status, are assessed while the history is obtained.
  - All women should be assessed for a history or risk of physical abuse, particularly because the likelihood of abuse by the partner increases during pregnancy. Pregnant women may report physical blows directed to the head, breasts, abdomen, and genitalia. Sexual assault by the partner also is common.
- *Review of systems.* During this portion of the interview, the woman is asked to identify and describe preexisting or concur-

rent problems in any of the body systems, and her mental status is assessed. For each sign or symptom described, the following additional data should be obtained: body location, quality, quantity, chronology, aggravating or alleviating factors, and associated manifestations (onset, character, and course).

- *Physical examination.* The initial physical examination begins with assessment of vital signs, height and weight, and blood pressure. Heart and lung sounds are evaluated, and extremities are examined. Distribution, amount, and quality of body hair are of particular importance because the findings reflect nutritional status, endocrine function, and attention to hygiene. The thyroid gland is assessed carefully.
  - One vaginal examination during pregnancy is recommended, but another is usually not done unless medically indicated.
- *Laboratory tests.* The laboratory data yielded by the analysis of the specimens obtained during the examination provide important information concerning the symptoms of pregnancy and the woman's health status (Table 7-1).

Follow-up visits

- The pattern of interviewing the woman first and then assessing physical changes and performing laboratory tests is maintained.
- At each visit, physical parameters are measured. Ideally, blood pressure is taken by using the same arm at every visit, with the woman sitting, using a cuff of appropriate size. Her weight is assessed, and the appropriateness of the gestational weight gain is evaluated in relationship to her body mass index (BMI). Urine may be checked by dipstick, and the presence and degree of edema are noted. For examination of the abdomen, the woman lies on her back with her arms by her side and head supported by a pillow. The bladder should be empty. Abdominal inspection is followed by measurement of the height of the fundus. While the woman lies on her back, the nurse should be alert for the occurrence of supine hypotension (see Emergency box). When a woman is lying in this position, the weight of abdominal contents may compress the vena cava and aorta, causing a decrease in blood pressure and a feeling of faintness.

TABLE 7-1

Laboratory Tests in Prenatal Period

LABORATORY TEST	PURPOSE
Hemoglobin, hematocrit, WBC, differential	Detects anemia; detects infection
Hemoglobin electrophoresis	Identifies women with hemoglobinopathies (e.g., sickle cell anemia, thalassemia)
Blood type, Rh, and irregular antibody	Identifies those fetuses at risk for developing erythroblastosis fetalis or hyperbilirubinemia in neonatal period
Rubella titer	Determines immunity to rubella
Tuberculin skin testing; chest film after 20 wk of gestation in women with reactive tuberculin tests	Screens for exposure to tuberculosis
Urinalysis, including microscopic examination of urinary sediment; pH, specific gravity, color, glucose, albumin, protein, RBCs, WBCs, casts, acetone; hCG	Identifies women with unsuspected diabetes mellitus, renal disease, hypertensive disease of pregnancy; infection; occult hematuria
Urine culture	Identifies women with asymptomatic bacteriuria
Renal function tests: BUN, creatinine, electrolytes, creatinine clearance, total protein excretion	Evaluates level of possible renal compromise in women with a history of diabetes, hypertension, or renal disease
Pap test	Screens for cervical intraepithelial neoplasia, herpes simplex type 2, and HPV

TABLE 7-1

Laboratory Tests in Prenatal Period—cont'd

LABORATORY TEST	PURPOSE
Vaginal or rectal smear for *Neisseria gonorrhoeae*, *Chlamydia*, HPV, GBS	Screens high risk population for asymptomatic infection; GBS done at 35-37 wk
RPR, VDRL, or FTA-ABS	Identifies women with untreated syphilis
HIV* antibody, hepatitis B surface antigen, toxoplasmosis	Screens for infection
1-hr glucose tolerance	Screens for gestational diabetes; done at initial visit for women with risk factors; done at 24-28 wk for all pregnant women
3-hr glucose tolerance	Screens for diabetes in women with elevated glucose level after 1-hr test; must have two elevated readings for diagnosis
Cardiac evaluation: ECG, chest x-ray film, and echocardiogram	Evaluates cardiac function in women with a history of hypertension or cardiac disease

*With patient permission.
BUN, Blood urea nitrogen; *ECG,* electrocardiogram; *FTA-ABS,* fluorescent treponemal antibody absorption test; *GBS,* group B streptococcus; *hCG,* human chorionic gonadotropin; *HIV,* human immunodeficiency virus; *HPV,* human papillomavirus; *RBC,* red blood cell; *RPR,* rapid plasma reagin; *VDRL,* Venereal Disease Research Laboratory; *WBC,* white blood cell.

- Individuals whose systolic blood pressure is 120 to 139 mm Hg or whose diastolic blood pressure is 80 to 89 mm Hg should be viewed as prehypertensive.
- An absolute systolic blood pressure of 140 mm Hg or more and a diastolic blood pressure of 90 mm Hg or more suggest

signs of
POTENTIAL COMPLICATIONS

First, Second, and Third Trimesters

FIRST TRIMESTER

Signs and Symptoms	Possible Causes
Severe vomiting	Hyperemesis gravidarum
Chills, fever	Infection
Burning on urination	Infection
Diarrhea	Infection
Abdominal cramping, vaginal bleeding	Miscarriage, ectopic pregnancy

SECOND AND THIRD TRIMESTERS

Signs and Symptoms	Possible Causes
Persistent, severe vomiting	Hyperemesis gravidarum, hypertension, preeclampsia
Sudden discharge of fluid from vagina before 37 weeks	Premature rupture of membranes (PROM)
Vaginal bleeding, severe abdominal pain	Miscarriage, placenta previa, abruptio placentae
Chills, fever, burning on urination, diarrhea	Infection
Severe backache or flank pain	Kidney infection or stones, preterm labor
Change in fetal movements: absence of fetal movements after quickening, any unusual change in pattern or amount	Fetal jeopardy or intrauterine fetal death
Uterine contractions, pressure, cramping before 37 weeks	Preterm labor
Visual disturbances: blurring, double vision, or spots	Hypertensive conditions, preeclampsia

Swelling of face or fingers and over sacrum	Hypertensive conditions, preeclampsia
Headaches: severe, frequent, or continuous	Hypertensive conditions, preeclampsia
Muscular irritability or convulsions	Hypertensive conditions, preeclampsia
Epigastric or abdominal pain (perceived as severe stomachache)	Hypertensive conditions, preeclampsia, abruptio placentae
Glycosuria, positive glucose tolerance test reaction	Gestational diabetes mellitus

the presence of hypertension. A systolic blood pressure of 125 mm Hg or more or a diastolic blood pressure of 75 mm Hg or more in midpregnancy or a systolic blood pressure of 130 mm Hg or more or a diastolic blood pressure of 85 mm Hg or more in later pregnancy is indicative of problems.

- A rise in systolic blood pressure of 30 mm Hg or more than the baseline pressure or a rise in the diastolic blood pressure of 15 mm Hg or more than the baseline pressure is also a significant finding regardless of the absolute values.
- The pregnant woman is monitored for a range of signs and symptoms that indicate potential complications in addition to hypertension (see Signs of Potential Complications box).
- Fetal heart tones (FHTs) are assessed at each visit usually after the first trimester when they can be heard with an ultrasound fetoscope.
- The fundal height, measurement of the height of the uterus above the symphysis pubis, is used as one indicator of fetal growth. The measurement also provides a gross estimate of the duration of pregnancy. From approximately 18 to 32 weeks of gestation, the height of the fundus in centimeters is approximately the same as the number of weeks of gestation (± 2) with an empty bladder at the time of measurement. A stable or decreased fundal height may indicate the presence of intrauterine growth restriction (IUGR); an excessive increase could indicate the presence of multifetal gestation (more than one fetus) or hydramnios.

- Fetal gestational age is determined from the menstrual history, contraceptive history, pregnancy test result, and the following findings obtained during the clinical evaluation:
  - First uterine evaluation: date, size
  - Fetal heart (FH) first heard: date, method (Doppler stethoscope, fetoscope)
  - Date of quickening
  - Current fundal height, estimated fetal weight (EFW)
  - Current week of gestation by history of LMP and/or ultrasound examination
  - Ultrasound examination: date, week of gestation, biparietal diameter (BPD)
  - Reliability of dates
- Quickening ("feeling of life") refers to the mother's first perception of fetal movement. It usually occurs between weeks 16 and 20 of gestation. Multiparas often perceive fetal movement earlier than primigravidas.
- Routine use of ultrasound examination in early pregnancy has been recommended. This procedure may be used to establish the duration of pregnancy if the woman cannot give a precise date for her LMP or if the size of the uterus does not conform to the EDB as calculated by Nägele's rule. Ultrasound also provides information about the well-being of the fetus.
- The assessment of fetal health status includes consideration of fetal movement. The mother is instructed to note the extent and timing of fetal movements and to report immediately if the pattern changes or if movement ceases. One method is for the woman to count fetal movements after a meal. A count of four or more kicks in 1 hour is reassuring.

Laboratory Tests

- The number of routine laboratory tests done during follow-up visits in pregnancy is limited. A clean-catch urine specimen is obtained to test for glucose, protein, nitrites, and leukocytes at each visit. Urine specimens for culture and sensitivity, as well as blood samples, are obtained only if signs and symptoms warrant.
- It is recommended that the maternal serum alpha-fetoprotein (MSAFP) screening be done between 15 and 22 weeks of gestation, ideally between 16 and 18 weeks of gestation. See Chapter 5.

- The multiple-marker, or triple-screen, blood test is also recommended between 16 and 18 weeks of gestation. See Chapter 5.
- A glucose challenge is usually done between 24 and 28 weeks of gestation. Testing may be done also at the initial physical for women with risk factors for gestational diabetes mellitus.
- Group beta streptococcus (GBS) testing is done between 35 and 37 weeks of gestation.
- Other diagnostic tests are available to assess the health status of both the pregnant woman and the fetus. See Table 7-1.

Interventions

Box 7-2 lists suggestions for how to include assessments and education in a timely way.

Education for self-care

The expectant mother needs information about many subjects. Several topics that may cause concerns in pregnant women are discussed in the following sections.

- *Nutrition.* Teaching may include discussion about foods high in iron, encouragement to take prenatal vitamins, and recommendations to moderate or limit caffeine intake. In some settings a registered dietitian conducts classes for pregnant women on the topics of nutritional status and nutrition during pregnancy or interviews them to assess their knowledge of these topics. Nurses can refer women to a registered dietitian if a need is revealed during the nursing assessment (see Chapter 6).
- *Personal hygiene.* During pregnancy, the sebaceous (sweat) glands are highly active because of hormonal influences, and women often perspire freely. Baths and warm showers can be therapeutic because they relax tense, tired muscles; help counter insomnia; and make the pregnant woman feel fresh.
- *Prevention of urinary tract infections.* Urinary tract infections are common, but they may be asymptomatic. Women should be instructed to inform their health care provider if blood or pain occurs with urination. The nurse can assess the woman's understanding and use of good handwashing techniques before and after urinating and of the importance of wiping

Text continued on p. 132.

BOX 7-2

Suggestions for Timely Prenatal Education

I. EARLY PREGNANCY (WEEKS 1-20)

		Testing: labs	Ultrasound
Fetal growth and development	_____	_____	_____
Maternal changes	_____		_____
Lifestyle: exercise/ stress/nutrition	_____	Possible complications:	
Drugs, OTC, tobacco, alcohol	_____	a. Threatened miscarriage	_____
STIs	_____	b. Diabetes	_____
Psychologic/social adjustments:	_____	c. Other _____	_____
Father of baby involved/accepts	_____	Introduction to breastfeeding	_____
		Acceptance of pregnancy	_____
		Dietary follow-up	_____

II. MIDPREGNANCY (WEEKS 21-27)

Fetal growth and development		Breastfeeding or bottle-feeding	_____
Maternal changes	_____	Birth plan initiated	_____
Daily fetal movement	_____	Dietary follow-up	_____
Possible complications:			
a. Preterm labor prevention	_____		
b. Preeclampsia symptoms	_____		
c. Other _____	_____		

III. LATE PREGNANCY (WEEKS 28-40)

Fetal growth and development	_____	Childbirth preparation	_____
Fetal evaluation:		S/S of labor; labor process	_____

BOX 7-2

Suggestions for Timely Prenatal Education—cont'd

Daily movement _____	NSTs _____	Pain management: natural childbirth, medications, epidural _____	
Kick counts _____	BPPs _____	Cesarean; VBAC _____	
Maternal changes _____		Birth plan complete _____	
Possible complications: review as needed		Review hospital policies (tour) _____	
a. Preterm labor prevention _____		Parenting preparation:	
b. Preeclampsia symptoms _____		Well-baby care _____	Car seat/ safety _____
c. Other _____ _____		Immunizations _____	Sibling preparation if applicable _____
Breastfeeding preparation:		Postpartum:	
Nipple assessment _____		Postpartum care and checkup _____	
Dietary follow-up _____		Emotional changes _____	
		Birth control options _____	
		Safer sex and STIs _____	

BPP, Biophysical profile; *NST,* nonstress test; *OTC,* over-the-counter preparations; *S/S,* signs and symptoms; *STI,* sexually transmitted infection; *VBAC,* vaginal birth after cesarean.

the perineum from front to back. Soft, absorbent toilet tissue, preferably white and unscented, should be used; harsh, scented, or printed toilet paper may cause irritation. Bubble bath or other bath oils should be avoided because these may irritate the urethra. Women should wear cotton crotch underpants and panty hose and avoid wearing tight-fitting slacks or jeans for long periods; anything that allows a buildup of heat and moisture in the genital area may foster the growth of bacteria. Advise the woman to drink at least 2 L (eight glasses) of liquid, preferably water, each day to maintain an adequate fluid intake that ensures frequent urination. Pregnant women should not limit fluids in an effort to reduce the frequency of urination. Women need to know that if urine looks dark (concentrated), they must increase their fluid intake. The consumption of yogurt and acidophilus milk also may help prevent urinary tract and vaginal infections.

- *Preparation for breastfeeding.* A woman's decision about the method of infant feeding often is made before pregnancy. If undecided, the pregnant woman and her partner are encouraged to choose which method of feeding is suitable for them. Breastfeeding should be encouraged.

  -Women with inverted nipples need special consideration if they are planning to breastfeed. The pinch test is done to determine whether the nipple is everted or inverted. The nurse shows the woman the way to perform the pinch test. It involves having the woman place her thumb and forefinger on her areola and gently press inward. This action will cause her nipple either to stand erect or to invert. Most nipples will stand erect.

  -The use of breast shells, small plastic devices that fit over the nipples, is suggested for women who have flat or inverted nipples. Breast shells should be worn for 1 to 2 hours daily during the last trimester of pregnancy.

  -The woman is taught to cleanse the nipples with warm water to keep the ducts from being blocked with dried colostrum. Soap, ointments, alcohol, and tinctures should not be applied because they remove protective oils that keep the nipples supple. The use of these substances may cause the nipples to crack during early lactation.

- *Dental care.* Dental care during pregnancy is especially important because nausea during pregnancy may lead to poor oral hygiene, allowing dental caries to develop. A fluoride toothpaste should be used daily. Dental surgery is not contraindicated during pregnancy. If dental treatment is necessary, the woman will be most comfortable having it done during the second trimester because the uterus is now outside the pelvis but not so large as to cause discomfort while she sits in a dental chair.

- *Physical activity.* Exercise tips for pregnancy are presented in the Patient Instructions for Self-Care box.
- *Posture and body mechanics.* Skeletal and musculature changes and hormonal changes (relaxing) in pregnancy may predispose the woman to backache and possible injury. Strategies to prevent or relieve backache are presented in the Patient Instructions for Self-Care box.
- *Rest and relaxation.* The pregnant woman is encouraged to plan regular rest periods, particularly as pregnancy advances. The side-lying position is recommended because it promotes uterine perfusion and fetoplacental oxygenation. Conscious relaxation is the process of releasing tension from the mind and body through deliberate effort and practice. The techniques for conscious relaxation are numerous and varied. Guidelines are given in Box 7-3.
- *Employment.* Employment of pregnant women usually has no adverse effects on pregnancy outcomes. Strategies to improve safety during pregnancy are described in the Patient Instructions for Self-Care box.

PATIENT INSTRUCTIONS FOR SELF-CARE

Exercise Tips for Pregnant Women

Consult your health care provider when you know or suspect you are pregnant. Discuss your medical and obstetric history, your current exercise regimen, and the exercises you would like to continue throughout pregnancy.

Seek help in determining an exercise routine that is well within your limit of tolerance, especially if you have not been exercising regularly.

Consider decreasing weight-bearing exercises (jogging, running) and concentrating on non–weight-bearing activ-

Continued

ities, such as swimming, cycling, or stretching. If you are a runner, starting in your seventh month, you may wish to walk instead.

Avoid risky activities such as surfing, mountain climbing, skydiving, and racquetball because such activities that require precise balance and coordination may be dangerous. Avoid activities that require holding your breath and bearing down (Valsalva maneuver). Jerky, bouncy motions also should be avoided.

Exercise regularly every day if possible, as long as you are healthy, to improve muscle tone and increase or maintain your stamina. Exercising sporadically may put undue strain on your muscles. Thirty minutes of moderate physical exercise is recommended. This activity can be broken up into shorter segments with rest in between. For example, exercise for 10 to 15 minutes, rest for 2 to 3 minutes, and then exercise for another 10 to 15 minutes.

Decrease your exercise level as your pregnancy progresses. The normal alterations of advancing pregnancy, such as decreased cardiac reserve and increased respiratory effort, may produce physiologic stress if you exercise strenuously for a long time.

Take your pulse every 10 to 15 minutes while you are exercising. If it is more than 140 beats/min, slow down until it returns to a maximum of 90 beats/min. You should be able to converse easily while exercising. If you cannot, you need to slow down.

Avoid becoming overheated for extended periods. It is best not to exercise for more than 35 minutes, especially in hot, humid weather. As your body temperature rises, the heat is transmitted to your fetus. Prolonged or repeated elevation of fetal temperature may result in birth defects, especially during the first 3 months. Your temperature should not exceed 38° C.

Avoid the use of hot tubs and saunas.

Warm-up and stretching exercises prepare your joints for more strenuous exercise and lessen the likelihood of strain or injury to your joints. After the fourth month of gestation, you should not perform exercises flat on your back.

A cool-down period of mild activity involving your legs after an exercise period will help bring your respiration, heart, and metabolic rates back to normal and prevent the pooling of blood in the exercised muscles.

Rest for 10 minutes after exercising, lying on your side. As the uterus grows, it puts pressure on a major vein in your abdomen, which carries blood to your heart. Lying on your side removes the pressure and promotes return circulation from your extremities and muscles to your heart, thereby increasing blood flow to your placenta and fetus. You should rise gradually from the floor to prevent dizziness or fainting (orthostatic hypotension).

Drink two or three 8-oz glasses of water after you exercise to replace the body fluids lost through perspiration. While exercising, drink water whenever you feel the need.

Increase your caloric intake to replace the calories burned during exercise and provide the extra energy needs of pregnancy. (Pregnancy alone requires an additional 300 kcal/day.) Choose high-protein foods, such as fish, milk, cheese, eggs, and meat.

Take your time. This is not the time to be competitive or train for activities requiring speed or long endurance.

Wear a supportive bra. Your increased breast weight may cause changes in posture and put pressure on the ulnar nerve.

Wear supportive shoes. As your uterus grows, your center of gravity shifts and you compensate for this by arching your back. These natural changes may make you feel off balance and more likely to fall.

Stop exercising immediately if you experience shortness of breath, dizziness, numbness, tingling, pain of any kind, more than four uterine contractions per hour, decreased fetal activity, or vaginal bleeding, and consult your health care provider.

Sources: American College of Obstetricians and Gynecologists (ACOG). (2002). Exercise during pregnancy and the postpartum period. ACOG Committee Opinion No. 267. *Obstetrics and Gynecology, 99*(1), 171-173; Artal, R., & Subak-Sharpe, G. (1998). *Pregnancy and exercise.* New York: Delacorte Press; Kramer, M. (2001). Regular aerobic exercise during pregnancy (Cochrane Review). In *The Cochrane Library,* issue 1. Oxford: Update Software; Morris, S., & Johnson, N. (2005). Exercise in pregnancy: A critical appraisal of the literature. *Journal of Reproductive Medicine, 50*(3), 181-188.

PATIENT INSTRUCTIONS FOR SELF-CARE

Posture and Body Mechanics

TO PREVENT OR RELIEVE BACKACHE
Do pelvic tilt:
- Pelvic tilt (rock) on hands and knees and while sitting in straight-back chair.
- Pelvic tilt (rock) in standing position against a wall or lying on floor.
- Perform abdominal muscle contractions during pelvic tilt while standing, lying, or sitting to help strengthen rectus abdominis muscle.
- Use good body mechanics.
- Use leg muscles to reach objects on or near floor. Bend at the knees, not from the back. Knees are bent to lower the body to squatting position. Feet are kept 12 to 18 inches apart to provide a solid base to maintain balance.
- Lift with the legs. To lift heavy object (e.g., young child), one foot is placed slightly in front of the other and kept flat as woman lowers herself onto one knee. She lifts the weight holding it close to her body and never higher than the chest. To stand up or sit down, she places one leg slightly behind the other as she raises or lowers herself.

TO RESTRICT THE LUMBAR CURVE
- For prolonged standing (e.g., ironing, employment), place one foot on low footstool or box; change positions often.
- Move car seat forward so that knees are bent and higher than hips. If needed, use a small pillow to support low back area.
- Sit in chairs low enough to allow both feet to be placed on floor, preferably with knees higher than hips.

TO PREVENT ROUND LIGAMENT PAIN AND STRAIN ON ABDOMINAL MUSCLES
- Implement suggestions given in Table 7-2 on p. 142.

- *Clothing.* Comfortable, loose clothing and shoes are recommended. Tight bras and belts, stretch pants, garters, tight-top knee socks, panty girdles, and other constrictive clothing should be avoided because tight clothing over the perineum encourages vaginitis and miliaria (heat rash), and impaired

BOX 7-3

Conscious Relaxation Tips

- *Preparation:* Loosen clothing, and assume a comfortable sitting or side-lying position with all parts of body well supported with pillows.
- *Beginning:* Allow yourself to feel warm and comfortable. Inhale and exhale slowly, and imagine peaceful relaxation coming over each part of the body, starting with the neck and working down to the toes. Often people who learn conscious relaxation speak of feeling relaxed even if some discomfort is present.
- *Maintenance:* Use imagery (fantasy or daydream) to maintain the state of relaxation. Using active imagery, imagine yourself moving or doing some activity and experiencing its sensations. Using passive imagery, imagine yourself watching a scene, such as a lovely sunset.
- *Awakening:* Return to the wakeful state gradually. Slowly begin to take in stimuli from the surrounding environment.
- *Further retention and development of the skill:* Practice regularly for some periods each day, for example, at the same hour for 10 to 15 minutes each day, to feel refreshed, revitalized, and invigorated.

circulation in the legs can cause varicosities. Platform shoes and high heels may cause the woman to lose her balance.

- *Travel.* Travel is not contraindicated in low risk pregnant women. However, women with high risk pregnancies are advised to avoid long-distance travel after fetal viability has been reached to avert possible economic and psychologic consequences of giving birth to a preterm infant far from home. Women who contemplate foreign travel should be aware that many health insurance carriers do not cover a birth in a foreign setting or even hospitalization for preterm labor. In addition, vaccinations for foreign travel may be contraindicated during pregnancy.
  - —Pregnant women who travel for long distances should schedule periods of activity and rest. While sitting, the woman can practice deep breathing, foot circling, and alternately

PATIENT INSTRUCTIONS FOR SELF-CARE

Safety during Pregnancy

Changes in the body resulting from pregnancy include relaxation of joints, alteration to center of gravity, faintness, and discomforts. Problems with coordination and balance are common. Therefore the woman should follow these guidelines:

- Use good body mechanics.
- Use safety features on tools and vehicles (safety seat belts, shoulder harnesses, headrests, goggles, and helmets) as specified.
- Avoid activities requiring coordination, balance, and concentration.
- Take rest periods; reschedule daily activities to meet rest and relaxation needs.

Embryonic and fetal development is vulnerable to environmental teratogens. Many potentially dangerous chemicals are present in the home, yard, and workplace: cleaning agents, paints, sprays, herbicides, and pesticides. The soil and water supply may be unsafe. Therefore the woman should follow these guidelines:

- Read all labels for ingredients and proper use of product.
- Ensure adequate ventilation with clean air.
- Dispose of wastes appropriately.
- Wear gloves when handling chemicals.
- Change job assignments or workplace as necessary.
- Avoid high altitudes (not in pressurized aircraft), which could jeopardize oxygen intake.

contracting and relaxing different muscle groups. Women riding in a car should wear automobile restraints and stop to walk every hour.

—Airline travel in large commercial jets usually poses little risk to the pregnant woman, but policies vary from airline to airline. The pregnant woman is advised to inquire about restrictions or recommendations from her carrier. Most health care providers allow air travel up to 36 weeks of gestation in women without medical or pregnancy complications.

- *Medications and herbal preparations.* The possible teratogenicity of many medications, both prescription and OTC, is still unknown. The use of all drugs, including OTC medications, herbs, and vitamins, should be limited and a careful record kept of all therapeutic and nontherapeutic agents used.
- *Immunizations.* Immunization with live or attenuated live viruses is contraindicated during pregnancy because of its potential teratogenicity. Live-virus vaccines include those for measles (rubeola and rubella), chickenpox, and mumps, as well as the Sabin (oral) poliomyelitis vaccine (no longer used in the United States). Vaccines consisting of killed viruses may be used. Those that may be administered during pregnancy include tetanus, diphtheria, recombinant hepatitis B, and rabies vaccines.
- *Alcohol, cigarette smoke, caffeine, and drugs.* A safe level of alcohol consumption during pregnancy has not yet been established; complete abstinence is strongly advised. Cigarette smoking or continued exposure to secondhand smoke is associated with fetal growth restriction (IUGR), an increased frequency of preterm labor, premature rupture of membranes (PROM), abruptio placentae, placenta previa, and fetal death. All women who smoke should be strongly encouraged to quit or at least reduce the number of cigarettes they smoke. Pregnant women are advised to limit their caffeine intake to no more than three cups of coffee or cola per day.
- *Normal discomforts.* Pregnant women have physical symptoms that would be considered abnormal in the nonpregnant state. Information about the physiology and prevention of and self-care for discomforts experienced during the three trimesters is given in Table 7-2.
- *Recognizing potential complications.* One of the most important responsibilities of care providers is to alert the pregnant woman to signs and symptoms that indicate a potential complication of pregnancy (see Signs of Potential Complications box on p. 126).
- *Recognizing preterm labor.* Teaching each expectant mother to recognize preterm labor is necessary for early diagnosis and treatment. Preterm labor occurs after the twentieth week but before the thirty-seventh week of pregnancy and consists of uterine contractions that, if untreated, cause the cervix to open earlier than normal and result in preterm birth. Warning signs and symptoms of preterm labor are given in the Patient Instructions for Self-Care box.

PATIENT INSTRUCTIONS FOR SELF-CARE

How to Recognize Preterm Labor

- Because the onset of preterm labor is subtle and often hard to recognize, it is important to know how to feel your abdomen for uterine contractions. You can feel for contractions in the following way. While lying down, place your fingertips on the top of your uterus. A contraction is the periodic tightening or hardening of your uterus. If your uterus is contracting, you will actually feel your abdomen get tight or hard and then feel it relax or soften when the contraction is over.

- If you think you are having any other signs and symptoms of preterm labor, empty your bladder, drink three or four glasses of water for hydration, lie down tilted toward your side, and place a pillow at your back for support.

- Check for contractions for 1 hour. To tell how often contractions are occurring, check the minutes that elapse from the beginning of one contraction to the beginning of the next.

- It is not normal to have frequent uterine contractions (every 10 minutes or more often for 1 hour).

- Contractions of labor are regular, frequent, and hard. They also may be felt as a tightening of the abdomen or a backache. This type of contraction causes the cervix to efface and dilate.

- Call your doctor, nurse-midwife, clinic, or labor and birth unit, or go to the hospital if any of the following signs occur:
  —You have uterine contractions every 10 minutes or more often for 1 hour, or
  —You have any of the other signs and symptoms for 1 hour, or
  —You have any bloody spotting or leaking of fluid from your vagina

- It is often difficult to identify preterm labor. Accurate diagnosis requires assessment by the health care provider, usually in the hospital or clinic.

- Post these instructions where they can be seen by everyone in the family.

PATIENT INSTRUCTIONS FOR SELF-CARE

Sexuality in Pregnancy

- Be aware that maternal physiologic changes, such as breast enlargement, nausea, fatigue, abdominal changes, perineal enlargement, leukorrhea, pelvic vasocongestion, and orgasmic responses, may affect sexuality and sexual expression.
- Discuss responses to pregnancy with your partner.
- Keep in mind that cultural prescriptions ("dos") and proscriptions ("don'ts") may affect your responses.
- Although your libido may be depressed during the first trimester, it often increases during the second and third trimesters.
- Discuss and explore with your partner:
  —Alternative behaviors (e.g., mutual masturbation, foot massage, cuddling)
  —Alternative positions (e.g., female superior, side-lying) for sexual intercourse
- Intercourse is safe as long as it is not uncomfortable. There is no correlation between intercourse and miscarriage, but observe the following precautions:
  —Abstain from intercourse if you experience uterine cramping or vaginal bleeding; report event to your caregiver as soon as possible.
  —Abstain from intercourse (or any activity that results in orgasm) if you have a history of cervical incompetence, until the problem is corrected.
- Continue to use "safer sex" behaviors. Women at risk for acquiring or conveying sexually transmitted infections (STIs) are encouraged to use condoms during sexual intercourse throughout pregnancy.

- *Sexual counseling.* Sexual counseling of expectant couples includes countering misinformation, providing reassurance of normality, and suggesting alternative behaviors (see Patient Instructions for Self-Care box). Because STIs may be transmitted to the woman and her fetus, the use of condoms is

Text continued on p. 155.

TABLE 7-2

Discomforts Related to Pregnancy

DISCOMFORT	PHYSIOLOGY	EDUCATION FOR SELF-CARE
FIRST TRIMESTER		
Breast changes, new sensation: pain, tingling, tenderness	Hypertrophy of mammary glandular tissue and increased vascularization, pigmentation, and size and prominence of nipples and areolae caused by hormonal stimulation	Wear supportive maternity bras with pads to absorb discharge, may be worn at night; wash with warm water and keep dry; breast tenderness may interfere with sexual expression or foreplay but is temporary
Urgency and frequency of urination	Vascular engorgement and altered bladder function caused by hormones; bladder capacity reduced by enlarging uterus and fetal presenting part	Empty bladder regularly; perform Kegel exercises; limit fluid intake before bedtime; wear perineal pad; report pain or burning sensation to primary health care provider
Languor and malaise; fatigue (early pregnancy, most commonly)	Unexplained; may be caused by increasing levels of estrogen, progesterone, and hCG or by elevated BBT; psychologic response to	Rest as needed; eat well-balanced diet to prevent anemia

Nausea and vomiting, morning sickness—occurs in 50%-75% of pregnant women; starts between first and second missed periods and lasts until about fourth missed period; may occur any time during day; fathers also may have symptoms

pregnancy and its required physical and psychologic adaptations

Cause unknown; may result from hormonal changes, possibly hCG; may be partly emotional, reflecting pride in, ambivalence about, or rejection of pregnant state

Avoid empty or overloaded stomach; maintain good posture—give stomach ample room; stop smoking; eat dry carbohydrate on awakening; remain in bed until feeling subsides, or alternate dry every other hour with fluids such as hot herbal decaffeinated tea, milk, or clear coffee until feeling subsides; eat five or six small meals per day; avoid fried, odorous, spicy, greasy, or gas-forming foods; consult primary health care provider if intractable vomiting occurs

Continued

BBT, Basal body temperature; *GI,* gastrointestinal; *hCG,* human chorionic gonadotropin.

TABLE 7-2

Discomforts Related to Pregnancy—cont'd

DISCOMFORT	PHYSIOLOGY	EDUCATION FOR SELF-CARE
Ptyalism (excessive salivation) may occur starting 2-3 wk after first missed period	Possibly caused by elevated estrogen levels; may be related to reluctance to swallow because of nausea	Use astringent mouthwash, chew gum, eat hard candy as comfort measures
Gingivitis and epulis (hyperemia, hypertrophy, bleeding, tenderness of the gums); condition will disappear spontaneously 1-2 mo after birth	Increased vascularity and proliferation of connective tissue from estrogen stimulation	Eat well-balanced diet with adequate protein and fresh fruits and vegetables; brush teeth gently and observe good dental hygiene; avoid infection; see dentist
Nasal stuffiness; epistaxis (nosebleed)	Hyperemia of mucous membranes related to high estrogen levels	Use humidifier; avoid trauma; normal saline nose drops or spray may be used
Leukorrhea: often noted throughout pregnancy	Hormonally stimulated cervix becomes hypertrophic and hyperactive, producing abundant amount of mucus	Not preventable; do not douche; wear perineal pads; perform hygienic practices such as wiping front to back;

		report to primary health care provider if accompanied by pruritus, foul odor, or change in character or color
Psychosocial dynamics, mood swings, mixed feelings	Hormonal and metabolic adaptations; feelings about female role, sexuality, timing of pregnancy, and resultant changes in life and lifestyle	Participate in pregnancy support group; communicate concerns to partner, family, and health care provider; request referral for supportive services if needed (financial assistance)
SECOND TRIMESTER		
Pigmentation deepens; acne, oily skin	Melanocyte-stimulating hormone (from anterior pituitary)	Not preventable; usually resolves during puerperium
Spider nevi (angiomas) appear over neck, thorax, face, and arms during second or third trimester	Focal networks of dilated arterioles (end-arteries) from increased concentration of estrogens	Not preventable; they fade slowly during late puerperium; rarely disappear completely

Continued

TABLE 7-2

Discomforts Related to Pregnancy—cont'd

DISCOMFORT	PHYSIOLOGY	EDUCATION FOR SELF-CARE
Palmar erythema occurs in 50% of pregnant women; may accompany spider nevi	Diffuse reddish mottling over palms and suffused skin over thenar eminences and fingertips; may be caused by genetic predisposition or hyperestrogenism	Not preventable; condition will fade within 1 wk after giving birth
Pruritus (noninflammatory)	Unknown cause; various types as follows: nonpapular; closely aggregated pruritic papules; increased excretory function of skin and stretching of skin possible factors	Keep fingernails short and clean; contact primary health care provider for diagnosis of cause; not preventable; use comfort measures for symptoms, such as Keri baths, distraction, tepid baths with sodium bicarbonate or oatmeal added to water, lotions and oils; change of soaps or reduction in use of soap; loose clothing; see health care provider if mild sedation is needed

Palpitations	Unknown; should not be accompanied by persistent cardiac irregularity	Not preventable; contact primary health care provider if accompanied by symptoms of cardiac decompensation
Supine hypotension (vena cava syndrome) and bradycardia	Induced by pressure of gravid uterus on ascending vena cava when woman is supine; reduces uteroplacental and renal perfusion	Side-lying position or semi-sitting posture, with knees slightly flexed (see discussion of supine hypotension)
Faintness and, rarely, syncope (orthostatic hypotension) may persist throughout pregnancy	Vasomotor lability or postural hypotension from hormones; in late pregnancy may be caused by venous stasis in lower extremities	Moderate exercise, deep breathing, vigorous leg movement; avoid sudden changes in position and warm, crowded areas; move slowly and deliberately; keep environment cool; avoid hypoglycemia by eating five or six small meals per day; wear elastic hose; sit as necessary; if symptoms are serious, contact primary health care provider

Continued

TABLE 7-2

Discomforts Related to Pregnancy—cont'd

DISCOMFORT	PHYSIOLOGY	EDUCATION FOR SELF-CARE
Food cravings	Cause unknown; craving influenced by culture or geographic area	Not preventable; satisfy craving unless it interferes with well-balanced diet; report unusual cravings to primary health care provider
Heartburn (pyrosis or acid indigestion): burning sensation, occasionally with burping and regurgitation of a little sour-tasting fluid	Progesterone slows GI tract motility and digestion, reverses peristalsis, relaxes cardiac sphincter, and delays emptying time of stomach; stomach displaced upward and compressed by enlarging uterus	Limit or avoid gas-producing or fatty foods and large meals; maintain good posture; sip milk for temporary relief; hot herbal tea; primary health care provider may prescribe antacid between meals; contact primary health care provider for persistent symptoms

Constipation	GI tract motility slowed because of progesterone, resulting in increased resorption of water and drying of stool; intestines compressed by enlarging uterus; predisposition to constipation because of oral iron supplementation	Drink six to eight glasses of water per day; include roughage in diet; moderate exercise; maintain regular schedule for bowel movements; use relaxation techniques and deep breathing; do not take stool softeners, laxatives, mineral oil, other drugs, or enemas without first consulting primary health care provider
Flatulence with bloating and belching	Reduced GI motility because of hormones, allowing time for bacterial action that produces gas; swallowing air	Chew foods slowly and thoroughly; avoid gas-producing foods, fatty foods, large meals; exercise; maintain regular bowel habits
Varicose veins (varicosities): may be associated with aching legs and tenderness; may be present in legs and vulva; hemorrhoids are varicosities in perianal area	Hereditary predisposition; relaxation of smooth muscle walls of veins because of hormones causing tortuous dilated veins in legs and pelvic vasocongestion; condition	Avoid obesity, lengthy standing or sitting, constrictive clothing, and constipation and bearing down with bowel movements; moderate exercise; rest with legs and

Continued

TABLE 7-2

Discomforts Related to Pregnancy—cont'd

DISCOMFORT	PHYSIOLOGY	EDUCATION FOR SELF-CARE
	aggravated by enlarging uterus, gravity, and bearing down for bowel movements; thrombi from leg varices rare but may occur in hemorrhoids	hips elevated; wear support stockings; thrombosed hemorrhoid may be evacuated; relieve swelling and pain with warm sitz baths, local application of astringent compresses
Leukorrhea: often noted throughout pregnancy	Hormonally stimulated cervix becomes hypertrophic and hyperactive, producing abundant amount of mucus	Not preventable; do not douche; maintain good hygiene; wear perineal pads; report to primary health care provider if accompanied by pruritus, foul odor, or change in character or color
Headaches (through wk 26)	Emotional tension (more common than vascular migraine headache); eye strain (refractory errors); vascular engorgement and congestion of sinuses resulting from hormone stimulation	Conscious relaxation; contact primary health care provider for constant "splitting" headache, to assess for preeclampsia

Carpal tunnel syndrome (involves thumb, second and third fingers, and lateral side of little finger)	Compression of median nerve resulting from changes in surrounding tissues; pain, numbness, tingling, burning; loss of skilled movements (typing); dropping of objects	Not preventable; elevate affected arm; splinting of affected hand may help; regressive after pregnancy; surgery is curative
Periodic numbness, tingling of fingers (acrodysesthesia) occur in 5% of pregnant women	Brachial plexus traction syndrome resulting from drooping of shoulders during pregnancy (occurs especially at night and early morning)	Maintain good posture; wear supportive maternity bra; condition will disappear if lifting and carrying baby does not aggravate it
Round ligament pain (tenderness)	Stretching of ligament caused by enlarging uterus	Not preventable; rest, maintain good body mechanics to avoid overstretching ligament; relieve cramping by squatting or bringing knees to chest; sometimes heat helps
Joint pain, backache, and pelvic pressure; hypermobility of joints	Relaxation of symphyseal and sacroiliac joints because of hormones, resulting in unstable pelvis; exaggerated	Maintain good posture and body mechanics; avoid fatigue; wear low-heeled shoes; abdominal supports may be

Continued

TABLE 7-2

Discomforts Related to Pregnancy—cont'd

DISCOMFORT	PHYSIOLOGY	EDUCATION FOR SELF-CARE
	lumbar and cervicothoracic curves caused by change in center of gravity resulting from enlarging abdomen	useful; conscious relaxation; sleep on firm mattress; apply local heat or ice; get back rubs; do pelvic tilt exercises; rest; condition will disappear 6-8 wk after birth
THIRD TRIMESTER Shortness of breath and dyspnea occur in 60% of pregnant women	Expansion of diaphragm limited by enlarging uterus; diaphragm is elevated about 4 cm; some relief after lightening	Good posture; sleep with extra pillows; avoid overloading stomach; stop smoking; contact health care provider if symptoms worsen to rule out anemia, emphysema, and asthma
Insomnia (later weeks of pregnancy)	Fetal movements, muscle cramping, urinary frequency, shortness of breath, or other discomforts	Reassurance; conscious relaxation; back massage or effleurage; support of body parts with pillows; warm milk or warm shower before retiring

Psychosocial responses: mood swings, mixed feelings, increased anxiety	Hormonal and metabolic adaptations; feelings about impending labor, birth, and parenthood	Reassurance and support from significant other and health care providers; improved communication with partner, family, and others
Urinary frequency and urgency return	Vascular engorgement and altered bladder function caused by hormones; bladder capacity reduced by enlarging uterus and fetal presenting part	Empty bladder regularly; Kegel exercises; limit fluid intake before bedtime; reassurance; wear perineal pad; contact health care provider for pain or burning sensation
Perineal discomfort and pressure	Pressure from enlarging uterus, especially when standing or walking; multifetal gestation	Rest, conscious relaxation, and good posture; contact health care provider for assessment and treatment if pain is present
Braxton Hicks contractions	Intensification of uterine contractions in preparation for work of labor	Reassurance; rest; change of position; practice breathing techniques when contractions are bothersome; effleurage; differentiate from preterm labor

Continued

TABLE 7-2
Discomforts Related to Pregnancy—cont'd

DISCOMFORT	PHYSIOLOGY	EDUCATION FOR SELF-CARE
Leg cramps (gastrocnemius spasm), especially when reclining	Compression of nerves supplying lower extremities because of enlarging uterus; reduced level of diffusible serum calcium or elevation of serum phosphorus; aggravating factors: fatigue, poor peripheral circulation, pointing toes when stretching legs or when walking, drinking more than 1 L (1 qt) of milk per day	Check for Homans sign; if negative, use massage and heat over affected muscle; dorsiflex foot until spasm relaxes; stand on cold surface; oral supplementation with calcium carbonate or calcium lactate tablets; aluminum hydroxide gel, 30 ml, with each meal removes phosphorus by absorbing it (consult primary health care provider before taking these remedies)
Ankle edema (nonpitting) to lower extremities	Edema aggravated by prolonged standing, sitting, poor posture, lack of exercise, constrictive clothing, or hot weather	Ample fluid intake for natural diuretic effect; put on support stockings before arising; rest periodically with legs and hips elevated, exercise moderately; contact health care provider if generalized edema develops; *diuretics are contraindicated*

recommended throughout pregnancy if the woman is at risk for acquiring an STI.

• *Psychosocial support.* Esteem, affection, trust, concern, consideration of cultural and religious responses, and listening are all components of the emotional support given to the pregnant woman and her family.

CHILDBIRTH AND PERINATAL EDUCATION

The goal of childbirth and perinatal education is to assist individuals and their family members to make informed, safe decisions about pregnancy, birth, and early parenthood. Perinatal

---

BOX 7-4

Questions to Ask When Choosing a Doula

To discover the specific training, experience, and services offered by anyone who provides labor support, potential patients, nursing supervisors, physicians, midwives, and others should ask the following questions of that person:

• What training have you had?
• Tell me about your experience with birth, personally and as a doula.
• What is your philosophy about childbirth and supporting women and their partners through labor?
• May we meet to discuss our birth plans and the role you will play in supporting me through childbirth?
• May we call you with questions or concerns before and after the birth?
• When do you try to join women in labor? Do you come to our home or meet us at the hospital?
• Do you meet with us after the birth to review the labor and answer questions?
• Do you work with one or more backup doulas for times when you are not available? May we meet them?
• What is your fee?

From Simkin, P., & Way, K. (1998). *DONA position paper: The doula's contributions to modern maternity care.* Seattle, WA: Doulas of North America.

education programs consist of a menu of class series and activities from preconception through the early months of parenting.

Current Practices in Childbirth Education

A variety of approaches to childbirth education have evolved as childbirth educators attempt to meet learning needs. In addition to classes designed specifically for pregnant adolescents, their partners, and parents, classes exist for other groups with special learning needs. These include classes for first-time mothers over 35 years, single women, adoptive parents, and parents of twins. Refresher classes for parents with children not only review coping techniques for labor and birth but also help couples prepare for sibling reactions and adjustments to a new baby. Cesarean birth classes are offered for couples who have this kind of birth scheduled because of breech position or other risk factors. Other classes focus on vaginal birth after cesarean (VBAC), because many women successfully give birth vaginally after previous cesarean birth. It is the responsibility of the nurse to be informed about childbirth methods so that she can provide support to the laboring couple.

Doulas

A doula is professionally trained to provide labor support, including physical, emotional, and informational support to women and their partners during labor and birth. Box 7-4 provides questions to ask when interviewing a prospective doula.

CHAPTER 8

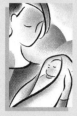

Complications of Pregnancy

HYPERTENSION IN PREGNANCY

Hypertension is the most common medical complication of pregnancy and includes both gestational and chronic hypertensive disorders. The classification system most commonly used in the United States today is based on reports from the American College of Obstetricians and Gynecologists (ACOG) and the National High Blood Pressure Education Program Working Group on High Blood Pressure in Pregnancy. This classification system is summarized in Table 8-1.

- *Gestational hypertension* is the onset of hypertension without proteinuria after week 20 of pregnancy. *Gestational hypertension* is a nonspecific term that replaces the term *pregnancy-induced hypertension (PIH)*.

- *Preeclampsia* is a hypertensive condition unique to human pregnancy; signs and symptoms usually develop only during pregnancy and disappear quickly after birth of the fetus and passage of placenta. The cause is unknown. No single patient profile identifies the woman who will have preeclampsia.

  –Certain high risk factors associated with the development of preeclampsia include primigravidity, multifetal presentation, preexisting diabetes mellitus, and African-American ethnicity (Box 8-1).

- *HELLP syndrome* is a laboratory diagnosis for a variant of severe preeclampsia that involves hepatic dysfunction, characterized by hemolysis (H) (burr cells on peripheral smear or elevated bilirubin [indirect] level), elevated liver enzymes (EL) (aspartate aminotransferase [AST] and alanine aminotransferase [ALT]), and low platelets (LP) (less than 100,000/mm^3).

TABLE 8-1

Classification of Hypertensive States of Pregnancy

TYPE	DESCRIPTION
GESTATIONAL HYPERTENSIVE DISORDERS	
Gestational hypertension	Development of mild hypertension during pregnancy in previously normotensive patient without proteinuria or pathologic edema
Gestational proteinuria	Development of proteinuria after 20 wk of gestation in previously nonproteinuric patient without hypertension
Preeclampsia	Development of hypertension and proteinuria in previously normotensive patient after 20 wk of gestation or in early postpartum period; in presence of trophoblastic disease it can develop before 20 wk of gestation
Eclampsia	Development of convulsions or coma in preeclamptic patient
CHRONIC HYPERTENSIVE DISORDERS	
Chronic hypertension	Hypertension and/or proteinuria in pregnant patient with chronic hypertension before 20 wk of gestation and persistent after 12 wk postpartum
Superimposed preeclampsia or eclampsia	Development of preeclampsia or eclampsia in patient with chronic hypertension before 20 wk of gestation

Modified from Gilbert, E., & Harmon, J. (2003). *Manual of high risk pregnancy and delivery* (3rd ed.). St. Louis: Mosby; Cunningham, F., Leveno, K., Bloom, S., Hauth, J., Gilstrap, L., & Wenstrom, K. (2005). *Williams obstetrics* (22nd ed.). New York: McGraw-Hill.

BOX 8-1

Risk Factors Associated with the Development of Preeclampsia

Chronic renal disease
Chronic hypertension
Family history of preeclampsia
Multifetal gestation
Primigravidity or new partner with multiparous woman
Extremes of maternal age: younger than 19 years or older than 40 years
Diabetes
Rh incompatibility
Obesity
African-American ethnicity
Insulin resistance
Limited sperm exposure with same partner
Preeclampsia in a previous pregnancy
Pregnancies after donor insemination, oocyte donation, or embryo donation
Maternal infections

Data from America College of Obstetricians and Gynecologists (ACOG). (2002). *Diagnosis and management of preeclampsia and eclampsia. ACOG Practice Bulletin No. 33.* Washington, DC: ACOG; Gilbert, E., & Harmon, J. (2003). *Manual of high risk pregnancy and delivery* (3rd ed.). St. Louis: Mosby; Sibai, B., Dekker, G., & Kupferminc, M. (2005). Pre-eclampsia. *Lancet, 365*(9461), 785-799.

CARE MANAGEMENT

Assessment

- The medical history is reviewed, especially the presence of diabetes mellitus, renal disease, and hypertension. Family history is explored for occurrence of preeclamptic or hypertensive conditions, diabetes mellitus, and other chronic conditions. A review of systems adds to the database for detecting BP changes from baseline and the presence of proteinuria. It is important to note whether the woman is having unusual, frequent, or severe headaches; visual disturbances; or epigastric pain. Abnormal amount and pattern of weight gain and increased signs of edema may be present even though they may not be specifically diagnostic signs of preeclampsia.

- Personnel caring for pregnant women need to be consistent in taking and recording BP measurements in the standardized manner. Electronic BP devices are less accurate in high-flow states such as pregnancy or in hypertensive or hypotensive states.

Physical Examination

- Edema that is observed is assessed for distribution, degree, and pitting. If periorbital or facial edema is not obvious, the pregnant woman is asked whether it was present when she awoke. Edema may be described as dependent or pitting. Dependent edema is edema of the lowest or most dependent parts of the body, where hydrostatic pressure is greatest. If a pregnant woman is ambulatory, this edema may first be evident in the feet and ankles. If the pregnant woman is confined to bed, the edema is more likely to occur in the sacral region. Pitting edema is edema that leaves a small depression or pit after finger pressure is applied to the swollen area. The pit, which is caused by movement of fluid to adjacent tissue away from the point of pressure, normally disappears within 10 to 30 seconds. Symptoms reflecting central nervous system (CNS) and visual system involvement usually accompany facial edema. Although it is not a routine assessment during the prenatal period, evaluation of the fundus of the eye yields valuable data. An initial baseline finding of normal eye grounds assists in differentiating preexisting disease from a new disease process.
- The presence of epigastric pain and oliguria is assessed.
- Respirations are assessed for crackles, which may indicate pulmonary edema.
- Deep tendon reflexes (DTRs) are evaluated if preeclampsia is suspected.
  - Normal response when the biceps reflex is elicited is flexion of the arm at the elbow, described as a 2+ response.
  - The patellar reflex is elicited with the woman's legs hanging freely over the end of the examining table or with the woman lying on her left side with the knee slightly flexed. Normal response is the extension or kicking out of the leg.
  - To assess for hyperactive reflexes (clonus) at the ankle joint, the examiner supports the leg with the knee flexed. With

one hand, the examiner sharply dorsiflexes the foot, maintains the position for a moment, and then releases the foot. Normal (negative clonus) response is elicited when no rhythmic oscillations (jerks) are felt while the foot is held in dorsiflexion. When the foot is released, no oscillations are seen as the foot drops to the plantar flexed position. Abnormal (positive clonus) response is recognized by rhythmic oscillations of one or more "beats" felt when the foot is in dorsiflexion and seen as the foot drops to the plantar flexed position.

- An important assessment is determination of fetal status. Uteroplacental perfusion is decreased in women with preeclampsia, placing the fetus in jeopardy. Fetal movement counts are assessed daily. Biophysical or biochemical monitoring, such as nonstress tests (NSTs), contraction stress testing, biophysical profile (BPP), and serial ultrasonography, may also be used to assess fetal status.

- The woman is checked for signs of progression of mild preeclampsia to severe preeclampsia or eclampsia.
  - Signs of worsening liver involvement, renal failure, worsening hypertension, cerebral involvement, and developing coagulopathies must be assessed and documented.
  - Respirations are assessed for crackles or diminished breath sounds, which may indicate pulmonary edema.
  - Noninvasive assessment parameters include level of consciousness (LOC), BP, hemoglobin oxygen saturation (pulse oximetry), electrocardiographic findings, and urine output.

- Blood and urine specimens are collected to aid in the diagnosis and treatment of preeclampsia, HELLP syndrome, and chronic hypertension. Baseline laboratory test information is useful in cases of early diagnosis of preeclampsia because it can be compared with later results to evaluate progression and severity of the disease (Table 8-2).
  - The hematocrit, hemoglobin, and platelet levels are monitored closely for changes indicating a worsening of patient status. Because hepatic involvement is a possible complication, serum glucose levels are monitored if liver function tests indicate elevated liver enzymes. Once the platelet count drops below 100,000/mm^3, coagulation profiles are needed to identify developing DIC.

TABLE 8-2

Common Laboratory Changes in Preeclampsia

	NORMAL (NONPREGNANT)	PREECLAMPSIA	HELLP
Hemoglobin; hematocrit	12-16 g/dl; 37%-47%	May ↑	↓
Platelets	150,000-400,000/mm³	Unchanged or <100,000/mm³	<100,000/mm³
Prothrombin time (PT); partial thromboplastin time (PTT)	12-14 sec; 60-70 sec	Unchanged	Unchanged
Fibrinogen	200-400 mg/dl	300-600 mg/dl	↓
Fibrin split products (FSP)	Absent	Absent or present	Present
Blood urea nitrogen (BUN)	10-20 mg/dl	↑	←
Creatinine	0.5-1.1 mg/dl	>1.2 mg/dl	←
Lactate dehydrogenase (LDH)*	45-90 units/L	↑	↑ (>600 units/L)
Aspartate aminotransferase (AST)	4-20 units/L	Unchanged to minimal ↑	↑ (>70 units/L)
Alanine aminotransferase (ALT)	3-21 units/L	Unchanged to minimal ↑	↑
Creatinine clearance	80-125 ml/min	130-180 ml/min	↓
Burr cells or schistocytes	Absent	Absent	Present
Uric acid	2-6.6 mg/dl	>5.9 mg/dl	>10 mg/dl
Bilirubin (total)	0.1-1 mg/dl	Unchanged or ↑	↑ (>1.2 mg/dl)

*LDH values differ according to the test/assays being done.
Sources: Cunningham, F., Leveno, K., Bloom, S., Hauth, J., Gilstrap, L., & Wenstrom, K. (2005). *Williams obstetrics* (22nd ed.). New York: McGraw-Hill; Dildy, G. (2004). Complications of preeclampsia. In G. Dildy, M. Belfort, G. Saade, J. Phelan, G. Hankins, & S. Clark (Eds.), *Critical care obstetrics* (4th ed.). Malden, MA: Blackwell Science; Roberts, J. (2004). Pregnancy-related hypertension. In R. Creasy, R. Resnik, & J. Iams (Eds.), *Maternal-fetal medicine: Principles and practice* (5th ed.). Philadelphia: Saunders.

- Urine output is assessed for volume of at least 30 ml/hr, or 120 ml/4 hr.
- Proteinuria is determined from dipstick testing of a clean-catch or catheterized urine specimen. A reading of 2+ or 3+ on two or more occasions, at least 6 hours apart, should be followed by a 24-hour urine collection. A 24-hour collection to test for protein and creatinine clearance is more reflective of true renal status.
- Renal laboratory assessments include monitoring trends in serum creatinine and blood urea nitrogen (BUN) levels. As renal function becomes compromised, renal excretion of creatinine and other waste products, including magnesium sulfate, decreases.
- Protein readings are designated as follows:

0	negative
Trace	trace
1+	30 mg/dl (equivalent to 0.3 g/L)
2+	100 mg/dl
3+	300 mg/dl
4+	1000 mg (1 g)/dl

Interventions

The most effective therapy is prevention. Early prenatal care, identification of pregnant women at risk, and recognition and reporting of physical warning signs are essential components for optimizing maternal and perinatal outcomes. The goals of therapy are maternal safety and a healthy newborn born as close to term as possible. At or near term, the plan of care for a woman with preeclampsia is most likely to be induction of labor, preceded, if necessary, by cervical ripening. When preeclampsia is diagnosed in a woman at less than 37 weeks of gestation, however, management depends on an evaluation of maternal and fetal condition.

Mild preeclampsia and home care

- If the woman at less than 37 weeks of gestation has mild preeclampsia (e.g., BP is stable, urine protein is less than 300 mg in a 24-hour collection, and woman has no subjective complaints), she may be managed expectantly, usually at home (Table 8-3). The maternal-fetal condition must be assessed two or three

TABLE 8-3

Differentiation Between Mild and Severe Preeclampsia

	MILD PREECLAMPSIA	SEVERE PREECLAMPSIA
MATERNAL EFFECTS		
Blood pressure (BP)	BP reading >140/90 mm Hg twice, 4-6 hr apart	Rise to ≥160/110 mm Hg on two separate occasions 4-6 hr apart with pregnant woman on bed rest
Mean arterial pressure (MAP)	>105 mm Hg	>105 mm Hg
Proteinuria		
—Qualitative dipstick	Proteinuria of ≥300 mg in a 24-hr specimen; ≥1+ on dipstick	Proteinuria of ≥2 g in 24 hr or ≥2+ on dipstick
—Quantitative 24-hr analysis		
Reflexes	May be normal	Hyperreflexia ≥3+, possible ankle clonus
Urine output	Output matching intake, ≥30 ml/hr or <650 ml/24 hr	<20 ml/hr or <400-500 ml/24 hr
Headache	Absent or transient	Persistent or severe
Visual problems	Absent	Blurred, photophobia, blind spots on funduscopy
Irritability or changes in affect	Transient	Severe

Epigastric pain	Absent	Present
Serum creatinine	Normal	Elevated, >1.2 mg/dl
Thrombocytopenia	Absent	Present, <100,000/mm^3
AST elevation	Normal or minimal	Marked
Pulmonary edema	Absent	Present
FETAL EFFECTS		
Placental perfusion	Reduced	Decreased perfusion expressing as IUGR in fetus; FHR: late decelerations
Premature placental aging	Not apparent	At birth placenta appearing smaller than normal for duration of pregnancy, premature aging apparent with numerous areas of broken syncytia, ischemic necroses (white infarcts) numerous, intervillous fibrin deposition (red infarcts)

AST, Aspartate aminotransferase; FHR, fetal heart rate; IUGR, intrauterine growth restriction.

Source: ACOG (2002). *Diagnosis and management of preeclampsia and eclampsia. ACOG Practice Bulletin number 33*, Washington, DC: ACOG; Cunningham, F., Leveno, K., Bloom, S., Hauth, J., Gilstrap, L., & Wenstrom, K. (2005). *Williams obstetrics* (22nd ed.). New York: McGraw-Hill.

times per week. If home nursing care is not an option, the woman may be asked to perform self-assessment daily, including weight, urine dipstick protein determinations, BP measurement, and fetal movement counting. She will be instructed to report the development of any subjective symptoms immediately to her health care provider and to return to the physician's office or high risk clinic for assessment as scheduled.

- The fetal condition also is closely monitored to allow additional time for fetal growth and maturation. An evaluation of fetal growth by ultrasound should be obtained every 3 weeks. Fetal movement is counted daily. Other fetal assessment tests include an NST once or twice per week and a BPP as needed. Fetal jeopardy as evidenced by inappropriate growth or abnormal test results necessitates induction of labor and birth or cesarean birth.

- Bed rest in the lateral recumbent position is a standard therapy for preeclampsia and may improve uteroplacental blood flow during pregnancy. Bed rest has been shown to be beneficial in decreasing BP and promoting diuresis. However, adverse physiologic outcomes related to complete bed rest, including cardiovascular deconditioning; diuresis with accompanying fluid, electrolyte, and weight loss; muscle atrophy; and psychologic stress, have been documented. Restricted activity, rather than strict bed rest, allows a woman with mild preeclampsia to be out of bed for brief periods. Gentle exercise (e.g., range of motion, stretching, Kegel exercises, and pelvic tilts) is important in maintaining muscle tone, blood flow, regularity of bowel function, and a sense of well-being. Relaxation techniques can help reduce the stress associated with the high risk condition and prepare the woman for labor and birth.

- Diet and fluid recommendations are much the same as for healthy pregnant women. Adequate fluid intake helps maintain optimum fluid volume and aids in renal perfusion and filtration.

Severe preeclampsia and HELLP syndrome and hospital care

- If the woman's condition worsens or she already has severe preeclampsia or HELLP syndrome and is critically ill, she should receive appropriate management (usually in a tertiary care center), ranging from immediate birth to conservative management of the pregnancy (see Table 8-3).

- The administration of magnesium sulfate as prophylaxis against seizures and an antihypertensive agent if diastolic BP is higher than 100 to 110 mm Hg is an important component of management.

- *Antepartum care* focuses on stabilization and preparation for birth. The woman may be admitted to an antepartum or a labor and birth unit, depending on the hospital. If the woman's condition is severe, she may be placed in a medical intensive care unit for hemodynamic monitoring.

  —Maternal and fetal surveillance, patient education regarding the disease process, and supportive measures directed toward the woman and her family are initiated.

  —Assessments include review of the cardiovascular system, pulmonary system, renal system, hematologic system, and CNS. Monitoring urinary output is critical because magnesium is excreted by the kidneys.

  —Fetal assessments for well-being (e.g., NST, BPP, and fetal movement counts) are important because of the potential for hypoxia related to uteroplacental insufficiency.

  —Baseline laboratory assessments include metabolic studies for liver enzyme (AST, ALT, and lactate dehydrogenase [LDH]) determination, complete blood count with platelets, coagulation profile to assess for DIC, and electrolyte studies to establish renal functioning.

  —Weight is measured on admission and daily.

  —An indwelling urinary catheter facilitates monitoring of renal function and effectiveness of therapy but is used only in women with severe preeclampsia, eclampsia, or HELLP syndrome.

  —If appropriate, vaginal examination may be done to check for cervical changes.

  —Abdominal palpation establishes uterine tonicity and fetal size, activity, and position.

  —Electronic monitoring to determine fetal status is initiated at least once each day.

  —Bed rest or restricted activity is commonly ordered.

  —The woman's room must be close to staff and emergency drugs, supplies, and equipment. Noise and external stimuli must be minimized.

—Seizure precautions are taken.

- *Intrapartum nursing care* of the woman with severe preeclampsia or HELLP syndrome involves continuous monitoring of maternal and fetal status as labor progresses. The assessment and prevention of tissue hypoxia and hemorrhage, both of which can lead to permanent compromise of vital organs, continue throughout the intrapartum and postpartum periods.

- One of the important goals of care for the woman with severe preeclampsia is prevention or control of convulsions. Magnesium sulfate is the drug of choice in the prevention and treatment of convulsions caused by preeclampsia or eclampsia.

  —Magnesium sulfate is administered as a secondary infusion (piggyback) to the main intravenous (IV) line by volumetric infusion pump. An initial loading dose of 4 to 6 g of magnesium sulfate per protocol or physician's order is infused over 15 to 20 minutes. This dose is followed by a maintenance dose of magnesium sulfate that is diluted in an IV solution per physician's order (e.g., 40 g of magnesium sulfate in 1000 ml of lactated Ringer's solution) and administered by infusion pump at 2 g/hr. This dose should maintain a therapeutic serum magnesium level of 4 to 7 mEq/L. Magnesium sulfate usually is continued intravenously for 24 hours postpartum (Box 8-2).

  —Magnesium sulfate interferes with the release of acetylcholine at the synapses, decreasing neuromuscular irritability, depressing cardiac conduction, and decreasing CNS irritability. Because magnesium circulates in a free state and unbound to protein and is excreted in the urine, accurate recordings of maternal urine output must be obtained and monitored. Diuresis is an excellent prognostic sign; however, if renal function declines, not all of the magnesium sulfate will be excreted, and this can cause magnesium toxicity.

  —Because magnesium sulfate is a CNS depressant, the nurse assesses for signs and symptoms of magnesium toxicity. Serum magnesium levels are obtained on the basis of the woman's response and when any signs of toxicity are present. Expected side effects of magnesium sulfate are a feeling of warmth, flushing, and nausea. Symptoms of mild toxicity include lethargy, muscle weakness, decreased deep tendon

BOX 8-2

Care of Patient with Preeclampsia Receiving Magnesium Sulfate

PATIENT AND FAMILY TEACHING

Explain Technique, Rationale, and Expected Reactions
- Route and rate
- Purpose of "piggyback"

Reasons for Use
- Tailor information to patient's readiness to learn
- Explain that magnesium sulfate is used to prevent disease progression
- Explain that magnesium sulfate is used to prevent seizures

Reactions to Expect from Medication
- Initially patient will feel flushed, hot, sedated, and nauseated and may experience burning at the IV site, especially during the bolus
- Sedation will continue

Monitoring to Anticipate
- Maternal: blood pressure, pulse, DTRs, level of consciousness, urine output (indwelling catheter), presence of headache, visual disturbances, epigastric pain
- Fetal: FHR and activity

ADMINISTRATION
- Verify physician order
- Position woman in side-lying position
- Prepare solution and administer with an infusion control device (pump)
- Piggyback a solution of 40 g magnesium sulfate in 1000 ml lactated Ringer's solution with an infusion control device at the ordered rate: loading dose—initial bolus of 4 to 6 g over 15 to 30 minutes; maintenance dose—1 to 3 g/hr

MATERNAL AND FETAL ASSESSMENTS
- Monitor blood pressure, pulse, respiratory rate, FHR, and contractions every 15 to 30 minutes, depending on patient condition

Continued

Care of Patient with Preeclampsia Receiving Magnesium Sulfate—cont'd

- Monitor intake and output, proteinuria, DTRs, presence of headache, visual disturbances, level of consciousness, and epigastric pain at least hourly
- Restrict hourly fluid intake to a total of 100 to 125 ml/hr; urinary output should be at least 30 ml/hr

REPORTABLE CONDITIONS

- Blood pressure: systolic ≥ 160 mm Hg, diastolic ≥ 110 mm Hg, or both
- Respiratory rate: less than or equal to 12 breaths/min
- Urinary output: less than 30 ml/hr
- Presence of headache, visual disturbances, or epigastric pain
- Increasing severity or loss of DTRs; increasing edema, proteinuria
- Any abnormal laboratory values (magnesium levels; platelet count; creatinine clearance; levels of uric acid, AST, ALT; prothrombin time; partial thromboplastin time; fibrinogen; fibrin split products)
- Any other significant change in maternal or fetal status

EMERGENCY MEASURES

- Keep emergency drug tray at bedside with calcium gluconate and intubation equipment
- Keep side rails up
- Keep lights dimmed, and maintain a quiet environment

DOCUMENTATION

- All of the above

ALT, Alanine aminotransferase; *AST,* aspartate aminotransferase; *DTRs,* deep tendon reflexes; *FHR,* fetal heart rate; *IV,* intravenous.

reflexes (DTRs), and slurred speech. Increasing toxicity may be indicated by maternal hypotension, bradycardia, bradypnea, and heart block.

NURSE ALERT *Loss of patellar reflexes, respiratory depression, oliguria, and decreased level of consciousness* *are signs of magnesium toxicity. Actions are needed to prevent respiratory or cardiac arrest. If magnesium toxicity is suspected, the infusion should be discontinued immediately. Calcium gluconate, the antidote for magnesium sulfate, may also be ordered (10 ml of a 10% solution, or 1 g) and given by slow IV push (usually by the physician) over at least 3 minutes to avoid undesirable reactions such as arrhythmias, bradycardia, and ventricular fibrillation.*

NURSE ALERT *Because magnesium sulfate is also a tocolytic agent, its use may increase the duration of labor. A preeclamptic woman receiving magnesium sulfate may need augmentation with oxytocin during labor. The amount of oxytocin needed to stimulate labor may be more than needed for a woman who is not receiving magnesium sulfate.*

Control of blood pressure

- For the severely hypertensive preeclamptic woman, antihypertensive medications may be ordered to lower the diastolic BP. Initiation of antihypertensive therapy reduces maternal morbidity and mortality rates associated with left ventricular failure and cerebral hemorrhage. Because a degree of maternal hypertension is necessary to maintain uteroplacental perfusion, antihypertensive therapy must not decrease the arterial pressure too much or too rapidly. The target range for the diastolic pressure is therefore less than 110 mm Hg and the systolic pressure less than 160 mm Hg.
  —IV hydralazine remains the antihypertensive agent of choice for the treatment of hypertension in severe preeclampsia. Labetalol hydrochloride, nifedipine, verapamil, and methyldopa are also used. The choice of agent used depends on patient response and physician preference. Table 8-4 compares antihypertensive agents used to treat hypertension in pregnancy.

Eclampsia

- If eclampsia develops the woman will have seizures. The convulsions that occur in eclampsia are frightening to observe. Increased hypertension and tonic contraction of all body muscles (seen as arms flexed, hands clenched, and legs

TABLE 8-4

Pharmacologic Control of Hypertension in Pregnancy

| ACTION | TARGET TISSUE | EFFECTS | | NURSING ACTIONS |
		MATERNAL	FETAL	
HYDRALAZINE (APRESOLINE, NEPRESOL)				
Arteriolar vasodilator	Peripheral arterioles: to decrease muscle tone, decrease peripheral resistance; hypothalamus and medullary vasomotor center for minor decrease in sympathetic tone	Headache, flushing, palpitation, tachycardia, some decrease in uteroplacental blood flow, increase in heart rate and cardiac output, increase in oxygen consumption, nausea and vomiting	Tachycardia; late decelerations and bradycardia if maternal diastolic pressure <90 mm Hg	Assess for effects of medications, alert mother (family) to expected effects of medications, assess blood pressure frequently because precipitous drop can lead to shock and perhaps abruptio placentae; assess urinary output; maintain bed

rest in a lateral position with side rails up; use with caution in presence of maternal tachycardia

LABETALOL HYDROCHLORIDE (NORMODYNE)

Beta-blocking agent causing vasodilation without significant change in cardiac output	Peripheral arterioles (see Hydralazine)	Minimal: flushing, tremulousness; minimal change in pulse rate	Minimal, if any	See Hydralazine; less likely to cause excessive hypotension and tachycardia; less rebound hypertension than hydralazine

METHYLDOPA (ALDOMET)

Maintenance therapy if needed: 250-500 mg orally every 8 hr (α_2-receptor agonist)	Postganglionic nerve endings: interferes with chemical neurotransmission	Sleepiness, postural hypotension, constipation; rare: drug-induced	After 4 mo maternal therapy, positive Coombs' test result in infant	See Hydralazine

CNS, Central nervous system.

Continued

TABLE 8-4

Pharmacologic Control of Hypertension in Pregnancy—cont'd

| ACTION | TARGET TISSUE | EFFECTS | | NURSING ACTIONS |
		MATERNAL	FETAL	
	to reduce peripheral vascular resistance, causes CNS sedation	fever in 1% of women and positive Coombs' test result in 20%		
NIFEDIPINE (PROCARDIA) Calcium channel blocker	Arterioles: to reduce systemic vascular resistance by relaxation of arterial smooth muscle	Headache, flushing; possible potentiation of effects on CNS if administered concurrently with magnesium sulfate; may interfere with labor	Minimal	See Hydralazine; use caution if patient also receiving magnesium sulfate

inverted) precede the tonic-clonic convulsions. During this stage, muscles alternately relax and contract. Respirations are halted and then begin again with long, deep, stertorous inhalations. Hypotension follows, and coma ensues. Nystagmus and muscular twitching persist for a time. Disorientation and amnesia cloud the immediate recovery. Oliguria and anuria are notable. Seizures may recur within minutes of the first convulsion, or the woman may never have another. Eclamptic seizures can result in tissue damage to the woman during the convulsion, especially if she is in a bed with unpadded side rails. During the convulsion the pregnant woman and fetus are not receiving oxygen, so eclamptic seizures produce a marked metabolic insult to both the woman and the fetus.

- The immediate care during a convulsion is to ensure a patent airway and maintain oxygenation. When convulsions occur, the woman is turned onto her side to prevent aspiration of vomitus and supine hypotension syndrome. After the convulsion ceases, food and fluid are suctioned from the glottis or trachea, and oxygen is administered by face mask. The drug of choice, magnesium sulfate (e.g., 2 to 4 g), is given by IV push and repeated every 15 minutes with a maximum of 6 g. Alternatively an anticonvulsant other than magnesium sulfate, such as diazepam, may be given. If an IV line is not already infusing then one is begun with a needle that is at least 18-gauge. Time, duration, and description of convulsions are recorded, and any urinary or fecal incontinence is noted. The fetus is monitored for adverse effects. Transient fetal bradycardia, decreased fetal heart rate (FHR) variability, and compensatory tachycardia are common.

- Aspiration is a leading cause of maternal morbidity and mortality after eclamptic seizure. After initial stabilization and airway management, the nurse should anticipate orders for a chest radiograph and possibly arterial blood gases (ABGs) to rule out the possibility of aspiration.

- A rapid assessment of uterine activity, cervical status, and fetal status is performed after a convulsion. During the convulsion, membranes may have ruptured; the cervix may have dilated because the uterus becomes hypercontractile and hypertonic; and birth may be imminent. If not, once a woman's seizure activity and BP are controlled, a decision should be made regarding whether birth should take place. The more serious the condition of the woman, the greater the need to proceed to birth either by labor induction or cesarean birth. Epidural anesthesia or systemic opioids are recommended for labor and birth pain management.

- Laboratory tests are ordered to assess for HELLP syndrome and to have blood typed and crossmatched for administration of packed red blood cells as needed. Blood is available for emergency transfusion because abruptio placentae, with accompanying hemorrhage and shock, often occurs in women with eclampsia.

Postpartum Nursing Care

After birth the symptoms of preeclampsia or eclampsia resolve quickly, usually within 48 hours. The hematopoietic and hepatic complications of HELLP syndrome may persist longer. Affected patients often show an abrupt decrease in platelet count, with a concomitant increase in LDH and AST levels, after a trend toward normalization of values has begun. Generally the laboratory abnormalities seen with HELLP syndrome resolve in 72 to 96 hours.

- Careful assessment of the woman with a hypertensive disorder continues throughout the postpartum period. Nursing care will include monitoring of vital signs, increased amounts of IV fluids intrapartally and postpartum and subsequent monitoring of intake and output and close monitoring of symptoms. Magnesium sulfate infusion may be continued 24 hours after the birth. Assessments for effects and side effects continue until the medication is discontinued. The woman is at risk for a boggy uterus and a large lochia flow as a result of the magnesium sulfate therapy. Uterine tone and lochial flow must be monitored closely.
- The preeclamptic woman is unable to tolerate excessive postpartum blood loss because of hemoconcentration. Oxytocin or prostaglandin products are used to control bleeding. Ergot products (e.g., Ergotrate, Methergine) are contraindicated because they can increase BP. The woman is asked to report symptoms such as headaches and blurred vision. The nurse assesses affect, LOC, BP, pulse, and respiratory status before an analgesic is given for headache. Magnesium sulfate potenti-

ates the action of narcotics, CNS depressants, and calcium channel blockers; these drugs must be administered with caution. The woman may need to continue an antihypertensive medication regimen if her diastolic BP exceeds 100 mm Hg at hospital discharge.

Chronic Hypertension

- Chronic hypertension in pregnancy is associated with an increased incidence of abruptio placentae, superimposed preeclampsia, and an increased perinatal death rate. Fetal effects include fetal growth restriction and small for gestational age (SGA) infants.
- Women who are at high risk are usually managed with antihypertensive therapy and frequent assessments of maternal and fetal well-being. Methyldopa (Aldomet) is usually the drug of choice, although beta-blockers and calcium channel blockers are also used. Women at low risk for complications may be monitored closely and antihypertensive therapy used as needed.
- As for any individual with hypertension, lifestyle changes are recommended. These changes include limiting sodium intake, performing exercise as appropriate, ingesting a balanced diet, limiting caffeine intake, and avoiding alcohol and tobacco. Women at low risk may be induced at approximately 40 weeks of gestation. In contrast, women at high risk are observed closely, and method and timing of birth depend on maternal and fetal status. In the postpartum period, women with chronic hypertension are at risk for complications such as renal failure, pulmonary edema, and heart failure. In addition, BP should be closely evaluated at the 6-week postpartal visit to ascertain need for antihypertensive therapy. Because all antihypertensive medications are found in breast milk, the drug of choice for women desiring to breastfeed is methyldopa.

HEMORRHAGIC COMPLICATIONS
Miscarriage

- Miscarriage is a pregnancy that ends before 20 weeks of gestation. Twenty weeks of gestation is considered the point of viability, or when the fetus is able to survive in an extrauterine environment. A fetal weight of less than 500 g may also be used to define miscarriage. A miscarriage or spontaneous abortion results from natural causes.

- The causes of early miscarriage (less than 8 weeks of gestation) include endocrine imbalance (as in women who have luteal phase defects or insulin-dependent diabetes mellitus with high blood glucose levels in the first trimester), immunologic factors (e.g., antiphospholipid antibodies), infections (e.g., bacteriuria and *Chlamydia trachomatis* infection), systemic disorders (e.g., lupus erythematosus), and genetic factors (e.g., congenital abnormalities).

- A late miscarriage (between 12 and 20 weeks of gestation) usually results from maternal causes, such as advancing maternal age and parity, chronic infections, premature dilation of the cervix and other anomalies of the reproductive tract, chronic debilitating diseases, poor nutrition, and recreational drug use.

- The types of miscarriage include threatened, inevitable, incomplete, complete, and missed. Signs and symptoms of miscarriage depend on the duration of pregnancy. Diagnosis of the type of miscarriage is based on the signs and symptoms present (Table 8-5).

- Whenever a woman with vaginal bleeding early in pregnancy seeks treatment, a thorough assessment should be performed (Box 8-3). Laboratory evaluation of human chorionic gonadotropin (hCG) levels is used in the diagnosis of pregnancy and pregnancy loss; low levels of hCG are characteristic of miscarriage. Ultrasonography can be used to determine the presence of a viable fetus within a gestational sac.

- Medical management (see Table 8-5) depends on the classification and on signs and symptoms. Traditionally, threatened miscarriages have been managed with bed rest and supportive care. Follow-up treatment depends on whether the threatened miscarriage progresses to actual miscarriage or symptoms subside and the pregnancy remains intact. Dilation and curettage (D&C) is a surgical procedure in which the cervix is dilated and a curette is inserted to scrape the uterine walls and remove uterine contents. A D&C is commonly performed to treat inevitable and incomplete miscarriage. The nurse

Text continued on p. 184.

August 9th —Due

TABLE 8-5

Assessing Miscarriage and the Usual Management

TYPE OF MISCARRIAGE	AMOUNT OF BLEEDING	UTERINE CRAMPING	PASSAGE OF TISSUE	CERVICAL DILATION	MANAGEMENT
Threatened	Slight, spotting	Mild	No	No	Bed rest (controversial), and avoidance of stress, sedation, sexual stimulation, and orgasm usually recommended. Acetaminophen-based analgesics may be given. Further treatment depends on woman's response to treatment.
Inevitable	Moderate	Mild to severe	No	Yes	Bed rest if no pain, fever, or bleeding. If pain, rupture of membranes,

From Cunningham, F., Leveno, K., Bloom, S., Hauth, J., Gilstrap, L., & Wenstrom, K. (2005). *Williams obstetrics* (22nd ed.). New York: McGraw-Hill; Gilbert, E., & Harmon, J. (2003). *Manual of high risk pregnancy and delivery* (3rd ed.). St. Louis: Mosby.

Continued

TABLE 8-5

Assessing Miscarriage and the Usual Management—cont'd

TYPE OF MISCARRIAGE	AMOUNT OF BLEEDING	UTERINE CRAMPING	PASSAGE OF TISSUE	CERVICAL DILATION	MANAGEMENT
					bleeding, or fever then prompt termination of pregnancy is accomplished, usually by dilation and curettage.
Incomplete	Heavy, profuse	Severe	Yes	Yes, with tissue in cervix	May or may not require additional cervical dilation before curettage. Suction curettage may be done.
Complete	Slight	Mild	Yes	No	No further intervention may be needed if uterine contractions are adequate to prevent hemorrhage and

| Missed | None, spotting | None | No | No | there is no infection. Suction or curettage may be performed to ensure no retained fetal or maternal tissue. If spontaneous evacuation of the uterus does not occur within 1 mo, pregnancy is terminated by method appropriate to duration of pregnancy. Blood clotting factors are monitored until uterus is empty. Disseminated intravascular coagulation and incoagulability of blood with uncontrolled |

Continued

TABLE 8-5

Assessing Miscarriage and the Usual Management—cont'd

TYPE OF MISCARRIAGE	AMOUNT OF BLEEDING	UTERINE CRAMPING	PASSAGE OF TISSUE	CERVICAL DILATION	MANAGEMENT
					hemorrhage may develop in cases of fetal death after the twelfth week, if products of conception are retained for longer than 5 wk. May be treated with dilation and curettage or 800 mcg of misoprostol.
Septic	Varies, usually malodorous	Varies	Varies	Yes, usually	Immediate termination of pregnancy by method appropriate to duration of pregnancy. Cervical culture and

					sensitivity studies are done, and broad-spectrum antibiotic therapy (e.g., ampicillin) is started. Treatment for septic shock is initiated if necessary.
Recurrent (generally defined as three or more consecutive abortions)	Varies	Varies	Yes	Yes, usually	Varies, depends on type. Prophylactic cerclage may be done if premature cervical dilation is the cause. Tests of value include parental cytogenetic analysis and lupus anticoagulant and anticardiolipin antibodies assays.

BOX 8-3

Assessment of Bleeding in Pregnancy

INITIAL DATABASE
- Chief complaint
- Vital signs
- Gravidity, parity
- Date of last menstrual period and estimated date of birth
- Pregnancy history (previous and current)
- Allergies
- Nausea and vomiting
- Pain (onset, quality, precipitating event, and location)
- Bleeding or coagulation problems
- Level of consciousness
- Emotional status

EARLY PREGNANCY
- Confirmation of pregnancy
- Bleeding (bright or dark, intermittent or continuous)
- Pain (type, intensity, persistence)
- Vaginal discharge

LATE PREGNANCY
- Estimated date of birth
- Bleeding (quantity, associated pain)
- Vaginal discharge
- Amniotic membrane status
- Uterine activity
- Abdominal pain
- Fetal status and viability

reinforces explanations, answers any questions or concerns, and prepares the woman for surgery. General preoperative and postoperative care is appropriate for the woman requiring surgical intervention for miscarriage. Analgesics or anesthesia appropriate to the procedure is used. For late incomplete or inevitable miscarriages and missed miscarriages (16 to 20 weeks of gestation), prostaglandins may be administered into the amniotic sac or by vaginal suppository to induce or augment labor and cause the products of conception to be expelled. IV oxytocin may also be used.

- Immediate nursing care focuses on physiologic stabilization. If the miscarriage is inevitable or incomplete, the woman may be prepared for labor induction or augmentation or manual or surgical evacuation of the uterus. After evacuation of the uterus the woman should be assessed for hemorrhage. For excessive bleeding after the miscarriage, ergot products such as ergonovine or a prostaglandin derivative such as carboprost tromethamine may be given to contract the uterus (see Medication Guide in Appendix B). Antibiotics are given as necessary. Analgesics, such as antiprostaglandin agents, may decrease discomfort from cramping. Transfusion therapy may be required for shock or anemia. The woman who is Rh negative and is not isoimmunized is given an intramuscular (IM) injection of $Rh_o(D)$ immune globulin within 72 hours of the miscarriage.
- Psychosocial aspects of care focus on what the pregnancy loss means to the woman and her family. Women experience feelings of grief and loss after a miscarriage. Discussions with the family must also be sensitive to the cultural beliefs of the mother and father specific to childbearing and grief. Explanations are provided regarding the nature of the miscarriage, expected procedures, and possible future implications for childbearing.
- Discharge teaching should emphasize the need for rest. If significant blood loss has occurred, iron supplementation may be ordered. Teaching includes information about normal physical findings, such as cramping, type and amount of bleeding, resumption of sexual activity, and family planning. Frequently, the woman and her family want to know when she may become pregnant again. Although this depends on the cause of the pregnancy loss, most health care providers suggest waiting approximately 2 to 3 months before becoming pregnant again, dependent on the provider and the woman. This time allowance facilitates physical and emotional healing.

Recurrent premature dilation of the cervix (incompetent cervix)

Passive and painless dilation of the cervical os without labor or contractions of the uterus (incompetent cervix) may occur in the second trimester or early in the third trimester of pregnancy. As a result, miscarriage or preterm birth may result.

- Conservative management consists of bed rest, hydration, progesterone, antiinflammatory drugs, and antibiotics.
- A cervical cerclage may be performed emergently or prophylactically.
  - Prophylactic cerclage is placed at 11 to 15 weeks of gestation, after which the woman is told to refrain from intercourse, prolonged (i.e., more than 90 minutes) standing, and heavy lifting. She is monitored during the course of her pregnancy with ultrasound scans to assess for cervical shortening and funneling.
  - The cerclage is electively removed (usually an office or a clinic procedure) when the woman reaches 37 weeks of gestation, or it may be left in place and a cesarean birth performed. If the cerclage is removed, placement must be repeated with each successive pregnancy.
  - If a cerclage is performed, the nurse monitors the woman postoperatively for contractions, rupture of membranes (ROM), and signs of infection. Discharge teaching focuses on continued monitoring of these aspects at home. The woman must understand the importance of activity restriction at home and the need for close observation and supervision. The woman should know the signs that would warrant immediate return to the hospital
- Strong contractions less than 5 minutes apart
- Rupture of membranes
- Severe perineal pressure
- An urge to push

Ectopic Pregnancy

- An ectopic pregnancy is one in which the fertilized ovum is implanted outside the uterine cavity, most often in the uterine tube. Abnormal vaginal bleeding, adnexal fullness, and pain are the classic symptoms of ectopic pregnancy. Women generally have abdominal pain as the primary presenting symptom at approximately 5 to 6 weeks of gestation. The tenderness can progress from a dull pain to a colicky pain when the tube stretches to sharp, stabbing pain.

- Differential diagnosis of ectopic pregnancy involves consideration of numerous disorders that share many signs and symptoms. Miscarriage, ruptured corpus luteum cyst, appendicitis, salpingitis, ovarian cysts, torsion of the ovary, and urinary tract infection must be considered (Table 8-6). Any woman with abdominal pain, vaginal spotting or bleeding, and a positive pregnancy test should undergo screening for ectopic pregnancy, including laboratory tests for β-hCG levels and a transvaginal ultrasound to confirm location of the gestational sac.

- Management may be surgical or medical. Removal of the ectopic pregnancy by salpingostomy is possible before rupture when the pregnancy is less than 2 cm in length and located in the ampulla. Postoperatively, residual tissue may be dissolved with a dose of methotrexate, an antimetabolite and folic acid antagonist that destroys rapidly dividing cells. General preoperative and postoperative care is appropriate for the woman with an ectopic pregnancy. Postoperatively, the nurse verifies the woman's Rh and antibody status and administers $Rh_o(D)$ immune globulin if appropriate. The woman should be encouraged to verbalize her feelings related to the loss. Referral to community resources may be appropriate.

- Hemodynamically stable women with ectopic pregnancies are eligible for methotrexate therapy if the mass is unruptured and measures less than 3.5 cm in diameter by ultrasound. After receiving the single methotrexate injection, the woman may return home but will need to return to the outpatient clinic or physician's office at least weekly for follow-up laboratory studies for 2 to 8 weeks or until the β-hCG level is less than 15 milliinternational units/ml. A repeat dose of methotrexate may be necessary if hCG titers do not drop to 25% by day 7. During this time of treatment, the woman is instructed to put nothing in her vagina (e.g., no tampons or douches and no sexual intercourse) and to avoid sun exposure because the drug may cause photosensitivity.

TABLE 8-6

Differential Diagnosis of Ectopic Pregnancy

	ECTOPIC PREGNANCY	APPENDICITIS	SALPINGITIS	RUPTURED OVARIAN CYST	MISCARRIAGE
Pain	Unilateral cramps and tenderness before rupture. May be colicky after rupture. Sudden sharp abdominal pelvic pain. Abdominal tenderness	Epigastric, periumbilical, then right lower quadrant pain, tenderness localizing at McBurney's point, rebound tenderness	Usually in both lower quadrants with or without rebound. Mild to severe pelvic pressure	Unilateral, becoming general with progressive bleeding, dull cramping	Mild uterine cramps to severe uterine pain
Nausea and vomiting	Occasionally before, frequently after rupture	Usual, precedes shift of pain to right lower quadrant	Infrequent	Rare	Almost never
Menstruation	Some aberration,	Unrelated to menses	Hypermenorrhea, metrorrhagia,	Period delayed,	Amenorrhea, then spotting,

	missed period, spotting		or both	then bleeding, often with pain	then brisk bleeding
Temperature, pulse, and blood pressure	37.2°-37.8°C, pulse variable, normal before and rapid after rupture, → BP after rupture	37.2°-37.8° C, pulse rapid	37.2°-40° C, pulse elevated in proportion to fever	Not over 37.2° C, pulse normal unless blood loss marked, then rapid	To 37.2° C Signs of shock related to obvious bleeding
Pelvic examination	Unilateral tenderness, especially on movement of cervix, crepitant mass on one side or in	No masses, rectal tenderness high on right side; no vaginal discharge	Bilateral tenderness on movement of cervix; purulent discharge	Tenderness over affected ovary, no masses	Cervix open or closed, uterus slightly enlarged, irregularly softened, tender with infection; vaginal bleeding

Continued

Modified from Gilbert, E., & Harmon, J. (2003). *Manual of high risk pregnancy and delivery* (3rd ed.). St. Louis: Mosby.
BP, Blood pressure; *WBC*, white blood cell.

TABLE 8-6

Differential Diagnosis of Ectopic Pregnancy—cont'd

	ECTOPIC PREGNANCY	APPENDICITIS	SALPINGITIS	RUPTURED OVARIAN CYST	MISCARRIAGE
	cul-de-sac; dark red or brown vaginal discharge				
Laboratory findings	WBC count to 15,000/mm³ Pregnancy test result is positive Ultrasound to rule out pregnancy after 6 wk	WBC count 10,000-18,000/mm³ (rarely normal) Pregnancy test result is negative	WBC count 15,000-30,000/mm³ Pregnancy test result is negative	WBC count normal to 10,000/mm³ Pregnancy test result is negative unless also pregnant Ultrasound will show ovarian cyst	WBC count normal Pregnancy test result is positive

NURSE ALERT *The woman receiving methotrexate therapy who consumes alcohol and takes vitamins containing folic acid (e.g., prenatal vitamins) increases her risk of experiencing side effects of the drug or exacerbating the ectopic rupture.*

- Future fertility should be discussed. Any woman who has been diagnosed with an ectopic pregnancy should be told of the increased risk for recurrent ectopic pregnancy. These women may need referral to grief or infertility support groups. In addition to the loss of the current pregnancy, they are faced with the possibility of future pregnancy losses or infertility.

Placenta Previa

Clinical manifestatons

In placenta previa, the placenta is implanted in the lower uterine segment near or over the internal cervical os. Sonographic diagnosis and increased understanding of the changes that occur in the relationship between the placental edge and the internal os as the pregnancy advances have led to a better classification of the types of placenta previa. This descriptive classification includes placenta previa (in the third trimester, the placenta covers the internal os) and marginal placenta previa (the distance of the placenta is 2 to 3 cm from the internal os and does not cover it). When the exact relationship of the os to the placenta has not been determined or in the case of apparent placenta previa in the second trimester, the term *low-lying placenta* is used.

- The most important risk factors are previous placenta previa, previous cesarean birth, and suction curettage for miscarriage or induced abortion, possibly related to endometrial scarring, multiple gestation (because of the larger placental area), closely spaced pregnancies, advanced maternal age (older than 35 years), African or Asian ethnicity, male fetal gender, cocaine use, multiparity, and tobacco use.
- Approximately 70% of women with placenta previa have painless vaginal bleeding; 20% have vaginal bleeding associated with uterine activity. Previa should be suspected whenever vaginal bleeding occurs after 20 weeks of gestation. Table 8-7 describes clinical manifestations of placenta previa.

TABLE 8-7

Summary of Findings: Abruptio Placentae and Placenta Previa

	ABRUPTIO PLACENTAE			
	GRADE 1 MILD SEPARATION (10%-20%)	GRADE 2 MODERATE SEPARATION (20%-50%)	GRADE 3 SEVERE SEPARATION (>50%)	PLACENTA PREVIA
Bleeding, external, vaginal	Minimal	Absent to moderate	Absent to moderate	Minimal to severe and life threatening
Total amount of blood loss	<500 ml	1000-1500 ml	>1500 ml	Varies
Color of blood	Dark red	Dark red	Dark red	Bright red
Shock	Rare, none	Mild shock	Common, often sudden, profound	Uncommon
Coagulopathy	Rare, none	Occasional DIC Increased, may be localized to one region or diffuse over uterus, uterus fails to relax	Frequent DIC Tetanic, persistent uterine contraction, boardlike uterus	None
Uterine tonicity	Normal			Normal

		between contractions Present		
Tenderness (pain)	Usually absent	Present	Agonizing, unremitting uterine pain	Absent
Ultrasonographic findings				
—Location of placenta	Normal, upper uterine segment	Normal, upper uterine segment	Normal, upper uterine segment	Abnormal, lower uterine segment
—Station of presenting part	Variable to engaged	Variable to engaged	Variable to engaged	High, not engaged
—Fetal position	Usual distribution*	Usual distribution*	Usual distribution*	Commonly transverse, breech, or oblique Usual distribution*
Gestational or chronic hypertension	Usual distribution*	Commonly present	Commonly present	Usual distribution*
Fetal effects	Normal fetal heart rate pattern	Nonreassuring fetal heart rate pattern	Nonreassuring fetal heart rate pattern, death can occur	Normal fetal heart rate pattern

DIC, Disseminated intravascular coagulation.

*Usual distribution refers to the usual variations of incidence seen when there is no concurrent problem.

- The maternal morbidity rate is approximately 5% and the infant mortality rate is less than 1% with placenta previa. Complications associated with placenta previa include premature rupture of membranes (PROM), preterm labor and birth, surgery-related trauma to structures adjacent to the uterus, anesthesia complications, blood transfusion reactions, over-infusion of fluids, abnormal placental attachments (e.g., placenta accreta), postpartum hemorrhage, thrombophlebitis, anemia, and infection.

Collaborative care

- A woman with third-trimester vaginal bleeding requires immediate evaluation. Necessary data from the history include gravidity, parity, estimated date of birth (EDB), general status, bleeding (i.e., quantity, quality, precipitating event, and associated pain), vital signs, and fetal status (see Box 8-3). Laboratory studies include a complete blood count, determination of blood type and Rh status, coagulation profile, and possible type and crossmatch. Placenta previa is diagnosed using transabdominal ultrasound. Management of placenta previa depends on the gestational age and condition of the fetus and the amount of bleeding present.
- Expectant management (observation and bed rest) is implemented if the fetus is not mature. Women may be placed in the hospital on complete bed rest or managed at home. If a woman is bleeding, she is usually placed in the labor and birth unit, where she and the fetus can be closely monitored.
  - Bleeding is assessed by checking the amount of bleeding on perineal pads, bed pads, and linens. Weighing pads, although not frequently used, is one way to more accurately assess blood loss: 1 g equals 1 ml of blood.
  - Ultrasonographic examinations may be done every 2 to 3 weeks.
  - Fetal surveillance may include an NST or BPP once or twice weekly.
  - Serial laboratory values are evaluated for decreasing hemoglobin and hematocrit levels and changes in coagulation values.

–Antepartum steroids (betamethasone) may be ordered to promote fetal lung maturity if gestation is less than 34 weeks.

–A vaginal speculum examination is postponed until fetal viability is reached (preferably after 34 weeks of gestation). If a pelvic examination is needed before that time, anticipate the possibility that an immediate cesarean birth may be required. The woman is taken to a delivery room or an operating room set up for cesarean birth because profound hemorrhage can occur during the examination. This type of vaginal examination, known as the *double-setup procedure,* is seldom performed.

–Once the woman reaches 37 weeks of gestation and fetal lung maturity is documented, cesarean birth can be scheduled.

• With active management, if the woman is at term and in labor or bleeding persistently, immediate intervention by cesarean birth is almost always indicated.

–During preparation for the surgery, maternal vital signs are assessed frequently for decreasing BP, increasing pulse rate, changes in LOC, and oliguria.

–Fetal assessment is maintained by continuous electronic fetal monitoring to assess for signs of hypoxia.

–Postoperatively, blood loss may continue. The large vascular channels in the lower uterine segment may continue to bleed because of the area's diminished muscle content. The natural mechanism to control bleeding–the interlacing muscle bundles contracting around open vessels (the "living ligature," characteristic of the upper part of the uterus)–is absent in the lower part of the uterus. Postpartum hemorrhage may therefore occur even if the fundus is contracted firmly.

• Emotional support for the woman and her family is extremely important. The actively bleeding patient is concerned not only for her own well-being but also for the well-being of her fetus. All procedures should be explained, and a support person should be present. The woman should be encouraged to express her concerns and feelings. If the woman and her support person or family desire spiritual support, the nurse can notify the hospital chaplain service or provide information about other supportive resources.

Premature Separation of Placenta

Clinical manifestations

Premature separation of the placenta, or abruptio placentae, is the detachment of part or all of the placenta from its implantation site. Separation occurs in the area of the decidua basalis after 20 weeks of gestation and before the birth of the infant.

- Maternal hypertension is probably the most consistently identified risk factor for abruption. Cocaine use is also a risk factor, believed to result in severe hypertension. Blunt external abdominal trauma, most often the result of motor vehicle accidents (MVAs) or maternal battering, is an increasingly significant cause of placental abruption. Other risk factors include cigarette smoking, previous abruption, preterm rupture of membranes, and twin gestation.
- The most common classification of placental abruption is according to type and severity. Clinical symptoms vary with degree of separation (see Table 8-7). Classic symptoms of abruptio placentae include vaginal bleeding, abdominal pain, and uterine tenderness and contractions.
- Maternal mortality rate approaches 1% for women with abruptio placentae. Maternal complications include hemorrhage, hypovolemic shock, hypofibrinogenemia, and thrombocytopenia. Renal failure and pituitary necrosis may result from ischemia. In rare cases, women who are Rh negative can become sensitized if fetal-to-maternal hemorrhage occurs and the fetal blood type is Rh positive. Perinatal deaths occur as a result of fetal hypoxia, preterm birth, and SGA status. Risks for neurologic defects are increased.

Collaborative care

- Abruptio placentae should be highly suspected in the woman with a sudden onset of intense, usually localized, uterine pain, with or without vaginal bleeding. Initial assessment is much the same as for placenta previa (see Table 8-7).
- Expectant management may be implemented if the abruption is mild and the fetus is less than 36 weeks of gestation and not in distress.

- —The woman is hospitalized and observed closely for signs of bleeding and labor.
- —The fetal status is also monitored with intermittent FHR monitoring and NSTs or BPPs until fetal maturity is determined or until the woman's condition deteriorates and immediate birth is indicated.
- —Use of corticosteroids to accelerate fetal lung maturity is appropriately included in the plan of care for expectant management.
- —Women who are Rh negative may be given Rh_o(D) immune globulin if fetal-to-maternal hemorrhage occurs.
- —If the mother is hemodynamically stable, a vaginal birth may be attempted if the fetus is alive and in no acute distress or if the fetus is dead. If vaginal birth is attempted, during labor, at least one large-bore (16- to 18-gauge) IV line should be started. Maternal vital signs are monitored frequently to observe for signs of declining hemodynamic status, such as increasing pulse rate and decreasing BP. Serial laboratory studies include hematocrit or hemoglobin determinations and clotting studies. Continuous electronic fetal monitoring is mandatory. An indwelling Foley catheter is inserted for continuous assessment of urine output, an excellent indirect measure of maternal organ perfusion.
- —In the presence of fetal compromise, severe hemorrhage, coagulopathy, poor labor progress, or increasing uterine resting tone, a cesarean birth is performed.
- Blood and fluid volume replacement will most likely be ordered, with a goal of maintaining the urine output at 30 ml/hr or greater and the hematocrit at 30% or greater. If this goal is not reached despite vigorous attempts at replacement, hemodynamic monitoring may be necessary. Fresh frozen plasma or cryoprecipitate may be given to maintain the fibrinogen level at a minimum of 100 to 150 mg/dl.

ENDOCRINE AND METABOLIC DISORDERS

Diabetes Mellitus

The key to an optimal pregnancy outcome is strict maternal glucose control before conception, as well as throughout the gestational period. Consequently, much emphasis is placed on preconception counseling for women with diabetes.

Clinical manifestations

Classifications. Diabetes mellitus refers to a group of metabolic diseases characterized by hyperglycemia resulting from defects in insulin secretion, insulin action, or both. The current classification system for diabetes includes four groups: type 1 diabetes, type 2 diabetes, other specific types (e.g., diabetes caused by infection or induced by drugs), and gestational diabetes mellitus (GDM).

—Type 1 diabetes includes those cases that are primarily caused by pancreatic islet beta cell destruction and that are prone to ketoacidosis. People with type 1 diabetes usually have an absolute insulin deficiency.

—Type 2 diabetes is the most prevalent form of the disease and includes individuals who have insulin resistance and usually relative (rather than absolute) insulin deficiency. Specific causes of type 2 diabetes are unknown at this time.

—Pregestational diabetes mellitus is the label sometimes given to type 1 or type 2 diabetes that existed before pregnancy.

—Gestational diabetes mellitus is any degree of glucose intolerance with the onset or first recognition occurring during pregnancy.

Pregestational Diabetes

• Women who have *pregestational diabetes* may have either type 1 or type 2 diabetes, which may or may not be complicated by vascular disease, retinopathy, nephropathy, or other diabetic sequelae. Almost all women with pregestational diabetes are insulin dependent during pregnancy. During the first trimester, when maternal blood glucose levels are normally reduced and the insulin response to glucose is enhanced, glycemic control is improved. The insulin dosage for the woman with well-controlled diabetes may need to be reduced to avoid hypoglycemia. Nausea, vomiting, and cravings typical of early pregnancy result in dietary fluctuations that influence maternal glucose levels and may also necessitate a reduction in insulin dosage. Because insulin requirements steadily increase after the first trimester, insulin dosage must be adjusted accordingly to prevent hyperglycemia. Insulin resistance begins as early as 14 to 16 weeks of gestation and continues to rise until it stabilizes during the last few weeks of pregnancy.

- *Maternal risks and complications.*
  - —Poor glycemic control later in pregnancy, particularly in women without vascular disease, increases the rate of fetal macrosomia and the risk of shoulder dystocia during birth. Women with diabetes therefore face an increased likelihood of cesarean birth because of failure to progress or operative vaginal birth (birth involving the use of episiotomy, forceps, or vacuum extractor).
  - —Hypertensive disorders, such as preeclampsia or eclampsia, occur more frequently during diabetic pregnancies. *Hydramnios (polyhydramnios)* (amniotic fluid in excess of 2000 ml) occurs approximately 10 times more often in diabetic pregnancies and is associated with PROM, onset of preterm labor, and postpartum hemorrhage.
  - —Infections are more common and more serious in pregnant women with diabetes. Vaginal infections, particularly monilial vaginitis, and urinary tract infections (UTIs) are more prevalent. Infection is serious because it causes increased insulin resistance and may result in ketoacidosis. Postpartum infection is more common among women who are insulin dependent.
  - —*Ketoacidosis* (ketone accumulation in the blood as a result of hyperglycemia) occurs most often during the second and third trimesters, when the diabetogenic effect of pregnancy is the greatest. When the maternal metabolism is stressed by illness or infection, the woman is at increased risk for diabetic ketoacidosis (DKA). DKA may also occur because of the woman's failure to take insulin appropriately. DKA may occur with blood glucose levels barely exceeding 200 mg/dl, compared with 300 to 350 mg/dl in the nonpregnant state. DKA can lead to preterm labor.
  - —The risk of hypoglycemia is also increased. Early in pregnancy, when hepatic production of glucose is diminished and peripheral use of glucose is enhanced, hypoglycemia occurs frequently, often during sleep. Later in pregnancy, hypoglycemia may also result as insulin doses are adjusted to maintain normoglycemia. Women with a prepregnancy

history of severe hypoglycemia are at increased risk for severe hypoglycemia during gestation. Table 8-8 compares signs and symptoms of hyperglycemia and hypoglycemia.

  —*Fetal and neonatal risks and complications.* The most important cause of perinatal loss in diabetic pregnancy is congenital malformations. Other complications include intrauterine growth restriction (IUGR), respiratory distress syndrome, sudden and unexplained stillbirth, risk of birth injuries related to increased fetal size, hypoglycemia, hypocalcemia, hypomagnesemia, hyperbilirubinemia, and polycythemia.

Collaborative care
Antepartum

- In addition to the routine prenatal assessment and examination, a detailed history regarding the onset and course of the diabetes and its management and the degree of glycemic control before pregnancy is obtained. Effective management of the diabetic pregnancy depends on the woman's adherence to a plan of care.

- Routine prenatal laboratory examinations are performed. At each visit urine may be tested for the presence of glucose, ketones, leukocytes, and protein.

- For the woman with pregestational type 1 or type 2 diabetes, laboratory tests may be done to assess past glycemic control, specifically over the last 4 to 6 weeks. At the initial prenatal visit, the *glycosylated hemoglobin A_{1c}* level may be measured. Values for the measurement of hemoglobin A_{1c} are as follows:
  - —Adult or elderly person without diabetes: 2.2% to 4.8%
  - —Person with good diabetic control: 2.5% to 5.9%
  - —Person with fair diabetic control: 6% to 8%
  - —Person with poor diabetic control: greater than 8%

- Fasting blood glucose or random (1 to 2 hours after eating) glucose levels may be assessed during antepartum visits. Blood glucose self-monitoring records may also be reviewed.

- During the first and second trimesters of pregnancy, routine prenatal care visits for the woman with pregestational diabetes will be scheduled every 1 to 2 weeks. In the last trimester she will likely be seen one or two times each week.

TABLE 8-8

Differentiation of Hypoglycemia (Insulin Shock) and Hyperglycemia (Diabetic Ketoacidosis)

CAUSES	ONSET	SYMPTOMS	INTERVENTIONS
HYPOGLYCEMIA (INSULIN SHOCK)			
Excess insulin	Rapid (regular insulin)	Irritability	Check blood glucose level when symptoms first appear.
Insufficient food (delayed or missed meals)	Gradual (modified insulin or oral hypoglycemic agents)	Hunger	Eat or drink 10-15 g simple carbohydrate immediately.
Excessive exercise or work		Sweating	Recheck blood glucose level in 15 min and eat or drink another 10-15 g simple carbohydrate if glucose remains low.
Indigestion, diarrhea, vomiting		Nervousness	Recheck blood glucose level in 15 min.
		Personality change	Notify primary health care provider if no change in glucose level.
		Weakness	
		Fatigue	
		Blurred or double vision	
		Dizziness	
		Headache	
		Pallor; clammy skin	
		Shallow respirations	
		Rapid pulse	
		Laboratory values	
		Urine: negative for sugar and acetone	

Continued

TABLE 8-8

Differentiation of Hypoglycemia (Insulin Shock) and Hyperglycemia (Diabetic Ketoacidosis)—cont'd

CAUSES	ONSET	SYMPTOMS	INTERVENTIONS
		Blood glucose: ≤60 mg/dl	If woman is unconscious, administer 50% dextrose IV push, 5%-10% dextrose in water IV drip, or glucagon. Obtain blood and urine specimens for laboratory testing.
HYPERGLYCEMIA (DKA) Insufficient insulin Excess or wrong kind of food	Slow (hours to days)	Thirst Nausea or vomiting Abdominal pain	Notify primary health care provider. Administer insulin in

Infection, injuries,
  illness
Emotional stress
Insufficient exercise

Constipation
Drowsiness
Dim vision
Increased urination
Headache
Flushed, dry skin
Rapid breathing
Weak, rapid pulse
Acetone (fruity)
  breath odor
Laboratory value
Urine: positive for sugar
  and acetone
Blood glucose: ≥200 mg/dl

accordance with blood
  glucose levels.
Give IV fluids such as
  normal saline solution or
  one-half normal saline
  solution; potassium when
  urinary output is
  adequate; bicarbonate
  for pH <7.
Monitor laboratory testing
  of blood and urine.

DKA, Diabetic ketoacidosis; *IV*, intravenous.

- Because the woman is at increased risk for infections, eye problems, and neurologic changes, foot care and general skin care are important.
- Dietary management during diabetic pregnancy must be based on blood (not urine) glucose levels. The dietary goals are to provide weight gain consistent with a normal pregnancy, to prevent ketoacidosis, and to minimize widely fluctuating blood glucose levels. For nonobese women, dietary counseling based on preconceptional body mass index (BMI) is 30 kcal/kg/day. In contrast, for obese women with a BMI greater than 30, it is recommended that the caloric intake total 25 kcal/kg/day. The average diet includes 2200 calories (first trimester) to 2500 calories (second and third trimesters). Total calories may be distributed among three meals and one evening snack or, more commonly, three meals and at least two snacks. Meals should be eaten on time and never skipped. A large bedtime snack of at least 25 g of carbohydrate with some protein is recommended to help prevent hypoglycemia and starvation ketosis during the night. Simple carbohydrates are limited; complex carbohydrates that are high in fiber content are recommended because the starch and protein in such foods help regulate the blood glucose level by more sustained glucose release.
- Any prescription of exercise during pregnancy for a woman with diabetes should be done by the primary health care provider and should be monitored closely to prevent complications, especially for women with vasculopathy. Exercise need not be vigorous to be beneficial: 15 to 30 minutes of walking four to six times each week is satisfactory for most pregnant women. Other exercises that may be recommended are non–weight-bearing activities, such as arm exercises or use of a recumbent bicycle. The best time for exercise is after meals, when the blood glucose level is rising. To monitor the effect of insulin on blood glucose levels, the woman can measure blood glucose before, during, and after exercise.
- Achieving and maintaining constant euglycemia are the primary goals of medical therapy. Blood glucose testing at home with a glucose reflectance meter or biosensor monitor

is the commonly accepted method for monitoring blood glucose levels. Blood glucose levels are routinely measured at various times throughout the day, such as before breakfast, lunch, and dinner; 2 hours after each meal; at bedtime; and in the middle of the night. Hyperglycemia will most likely be identified in 2-hour postprandial values, because blood glucose levels peak approximately 2 hours after a meal. Acceptable fasting levels are generally between 65 and 105 mg/dl, and 2-hour postprandial levels should be less than 130 mg/dl (Table 8-9).

- Insulin requirements during pregnancy change dramatically as the pregnancy progresses, necessitating frequent adjustments in insulin dosage. In the first trimester, from 3 to 7 gestational weeks there is an increase in insulin requirements, followed by a decrease between 7 and 15 gestational weeks. However, insulin dosage may need to be decreased because of hypoglycemia. Many types of biosynthetic human insulin preparations are available, including rapid acting (Lispro), short acting (regular), intermediate acting (NPH, Lente), and long acting (ultralente and Lantus [insulin glargine]). Lantus is categorized as a pregnancy category C drug by the U.S. Food and Drug Administration (FDA). This insulin preparation is most often used with women with insulin-resistant diabetes (type 2) requiring high doses of long-acting insulin. Table 8-10 compares insulin administration and action times.

TABLE 8-9

Target Blood Glucose Levels During Pregnancy

TIME OF DAY	TARGET GLUCOSE LEVEL (MG/DL)
Premeal	>65 but <105
Postmeal (1 hr)	<130-155
Postmeal (2 hr)	<130

From American Diabetes Association (ADA). (2004). Gestational diabetes mellitus. *Diabetes Care 27 (Suppl 1)*. S88-S90. Moore, T. (2004). Diabetes in pregnancy. In R. Creasy, R. Resnik, & J. Iams (Eds.). *Maternal-fetal medicine: Principles and practice* (5th ed.). Philadelphia: Saunders.

TABLE 8-10

Insulin Administration During Pregnancy: Expected Time of Action

TYPE OF INSULIN	ONSET	PEAK	DURATION
Lispro (short acting)	Within 15 min	30-90 min	6-8 hr
Regular (short acting)	30 min-1 hr	2-4 hr	8-12 hr
Intermediate acting	1-2½ hr	4-15 hr	12-24 hr
Long acting	4-8 hr	14-24 hr	24-36 hr
Lantus (long acting)	60-70 min	No pronounced peak	24 hr

Reference: Facts and Comparisons (2003). St. Louis: Wolters Kluwer Co.

- Most women with insulin-dependent diabetes are managed with two or three injections per day, also known as *multiple injection therapy* (MIT). Usually, two thirds of the daily insulin dose, with longer-acting and shorter-acting insulin combined in a 2 : 1 ratio, is given before breakfast. The remaining one third, again a combination of longer- and short-acting insulin, is administered in the evening before dinner. To reduce the risk of hypoglycemia during the night, separate injections often are administered, with short-acting insulin given before dinner, followed by longer-acting insulin at bedtime.
  - Urine testing for ketones may also be done if a meal is missed or delayed, when illness occurs, or when the blood glucose level is greater than 200 mg/dl. Spilling a trace or a small amount of ketones requires no treatment. However, if ketones appear repeatedly at the same time each day, some adjustment in diet may be needed. If testing shows a large amount of ketones, the health care provider should be contacted immediately.
  - Diagnostic techniques for fetal surveillance are often performed to assess fetal growth and well-being. A baseline sonogram is done during the first trimester to assess gestational age. Follow-up ultrasound examinations are usually performed during the pregnancy (as often as every 4 to 6 weeks) to monitor fetal growth; estimate fetal weight; and detect hydramnios, macrosomia, and congenital anomalies. The majority of fetal surveillance measures are concentrated in the third trimester, when the risk of fetal compromise is greatest. Pregnant women should be taught how to do daily fetal movement counts from 28 weeks of gestation. The NST used to evaluate fetal well-being may be used weekly or more often twice weekly, typically beginning around 28 weeks of gestation.

Intrapartum. Vaginal births are expected for most women with pregestational diabetes, although elective induction between 38 and 40 weeks of gestation is common. During the intrapartum period the woman must be monitored closely to prevent complications related to dehydration, hypoglycemia, and hyperglycemia.

- Blood glucose levels and hydration must be carefully controlled during labor. An IV line is inserted for infusion of a maintenance fluid, such as lactated Ringer's solution or 5% dextrose in lactated Ringer's solution.
- Most commonly, insulin is administered by continuous infusion. Only regular insulin may be administered intravenously.
- Determinations of blood glucose levels are made every hour, and fluids and insulin are adjusted to maintain blood glucose levels between 80 and 120 mg/dl. It is essential that these target glucose levels be maintained because hyperglycemia during labor can precipitate metabolic problems in the neonate, particularly hypoglycemia.
  - During labor, continuous fetal heart monitoring is necessary. A neonatologist, pediatrician, or neonatal nurse practitioner may be present at the birth to initiate assessment and neonatal care.
  - If a cesarean birth is planned, it should be scheduled in the early morning to facilitate glycemic control. The morning dose of insulin may be withheld, and the woman is given nothing by mouth. Epidural anesthesia is recommended because hypoglycemia can be detected earlier if the woman is awake. After surgery, glucose levels should be closely monitored at least every 2 hours with a target plasma glucose between 80 and 160 mg/dl and an IV solution containing 5% dextrose is infused.

Postpartum

- In the immediate 24 hours postpartum, insulin requirements decrease substantially because the major source of insulin resistance, the placenta, has been removed. Blood glucose levels are monitored in the postpartum period, and insulin dosage is adjusted using a sliding scale. Some women may not require insulin for 24 to 72 hours postpartum. Women with type 2 diabetes are soon able to maintain euglycemia through diet alone or with oral hypoglycemics.
- Possible postpartum complications include preeclampsia-eclampsia, hemorrhage, and infection.
- Mothers are encouraged to breastfeed. In addition to the advantages of maternal satisfaction and pleasure, breastfeeding has an antidiabetogenic effect for the children of women with diabetes and for women with gestational diabetes.

- The risks and benefits of contraceptive methods should be discussed with the mother and her partner before discharge from the hospital. Barrier methods are often recommended as safe, inexpensive options that have no inherent risks for women with diabetes. Use of oral contraceptives by diabetic women is controversial because of the risk of thromboembolic and vascular complications and the effect on carbohydrate metabolism. In women without vascular disease or other risk factors, combination low-dose or progestin-only oral contraceptives may be prescribed. Opinion is divided about the use of long-acting parenteral progestins. Transdermal (patch) administration and transvaginal (vaginal ring) administration are newer contraceptive methods and lack data about use with women who have diabetes. Sterilization may be an option for the woman who has completed her family, who has poor glycemic control, or who has significant vascular problems.

Gestational Diabetes Mellitus

Clinical manifestations

- Classic risk factors for GDM include maternal age above 25 years; obesity; family history of type 2 diabetes; an obstetric history of an infant weighing more than 4500 g, hydramnios, unexplained stillbirth, miscarriage, or an infant with congenital anomalies. Women at high risk for GDM are often screened at their initial prenatal visit and then rescreened later (at 24 to 28 weeks of gestation) in pregnancy if the initial screen is negative.
- *Maternal risks* include hypertensive disorders and fetal macrosomia, which can lead to increased rates of perineal lacerations, episiotomy, and cesarean birth.
- *Fetal risks* are similar to those listed for the fetus of a mother who has pregestational diabetes except that the incidence of congenital anomalies is not increased.

Collaborative care
Screening for gestational diabetes mellitus

- ACOG recommends that all pregnant women be screened for GDM by history, clinical risk factors, or laboratory screening of blood glucose levels. Women at high risk for developing

GDM should be screened at the first prenatal visit and again at 24 to 28 weeks of gestation. Screening and diagnosis of gestational diabetes are depicted in Fig. 8-1.

Antepartum Care

- As with pregestational diabetes, the aim of therapy in women with GDM is strict blood glucose control. Fasting blood glucose levels should range from 65 to 105 mg/dl, and 1-hour postprandial blood levels should be less than 130 to 155 mg/dl.

  –Dietary modification is the mainstay of treatment for GDM. The woman with GDM is placed on a standard diabetic diet. The usual prescription is for 30 kcal/kg/day based on preconceptional weight for women with a normal BMI and 25 kcal/kg/day for obese women, which translates into 1500 to 2000 kcal/day for most women. Carbohydrate intake is restricted to approximately 35% to 40% of caloric intake. Dietary counseling by a nutritionist is recommended.

  –Exercise in women with GDM helps lower blood glucose levels and may be instrumental in decreasing the need for

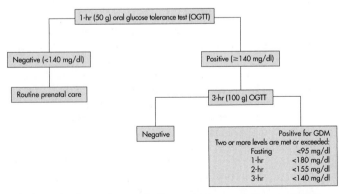

Fig. 8-1 Screening and diagnosis for gestational diabetes. (From American Diabetes Association [ADA]. [2004]. Position statement: Gestational diabetes mellitus. *Diabetes Care, 27* [Suppl 1], S88-S90.)

insulin. Women with GDM who already have an active lifestyle should be encouraged to continue an exercise program.

—Blood glucose monitoring is necessary to determine whether euglycemia can be maintained by diet and exercise. Women are encouraged to monitor their blood sugar daily. Women with GDM may perform self-monitoring at home, or monitoring may be done at the clinic or office visit.

—Up to 20% of women with GDM will require insulin during the pregnancy to maintain adequate blood glucose levels, despite compliance with the prescribed diet.

—There is no standard recommendation for fetal surveillance in pregnancies complicated by GDM. Women whose blood glucose levels are well controlled by diet are at low risk for fetal complications. Daily fetal kick counts may be done beginning at 28 weeks of gestation, and NSTs are done twice weekly beginning at 36 weeks of gestation. Usually these women progress to term and spontaneous labor without intervention. Women with GDM whose blood glucose levels are poorly controlled or who require insulin therapy, have hypertension, or have a history of previous stillbirth generally receive more intensive fetal biophysical monitoring.

Intrapartum Care. During the labor and birth process, blood glucose levels are monitored at least every 2 hours to maintain levels at 80 to 120 mg/dl. Glucose levels within this range will decrease the incidence of neonatal hypoglycemia. IV fluids containing glucose are not commonly given during labor. Although gestational diabetes is not an indication for cesarean birth, it may be necessary in the presence of preeclampsia or macrosomia.

Postpartum Care. Most women with GDM will return to normal glucose levels after childbirth. However, GDM is likely to recur in future pregnancies, and women with GDM are at significant risk for developing glucose intolerance later in life, so they should be screened at the 6-week postpartum examination. Women with gestational diabetes are encouraged to breastfeed.

Hyperemesis Gravidarum

Nausea and vomiting complicate approximately 70% of all pregnancies, beginning typically at 4 to 6 weeks of gestation, and are generally confined to the first trimester. Although these manifestations are distressing, they are typically benign, with no significant metabolic alterations or risks to the mother or fetus. When vomiting during pregnancy becomes excessive enough to cause weight loss of at least 5% of prepregnancy weight and is accompanied by dehydration, electrolyte imbalance, ketosis, and acetonuria, the disorder is termed *hyperemesis gravidarum*. Hyperemesis gravidarum has been associated with women who are nulliparous, have increased body weight, have a history of migraines, or are pregnant with twins. In addition, an interrelated psychologic component has been associated with hyperemesis and must be assessed.

Clinical manifestations

The woman with hyperemesis usually has significant weight loss and dehydration. She may have a decreased BP, increased pulse rate, and poor skin turgor. She frequently is unable to keep down even clear liquids taken by mouth. Laboratory tests may reveal electrolyte imbalances.

Collaborative management

- The assessment should include frequency, severity, and duration of episodes of nausea and vomiting. If the woman reports vomiting, then the assessment should also include the approximate amount and color of the vomitus. Other symptoms, such as diarrhea, indigestion, and abdominal pain or distention, are also identified. The woman is asked to report any precipitating factors relating to the onset of her symptoms. Any pharmacologic or nonpharmacologic treatment measures should be recorded. Prepregnancy weight and documented weight gain or loss during pregnancy are important to note.
- The woman's weight and vital signs are measured, and a complete physical examination is performed, with attention to signs of fluid and electrolyte imbalance and nutritional status. The most important initial laboratory test to be obtained is a dipstick determination of ketonuria. Other laboratory tests that may be ordered are a urinalysis, a complete blood cell

count, electrolytes, liver enzymes, and bilirubin levels to rule out other underlying diseases such as pyelonephritis, pancreatitis, cholecystitis, and hepatitis. Because of the association between hyperemesis gravidarum and hyperthyroidism, thyroid levels may also be measured.

- Psychosocial assessment includes asking the woman about anxiety, fears, and concerns related to her own health and the effects on pregnancy outcome. Family members should be assessed both for anxiety and with regard to their role in providing support for the woman.

- Initially, the woman who is unable to keep down clear liquids by mouth will require IV therapy for correction of fluid and electrolyte imbalances. She should be kept on nothing-by-mouth (NPO) status until dehydration has been resolved and for at least 48 hours after vomiting has stopped to prevent rapid recurrence of the problem. Medications may be used if nausea and vomiting are uncontrolled. The most frequently used drugs include pyridoxine (vitamin B_6) (25 to 75 mg daily) alone or in combination with doxylamine (Unisom) (25 mg), promethazine (Phenergan), and metoclopramide (Reglan). Other less commonly used drugs include meclizine (Antivert), dimenhydrinate (Dramamine), diphenhydramine (Benadryl), prochlorperazine (Compazine), and ondansetron (Zofran). Enteral or parenteral nutrition may be used for women nonresponsive to other medical therapies. In addition to medical management, some women can also benefit from psychotherapy or stress reduction techniques. Once the vomiting has stopped, feedings are started in small amounts at frequent intervals, and the diet is slowly advanced as tolerated until the woman can consume a nutritionally sound diet.

  - Nursing care of the woman with hyperemesis gravidarum involves implementing the medical plan of care. Interventions may include initiating and monitoring IV therapy, administering drugs and nutritional supplements, and monitoring the woman's response to interventions. The nurse observes the woman for any signs of complications, such as metabolic acidosis (secondary to starvation), jaundice, or hemorrhage. Accurate measurement of intake and output, including the amount of emesis, is an important aspect of care. Oral hygiene while the woman is receiving nothing by mouth, and after episodes of vomiting, helps allay associated discomforts. Assistance with positioning and providing a quiet, restful environment, free from odors, may increase the woman's comfort. When the woman begins responding to therapy, the diet progresses slowly as tolerated by the woman until she is able to consume a nutritional diet. Because sleep disturbances may accompany hyperemesis gravidarum, promoting adequate rest is important. The nurse can assist in coordinating treatment measures and periods of visitation to provide opportunity for rest periods.

Hyperthyroidism

- Graves' disease is the most common cause of hyperthyroidism. Clinical manifestations of hyperthyroidism include tachycardia, fatigue, heat intolerance, emotional lability, weight loss, and severe nausea and vomiting. Exophthalmos and enlargement of the thyroid gland (goiter) may also occur. Many of these symptoms also occur with pregnancy, so the disorder can be difficult to diagnose. Laboratory findings include elevated free thyroxine (T_4) and triiodothyronine (T_3) levels and suppressed thyroid-stimulating hormone (TSH) levels.

  - The primary treatment of hyperthyroidism during pregnancy is drug therapy; the medication of choice is propylthiouracil (PTU). Women generally show clinical improvement within 2 weeks of beginning therapy, but the medication requires 6 to 8 weeks to reach full effectiveness. PTU is well tolerated by most women.

  - Maternal side effects include pruritus, skin rash, fever, a metallic taste, nausea, bronchospasm, oral ulcerations, hepatitis, and a lupuslike syndrome. PTU readily crosses the placenta and may induce fetal hypothyroidism and goiter. Radioactive iodine must not be used in diagnosis or treatment of hyperthyroidism in pregnancy because it may compromise the fetal thyroid.

  - Mothers choosing to breastfeed who are also taking hyperthyroid medication need to be instructed that small amounts are excreted in the breast milk, but PTU has not been found to adversely affect the neonate's thyroid function.

Hypothyroidism

- Hypothyroidism during pregnancy is less common than hyperthyroidism. It is often associated with menstrual and fertility problems and an increased risk of miscarriage. Characteristic symptoms of hypothyroidism include weight gain; fatigue; cold intolerance; constipation; cool, dry skin; coarsened hair; and muscle weakness. Laboratory values in pregnancy include low or low-normal T_3 and T_4 levels and elevated levels of TSH.
  - —Pregnant women with untreated hypothyroidism are at increased risk for preeclampsia, placental abruption, and stillbirth. Infants born to mothers with hypothyroidism may be of low birth weight, but for the most part if such women are treated before conception or early in the pregnancy, the infants are healthy and without evidence of thyroid dysfunction.
  - —Thyroid hormone supplements are used to treat hypothyroidism. Levothyroxine (e.g., l-thyroxine [Synthroid]) is most often prescribed during pregnancy.

CARDIOVASCULAR DISORDERS

Heart disease is the leading cause of nonobstetric maternal death. Rheumatic fever is responsible for about 50% of cardiac complications; congenital diseases and mitral valve disease are the next most common causes. A maternal mortality rate of up to 50% is anticipated in women with persistent cardiac decompensation.

- The degree of disability experienced by the woman with cardiac disease often is more important in the treatment and prognosis during pregnancy than is the diagnosis of the type of cardiovascular disease. The New York Heart Association's (NYHA's) functional classification of organic heart disease, a widely accepted standard, is as follows:

  Class I: asymptomatic without limitation of physical activity

  Class II: symptomatic with slight limitation of activity

  Class III: symptomatic with marked limitation of activity

  Class IV: symptomatic with inability to carry on any physical activity without discomfort

- The functional classification of the disease is determined at 3 months and again at 7 or 8 months of gestation. Pregnant women may progress from class I or II to III or IV during pregnancy. The incidence of miscarriage is increased, and preterm labor and birth are more prevalent in pregnant women with cardiac problems. In addition, IUGR is common, probably because of low oxygen pressure (Po_2) in the mother. The incidence of congenital heart lesions is increased (2% to 3%) in children of mothers with congenital heart disease. Therefore preconceptional counseling is essential for positive pregnancy outcomes.

Rheumatic Heart Disease

- Episodes of rheumatic fever create an autoimmune reaction in the heart tissue, leading to permanent damage of heart valves. Heart murmurs resulting from stenosis, valvular insufficiency, or thickening of the walls of the heart characterize rheumatic heart disease (RHD), and symptoms include cardiac murmurs, congestive heart failure, and an enlarged heart. Recurrences of rheumatic fever are common, each with the potential to increase the severity of heart damage.
- For women with a history of rheumatic fever, the American Heart Association recommends lifelong prophylaxis with benzathine G penicillin, even during pregnancy. For those women with penicillin allergies, erythromycin is an acceptable alternative during pregnancy.
- Treatment also includes limited physical activity, diuretics, sodium restriction, and medications such as digoxin, betablockers, and calcium channel blockers. It is recommended that affected women give birth vaginally, with use of an epidural anesthetic and strict monitoring of their fluid intake.
  - *Mitral valve stenosis* is a narrowing of the opening of the mitral valve caused by stiffening of valve leaflets, which obstructs blood flow from the atrium to the ventricle and is the characteristic lesion resulting from RHD. The care of the woman with mitral stenosis typically is managed by reducing her activity, restricting dietary sodium, and increasing bed rest.

Mitral Valve Prolapse

Mitral valve prolapse (MVP) is a common, usually benign, condition in which the mitral valve leaflets prolapse into the left atrium during ventricular systole, allowing some backflow of blood. Midsystolic click and late systolic murmur are hallmarks of this syndrome. Most cases are asymptomatic.

• A few women have atypical chest pain (sharp and located in the left side of the chest) that occurs at rest and does not respond to nitrates. They may also have anxiety, palpitations, dyspnea on exertion, and syncope.

• Women usually are treated with beta-blockers, such as propranolol (Inderal). Pregnancy and its associated hemodynamic changes may change or alleviate the murmur and click of MVP, as well as symptoms.

Congenital Heart Defects

• Some congenital heart disorders are associated with a normal pregnancy outcome, because the woman has had corrective surgery. These include atrial septal defect (ASD), an abnormal opening between the atria. It is one of the causes of a left-to-right shunt and is the most common congenital defect seen during pregnancy. This defect may go undetected because the woman usually is asymptomatic. The pregnant woman with an ASD will most likely have an uncomplicated pregnancy even without corrective surgery, unless she has pulmonary hypertension. With complicated ASDs some women may have right-sided heart failure or arrhythmias as the pregnancy progresses as a result of increased plasma volume.

–Tetralogy of Fallot is the most common cyanotic heart disease present during pregnancy. Other cyanotic congenital heart diseases are rarely seen during pregnancy because women with these conditions rarely survive to adulthood. Components of tetralogy of Fallot include a ventricular septal defect (VSD), pulmonary stenosis, overriding aorta, and right ventricular hypertrophy, leading to a right-to-left shunt. Medical management for women with uncorrected tetralogy of Fallot includes monitoring maternal hematocrits, hypotension during labor, anticoagulant therapy, high-concentration oxygen administration, and hemodynamic monitoring during labor and birth. Complications include right-sided heart failure, arrhythmias, and conduction defects, with the most dangerous time being the late third trimester and early postpartum period. Women with tetralogy of Fallot are counseled before conception to have surgical repair.

Collaborative Care

Assessment

• The woman is assessed for factors that would increase stress on the heart, such as anemia, infection, and edema, and how she is adapting to the physiologic changes of pregnancy. Special attention is given to the review of the cardiovascular and pulmonary systems. The nurse should determine whether the woman has experienced chest pain at rest or on exertion; edema of the face, hands, or feet; hypertension; heart murmurs; palpitations; paroxysmal nocturnal dyspnea; diaphoresis; pallor; or syncope. Pulmonary signs and symptoms such as cough, hemoptysis, shortness of breath, and orthopnea can indicate cardiac disease. Table 8-11 lists normal and abnormal cardiovascular signs and symptoms during pregnancy.

–Routine assessments continue during the prenatal period, including monitoring the amount and pattern of weight gain, edema, vital signs, and discomforts of pregnancy. In addition, the woman is observed for signs of cardiac decompensation, that is, progressive generalized edema, crackles at the base of the lungs, or pulse irregularity (see Signs of Potential Complications box). Symptoms of cardiac decompensation may appear abruptly or gradually. Medical intervention must be instituted immediately to maintain optimal cardiac status.

–Routine urinalysis and blood work (complete blood cell count and blood chemistry) are done during the initial visit. The woman with cardiac impairment requires a baseline electrocardiogram (ECG) at the beginning of her pregnancy, if not before pregnancy, which permits vital diagnostic comparisons of subsequent ECGs.

TABLE 8-11

Cardiovascular Signs and Symptoms During Pregnancy

NORMAL	ABNORMAL
SIGNS	
Neck vein pulsation	Neck vein distention
Diffuse or displaced apical pulse	Cardiomegaly; heave
Split S_1, accentuated S_2	Loud P_2; wide split of S_2
Third heart sound—loud	Summation gallop
Systolic murmur (1-2/6) (92%-95%)	Loud systolic murmur (4-6/6)
Venous hum	Diastolic murmur
Sinus arrhythmia	Sustained arrhythmia
Peripheral edema, particularly lower extremities	Clubbing or cyanosis
SYMPTOMS	
Fatigue	Symptoms at rest
Chest pain	Exertional chest pain
Dyspnea	Exertional severe dyspnea
Orthopnea	Orthopnea (progressive)
Hyperpnea	Paroxysmal nocturnal dyspnea
Palpitations	Tachycardia (>120 beats/min); arrhythmia
Syncope (vasovagal)	Exertional syncope

Adapted from Blackburn, S. (2003). *Maternal, fetal, & neonatal physiology: A clinical perspective* (2nd ed.). St. Louis: Saunders.

Interventions
Antepartum
• Therapy for the pregnant woman with heart disease is focused on minimizing stress on the heart, which is greatest between 28 and 32 weeks as the hemodynamic changes reach their maximum.
  –The woman with class I or II heart disease requires 8 to 10 hours of sleep every day and should take 30-minute naps after

signs of
POTENTIAL COMPLICATIONS

Cardiac Decompensation

PREGNANT WOMAN: SUBJECTIVE SYMPTOMS
- Increasing fatigue or difficulty breathing, or both, with her usual activities
- Feeling of smothering
- Frequent cough
- Palpitations; feeling that her heart is "racing"
- Generalized edema: swelling of face, feet, legs, and fingers (e.g., rings do not fit anymore)

NURSE: OBJECTIVE SIGNS
- Irregular, weak, rapid pulse (>100 beats/min)
- Progressive, generalized edema
- Crackles at base of lungs after two inspirations and exhalations that do not clear after coughing
- Orthopnea; increasing dyspnea
- Rapid respirations (greater than or equal to 25 breaths/min)
- Moist, frequent cough
- Cyanosis of lips and nail beds

eating. Her activities are restricted, with housework, shopping, and exercise limited to the amount allowed for the functional classification of her heart disease. Information on how to cope with activity limitations is important in meeting emotional needs of the woman. Referral to a support group may help the woman and her family handle stress.

–The pregnant woman with class II cardiac disease should avoid heavy exertion and should stop any activity that causes even minor signs and symptoms of cardiac decompensation. She may be admitted to the hospital near term (earlier if signs of cardiac overload or arrhythmia develop) for evaluation and treatment.

–Bed rest for much of each day is necessary for pregnant women with class III cardiac disease. Approximately 30% of these women experience cardiac decompensation during pregnancy. With this possibility the woman may require hospitalization for the remainder of the pregnancy. Because decompensation occurs even at rest in persons with class IV cardiac disease, a major initial effort must be made to improve the cardiac status of the pregnant woman in this category.

- Infections are treated promptly. Women with valvular dysfunction may receive prophylactic antibiotics.

  – The pregnant woman needs a well-balanced diet, high in iron and folic acid supplementation, with high protein and adequate calories to gain weight. The iron supplements tend to cause constipation. Therefore the pregnant woman should increase her intake of fluids and fiber, and a stool softener may be prescribed. It is important for the pregnant woman with cardiac disease to avoid straining during defecation, thus causing the Valsalva maneuver (forced expiration against a closed airway, which when released causes blood to rush to the heart and overload the cardiac system). For some women, sodium restriction may be necessary, but the amount of sodium should not be less than 2.5 g/day. The woman's intake of potassium is monitored to prevent hypokalemia, especially if she is taking diuretics. A referral to a registered dietitian is recommended.

  – Cardiac medications are prescribed as needed for the pregnant woman. If anticoagulant therapy is required during pregnancy, heparin should be used, because this large-molecule drug does not cross the placenta. The nurse should closely monitor the woman's blood work, specifically the partial thromboplastin time (PTT). The woman needs specific nutritional teaching to avoid foods high in vitamin K, such as raw dark green and leafy vegetables, which counteract the effects of the heparin. In addition, she will require a folic acid supplement.

  – Tests for fetal maturity and well-being, as well as placental sufficiency, may be necessary.

Intrapartum

- Labor and giving birth place an additional burden on the woman's already compromised cardiovascular system. Assessments include the routine assessments for all laboring women, as well as assessments for cardiac decompensation. In addition, ABGs may be needed to assess for adequate oxygenation. A Swan-Ganz catheter may be inserted to accurately monitor hemodynamic status during labor and birth. ECG monitoring and continuous monitoring of blood pressure and pulse oximetry are usually instituted for the woman, and the fetus is continuously monitored electronically.

–Nursing care during labor and birth focuses on the promotion of cardiac function. Anxiety is minimized by maintaining a calm atmosphere in the labor and birth rooms. Nursing techniques that promote comfort, such as back massage, are used.

• Cardiac function is supported by keeping the woman's head and shoulders elevated and body parts resting on pillows. The side-lying position usually facilitates hemodynamics during labor. Discomfort is relieved with medication and supportive care. Epidural regional anesthesia provides better pain relief than narcotics and causes fewer alterations in hemodynamics. Maternal hypotension must be avoided.

–The woman may require other types of medication (e.g., anticoagulants or prophylactic antibiotics). If evidence of cardiac decompensation appears, the physician may order deslanoside (Cedilanid-D) for rapid digitalization, furosemide (Lasix) for rapid diuresis, and oxygen by intermittent positive pressure to decrease the development of pulmonary edema.

–If there are no obstetric problems, vaginal birth is recommended and may be accomplished with the woman in the side-lying position to facilitate uterine perfusion. If the supine position is used, a pad is positioned under the hip to displace the uterus laterally and minimize the danger of supine hypotension. Open glottis pushing is recommended, and the Valsalva maneuver must be avoided when pushing because it reduces diastolic ventricular filling and obstructs left ventricular outflow. Mask oxygen is important. Episiotomy and vacuum extraction or outlet forceps may be used because these procedures decrease the second stage of labor and decrease the workload of the heart in second-stage labor. Cesarean birth is not routinely recommended for women who have cardiovascular disease because there is risk of dramatic fluid shifts, sustained hemodynamic changes, and increased blood loss.

–Penicillin prophylaxis may be ordered for pregnant women with class II or higher cardiac disease to protect against bacterial endocarditis in labor and during the early puerperium. Dilute IV oxytocin immediately after birth may be employed to prevent hemorrhage. Ergot products should not be used because they increase blood pressure.

Postpartum

- Monitoring for cardiac decompensation in the postpartum period is essential. The first 24 to 48 hours postpartum are the most difficult in terms of hemodynamics for the woman. Hemorrhage or infection, or both, may worsen the cardiac condition. The woman with a cardiac disorder may continue to require a Swan-Ganz catheter and ABG monitoring.
  - –Care in the postpartum period is tailored to the woman's functional capacity. Routine postpartum assessments are done. The head of the bed is elevated, and the woman is encouraged to lie on her side. Progressive ambulation may be permitted as tolerated. The nurse may need to help the woman meet her grooming and hygiene needs and other activities. Bowel movements without stress or strain for the woman are promoted with stool softeners, diet, and fluids.
  - –The woman may need help in the care of the infant. Breastfeeding is not contraindicated, but not all women with heart disease will be able to nurse their infants. The woman may need assistance in positioning herself or the infant for feeding. To further conserve the woman's energy, the infant may need to be brought to the mother and taken from her after the feeding. Preparation for discharge is carefully planned with the woman and family. Maternal cardiac output is usually stabilized by 2 weeks postpartum.

Cardiopulmonary Resuscitation of the Pregnant Woman

Cardiac arrest in a pregnant woman is most often related to events at the time of birth, such as amniotic fluid embolism, eclampsia, and drug toxicity. Various protocols exist for cardiopulmonary resuscitation (CPR) during pregnancy. The most widely used guide is the American Heart Association (AHA) Guidelines for Cardiopulmonary Resuscitation and Emergency Cardiovascular Care. Standard resuscitative efforts with a few modifications are implemented. To prevent supine hypotension, the pregnant woman is placed on a flat, firm surface with the uterus displaced laterally either manually or with a wedge or rolled blanket or towel under her right hip. If defibrillation is needed, the paddles need to be placed one rib interspace higher than usual because the heart is displaced slightly by the enlarged uterus. If possible, the fetus should be monitored during the cardiac arrest.

Anemia

- Anemia is the most common medical disorder of pregnancy. Anemia results in reduction of the oxygen-carrying capacity of the blood. Because the oxygen-carrying capacity of the blood is decreased, the heart tries to compensate by increasing the cardiac output. This effort increases the workload of the heart and stresses ventricular function. Therefore anemia that occurs with any other complication (e.g., preeclampsia) may result in congestive heart failure.
  - An indirect index of the oxygen-carrying capacity is the packed red blood cell (RBC) volume, or hematocrit level. At or near sea level, the pregnant woman is anemic when her hemoglobin level is less than 11 g/dl or hematocrit is less than 33%.
  - When a woman has anemia during pregnancy, the loss of blood at birth, even if minimal, is not well tolerated. She is at an increased risk for requiring blood transfusions. Women with anemia have a higher incidence of puerperal complications, such as infection, than do pregnant women with normal hematologic values.
  - Nursing care of the anemic pregnant woman requires that the nurse be able to distinguish between the normal physiologic anemia of pregnancy and the disease states. Approximately 90% of cases of anemia in pregnancy are of the iron deficiency type. The remaining 10% of cases embrace a considerable variety of acquired and hereditary anemias, including folic acid deficiency, sickle cell anemia, and thalassemia.

—Because of the increased iron needs necessitated for fetal development and maternal stores, pregnant women even with good nutrition can become iron deficient without iron therapy. If *iron deficiency anemia* is diagnosed, increased iron dosages are recommended (elemental iron, 60 to 120 mg/day).

—Even in well-nourished women, it is common to have a folate deficiency. Women with megaloblastic anemia caused by folic acid deficiency have the usual presenting symptoms and signs of anemia: pallor, fatigue, and lethargy, as well as glossitis and skin roughness. Folic acid deficiency anemia is common in multiple gestations. Folate deficiency during conception has been associated with increases in the incidence of neural tube defects, cleft lip, and cleft palate. During pregnancy the recommended daily intake is 400 mcg of folic acid per day. Women are instructed to consume foods high in folic acid (fresh, green, leafy vegetables and legumes).

—Sickle cell hemoglobinopathy is a disease caused by the presence of abnormal hemoglobin in the blood. Sickle cell trait (SA hemoglobin pattern) is sickling of the RBCs but with a normal RBC life span. It usually causes only mild clinical symptoms. Sickle cell anemia (sickle cell disease) is a recessive, hereditary, familial hemolytic anemia that affects those of African-American or Mediterranean ancestry. These individuals usually have abnormal hemoglobin types (SS or SC). Beginning in childhood, persons with sickle cell anemia have recurrent attacks (crises) of fever and pain in the abdomen or extremities. Women with sickle cell trait usually do well in pregnancy, although they are at increased risk for urinary tract infections (UTIs) and may be deficient in iron. If the woman has sickle cell anemia, the anemia that occurs in normal pregnancies may aggravate the condition and bring on more crises. These women are prone to pyelonephritis, UTIs and hematuria, leg ulcers, intense bone pain, strokes, cardiomyopathy, congestive heart failure, acute chest syndrome, and preeclampsia. Transfusions of the woman have been the usual treatment for symptomatic patients; however, prophylactic red cell transfusions are common as well and significantly reduce the number of painful crises.

–Thalassemia (Mediterranean or Cooley's anemia) is a relatively common hereditary anemia that involves the abnormal synthesis of the alpha or beta chains of hemoglobin. Beta thalassemia is the more common variety in the United States and often is diagnosed in persons of Mediterranean, North African, African-American, Middle Eastern, or Asian descent. The unbalanced synthesis of hemoglobin leads to premature RBC death, resulting in severe anemia. Couples with the thalassemia trait should seek genetic counseling. Women with thalassemia major often have problems conceiving. During pregnancy, women with thalassemia minor may demonstrate a mild persistent anemia, but the RBC level may be normal or even elevated. Supplemental iron and folic acid should be administered.

PULMONARY DISORDERS

Asthma

- Bronchial asthma is an acute respiratory illness characterized by periods of exacerbations and remissions. Exacerbations are triggered by allergens, marked change in ambient temperature, or emotional tension. In response to stimuli, there is widespread but reversible narrowing of the hyperreactive airways, making it difficult to breathe. The clinical manifestations are expiratory wheezing, productive cough, thick sputum, and dyspnea.

  –The effect of asthma on pregnancy is unpredictable although IUGR and preterm birth occur. Women often experience few symptoms of asthma in the first trimester and in the last weeks of pregnancy. The severity of symptoms usually peaks between 29 and 36 weeks of gestation.

  –Therapy for asthma has three objectives: (1) relief of the acute attack, (2) prevention or limitation of later attacks, and (3) adequate maternal and fetal oxygenation. These goals can be achieved in pregnancy by eliminating environmental triggers (e.g., dust mites, animal dander, and pollen), drug therapy (e.g., inhaled beta-agonists, inhaled cromolyn, corticosteroids, or antiinflammatory agents), and patient education. Respiratory infections should be treated and mist or steam inhalation employed to aid expectoration of mucus. Acute episodes may require albuterol, steroids, aminophylline, beta-adrenergic agents, and oxygen. Almost all asthma medications are considered safe in pregnancy.

—Asthma attacks can occur in labor; therefore medications for asthma are continued in labor and postpartum. Pulse oximetry should be instituted during labor. Epidural anesthesia reduces oxygen consumption and is recommended for pain relief. Fentanyl, a non–histamine-releasing narcotic, may be used also for pain control and is not associated with bronchospasm. During the postpartum period, women in whom excessive bleeding occurs will receive prostaglandin E_2. The woman usually returns to her prepregnancy asthma status within 3 months after giving birth.

NEUROLOGIC DISORDERS

The pregnant woman with a neurologic disorder needs to deal with potential teratogenic effects of prescribed medications, changes of mobility during pregnancy, and impaired ability to care for the baby. The nurse should be aware of all drugs the woman is taking and the associated potential for producing congenital anomalies. As the pregnancy progresses, the woman's center of gravity shifts and causes balance and gait changes.

Epilepsy

• Epilepsy is a disorder of the brain that causes recurrent seizures and is the most common neurologic disorder accompanying pregnancy. Epilepsy may result from developmental abnormalities or injury, or it may have no known cause.

• The differential diagnosis between epilepsy and eclampsia may pose a problem. Epilepsy and eclampsia can coexist. However, a history of seizures and a normal plasma uric acid level, as well as the absence of hypertension, generalized edema, or proteinuria, point to epilepsy.

—During pregnancy, the risk of vaginal bleeding is doubled, and there is a threefold risk of abruptio placentae. Abnormal presentations are more common in labor and birth, and there is an increased possibility that the fetus will experience seizures in utero.

–Teratogenicity of antiepileptic drugs (AEDs) is well documented. Therefore polytherapy and the use of the smallest dose possible to control seizures during pregnancy are recommended. AEDs prescribed in pregnancy should also be administered with folic acid because of the depletion that occurs when anticonvulsants are taken. Congenital anomalies that can occur with AEDs include cleft lip or palate, congenital heart disease, urogenital defects, and neural tube defects.

Bell Palsy

• The incidence of Bell palsy (idiopathic facial paralysis) usually peaks during the third trimester and the puerperium. The clinical manifestations include the sudden development of a unilateral facial weakness, with maximal weakness within 48 hours after onset, pain surrounding the ear, difficulty closing the eye on the affected side, and hyperacusis (sensitivity to normal sounds). In addition, taste on the anterior two thirds of the tongue may be lost, depending on the location of the lesion.

• Antiviral therapy and steroids may be prescribed, although controversy exists regarding whether they hasten recovery. Treatment includes prevention of injury to the exposed cornea, facial muscle massage, careful chewing and manual removal of food from inside the affected cheek, and reassurance that return of normal neurologic function is likely in 85% of affected women.

AUTOIMMUNE DISORDERS

Autoimmune disorders make up a large group of diseases that disrupt the function of the immune system of the body. In these types of disorders the body develops antibodies that attack its normally present antigens, causing tissue damage. Autoimmune disorders have a predilection for women in their reproductive years; therefore associations with pregnancy are not uncommon. Pregnancy may affect the disease process. Some disorders adversely affect the course of pregnancy or are detrimental to the fetus. Autoimmune disorders of concern in pregnancy are systemic lupus erythematosus (SLE) and rheumatoid arthritis.

Systemic Lupus Erythematosus

- One of the most common serious disorders of childbearing age, SLE is a chronic, multisystem inflammatory disease characterized by autoimmune antibody production that affects the skin, joints, kidneys, lungs, CNS, liver, and other body organs. Early symptoms, such as fatigue, weight loss, skin rashes, and arthralgias, may be overlooked. Anemia and leukopenia are common. Eventually all organs become involved. The condition is characterized by a series of exacerbations and remissions.

  - A woman with SLE is advised to wait until she has been in remission for at least 6 months before attempting to get pregnant. An exacerbation of SLE during pregnancy or postpartum occurs in approximately one third of women with SLE. Women are at increased risk for complications such as preeclampsia, renal disease, and preterm birth.

  - Medical therapy is kept to a minimum in women who are in remission or who have a mild form of SLE. Antiinflammatory drugs, such as prednisone and aspirin, may be used. It is recommended that aspirin not be used after 24 weeks of gestation because of an increased risk of premature closure of the fetal ductus arteriosus. Immunosuppressive drugs are not recommended during pregnancy.

  - Nursing care focuses on early recognition of signs of SLE exacerbation and pregnancy complications, education and support of the woman and her family, and assessment of fetal well-being.

  - Vaginal birth is preferred, but cesarean birth is common because of maternal and fetal complications. During the postpartum period, the mother should rest as much as possible to prevent an exacerbation of SLE. Adverse perinatal outcomes include preterm births, fetal growth restriction, stillbirth, and neonatal lupus. Breastfeeding is encouraged unless the mother is taking immunosuppressive agents.

GASTROINTESTINAL DISORDERS

Compromise of gastrointestinal function during pregnancy is a concern. Obvious physiologic alterations, such as the greatly enlarged uterus, and less apparent changes, such as hormonal differences and hypochlorhydria (deficiency of hydrochloric acid in the stomach's gastric juice), require understanding for proper diagnosis and treatment. Gallbladder disease and inflammatory bowel disease are two gastrointestinal disorders that may occur during pregnancy.

Cholelithiasis and Cholecystitis

- Women are more likely to have cholelithiasis (presence of gallstones in the gallbladder) than men, and pregnancy seems to make the woman more vulnerable to gallstone formation and the development of cholecystitis (inflammation of the gallbladder). Women with acute cholecystitis usually have colicky abdominal pain in the right upper quadrant and nausea and vomiting, especially after eating a meal high in fat. Fever and an increased leukocyte count may also be present. Ultrasound is often used to detect the presence of stones or for dilation of the common bile duct.
  - The woman with cholelithiasis or cholecystitis in the first trimester should be treated conservatively with IV fluids, bowel rest, nasogastric suctioning, and antibiotics. Meperidine or atropine alleviates ductal spasm and pain. Generally, gallbladder surgery is postponed until the puerperium in nonacute disease. Laparoscopic cholecystectomy is the preferred surgery and may be performed throughout the pregnancy, preferably in the first or second trimester.

SURGICAL EMERGENCIES DURING PREGNANCY

The need for abdominal surgery occurs as frequently among pregnant women as among nonpregnant women of comparable age. Common conditions necessitating abdominal surgery during pregnancy include cerclage, ovarian cystectomy, and appendectomy. Fetal concerns include teratogenic effects secondary to the anesthetic drugs used, intrauterine fetal death, and premature labor. Regional anesthesia is preferred, with intensive fetal and maternal monitoring. After 24 weeks of gestation, lateral displacement of the uterus facilitates uteroplacental perfusion.

Appendicitis

- The diagnosis of appendicitis is often delayed because the usual signs and symptoms mimic some normal changes of pregnancy, such as nausea and vomiting and increased white blood cell (WBC) count. As pregnancy progresses, the appendix is pushed upward and to the right of its usual anatomic location. Because of these changes, rupture of the appendix and the subsequent development of peritonitis occur two to three times more often in pregnant women than in nonpregnant women.
  - The woman with appendicitis most commonly has right lower quadrant abdominal pain, nausea and vomiting, and loss of appetite. Approximately one half of these affected women have muscle guarding. Moving the uterus tends to increase the pain. Temperature may be normal or mildly increased (to 38.3°C). Because of the physiologic increase in WBCs that occurs in pregnancy, elevated WBC counts are not clear indicators of appendicitis. Significant increases associated with appendicitis must be monitored either by rising levels on serial samples or by an increasing left shift.
  - The diagnosis of appendicitis requires a high level of suspicion because the typical signs and symptoms are similar to those found in many other conditions, including pyelonephritis, round ligament pain, placental abruption, torsion of an ovarian cyst, cholecystitis, and preterm labor (see Table 8-6).
  - Appendectomy before rupture usually does not require either antibiotic or tocolytic therapy. If surgery is delayed until after rupture, multiple antibiotics are ordered. Rupture is likely to result in preterm labor, necessitating the use of tocolytic agents.

Gynecologic Problems

Pregnancy predisposes a woman to ovarian problems, especially during the first trimester. Ovarian cysts and twisting (torsion) of ovarian cysts or twisting of adnexal tissues may occur. Other problems include retained or enlarged cystic corpus luteum of pregnancy and bacterial invasion of reproductive or other intraperitoneal organs. Serial ultrasounds, magnetic resonance images (MRIs), and transvaginal color Doppler are used to diagnose most ovarian abnormalities. Ovarian masses generally regress by 16 to 20 weeks of gestation, but if they do not regress then elective surgery may be done to remove masses.

Collaborative Care

- The extent of preoperative assessment is determined by the immediacy of surgical intervention and the specific condition that necessitates surgery.
- Preoperative care for a pregnant woman differs from that for a nonpregnant woman in one significant aspect: the presence of at least one other person, the fetus.
- Continuous fetal heart rate (FHR) and uterine contraction monitoring should be performed if the fetus is considered viable.
- Procedures such as preparation of the operative site and time of insertion of IV lines and urinary retention catheters vary with the physician and the facility.
- Solid foods and liquids are restricted before surgery. If the woman experiences a prolonged NPO status, IV fluids with dextrose should be given. To decrease the risk of vomiting and aspiration, special precautions are taken before anesthetic is administered (e.g., administering an antacid).
- During surgery, perinatal nurses may collaborate with the surgical staff to provide for the special needs of pregnant women undergoing surgery.
- To improve fetal oxygenation, the woman is positioned on the operating table with a lateral tilt to avoid maternal compression of the vena cava.
- During abdominal surgery, uterine contractions may be palpated manually.
- In the immediate recovery period, general observations and care pertinent to postoperative recovery are initiated.

- Continuous fetal and uterine monitoring will likely be initiated or resumed because of the increased risk of preterm labor.
- Plans for the woman's return home and for convalescent care should be completed as early as possible before discharge.

INFECTIONS ACQUIRED DURING PREGNANCY

Sexually Transmitted Infections

This discussion focuses only on the effects of several common STIs on pregnancy and the fetus (Table 8-12). Effects on pregnancy and the fetus also vary according to whether the infection has been treated at the time of labor and birth.

- The most common STIs in women are chlamydia, human papillomavirus, gonorrhea, herpes simplex virus type 2, syphilis, and human immunodeficiency virus (HIV) infection. Risk factors are the same as for the nonpregnant woman.
- Physical examination and laboratory studies to determine the presence of STIs in the pregnant woman are the same as those done in nonpregnant women.
- Treatment of specific STIs may be different for the pregnant woman and may even be different at different stages of pregnancy. Table 8-13 describes the maternal, fetal, and neonatal effects and treatment of common STIs during pregnancy. Infected women need instruction regarding how to take prescribed medications, information on whether their partner or partners also need to be evaluated and treated, and a review of preventive measures to avoid reinfection.

HIV AND AIDS

- Pregnancy is not encouraged in HIV-positive women. Preconception counseling is recommended because exposure to the virus has a significant impact on the pregnancy, neonatal feeding method, and neonatal health status. HIV-positive women should be counseled about use of antiretroviral therapy (ART) or highly active antiretroviral therapy (HAART), the risk of perinatal transmission, and

Text continued on p. 240.

TABLE 8-12

Pregnancy and Fetal Effects of Common Sexually Transmitted Infections

INFECTION	PREGNANCY EFFECTS	FETAL EFFECTS
Chlamydia	Premature rupture of membranes Preterm labor Intraamniotic infection	Preterm birth Conjunctivitis Pneumonia
Gonorrhea	Preterm labor Premature rupture of membranes Postpartum endometritis Miscarriage	Preterm birth Sepsis Conjunctivitis
Group B streptococcus	Preterm labor Premature rupture of membranes Chorioamnionitis Postpartum sepsis Urinary tract infections	Preterm birth Early-onset sepsis
Herpes simplex	Rare—infection Dystocia from large lesions Excessive bleeding from lesions after birth trauma	Systemic infection
Human papillomavirus (HPV)		Respiratory papillomatosis (rare)
Syphilis	Preterm labor Miscarriage	Preterm birth Stillbirth Congenital infection

Data from Cunningham, F., Leveno, K., Bloom, S., Hauth, J., Gilstrap, L., & Wenstrom, K. (2005). *Williams obstetrics* (22nd ed.). New York: McGraw-Hill; Gilbert, E., & Harmon, J. (2003). *Manual of high risk pregnancy and delivery* (3rd ed.). St. Louis: Mosby.

TABLE 8-13

Treatment of Common Sexually Transmitted Infections in Pregnancy

SEXUALLY TRANSMITTED INFECTION	TREATMENT	NURSING CONSIDERATIONS
Chlamydia	Erythromycin, 500 mg PO four times per day × 7 days; or amoxicillin, 500 mg PO three times per day × 7 days	Instruct woman to take after meals and with 8 oz water; instruct partner to be tested and treated if needed.
Herpes	Acyclovir is used in pregnancy only if the potential benefit outweighs the potential risk to the fetus. Analgesics and topical anesthetics may be ordered for severe discomfort.	Instruct woman in comfort measures: keep lesions clean and dry; use compresses on lesions (cold milk, colloidal oatmeal) q2-4h, sitz baths; patient should abstain from intercourse while lesions are present; if woman has active lesions at time of labor, a cesarean birth will usually be performed to prevent perinatal transmission.

Continued

TABLE 8-13

Treatment of Common Sexually Transmitted Infections in Pregnancy—cont'd

SEXUALLY TRANSMITTED INFECTION	TREATMENT	NURSING CONSIDERATIONS
Gonorrhea	Ceftriaxone, 125 mg IM × one dose, or cefixime, 400 mg PO × one dose, or spectinomycin, 2 g IM as single dose plus treatment for chlamydial infection	Screening is done at first prenatal visit; repeated in third trimester if high risk. Instruct partner to be tested and treated if needed. Infants are treated within 1 hr of birth with ophthalmic erythromycin or tetracycline ointment.
Group B streptococcus	Penicillin G, 5 million units IV initial dose followed by 2.5 million units IV q4h during labor, or ampicillin, 2 g IV initial dose followed by 1 g IV q4h	Pregnant women should be screened at 36-37 wk of gestation; if positive or status unknown at time of labor, the woman is treated.

| Hepatitis B | For exposure, hepatitis B immune globulin, 0.06 mg/kg IM; repeat in 1 mo, followed by hepatitis B vaccine series | Screening should be at first prenatal visit, with rescreening in third trimester for high risk patients; treatment is supportive—bed rest, high-protein, low-fat diet, increased fluid intake; the woman should avoid medications that are metabolized in the liver. |
| Human papillomavirus | Trichloracetic acid (TCA) or bichloracetic acid (BCA) 80% to 90% applied topically to warts one to three times per week; lidocaine (Xylocaine) jelly applied for burning sensations; cryotherapy with liquid nitrogen in second and third trimesters; CO_2 laser ablation therapy | Podophyllum and 5-fluorouracil are possibly teratogenic and should not be used in pregnancy; inform partners to be tested and treated if needed; couples should use condoms for intercourse; inform patients that smoking can decrease effects of therapy. |

Continued

IM, Intramuscularly; *IV,* intravenously; *PO,* by mouth.

TABLE 8-13

Treatment of Common Sexually Transmitted Infections in Pregnancy—cont'd

SEXUALLY TRANSMITTED INFECTION	TREATMENT	NURSING CONSIDERATIONS
Syphilis	Benzathine penicillin G, 2.4 million units IM once; if syphilis of more than 1 yr duration then 2.4 million units IM (one dose per wk × 3 wk) No proven alternatives to penicillin in pregnancy; women who have a history of allergy to penicillin should be desensitized and treated with penicillin	Treatment cures maternal infection and prevents congenital syphilis 98% of the time; routine screening during pregnancy should be at the first prenatal visit and in the third trimester in women at high risk; partners should be tested and treated if needed.

Trichomonas	Metronidazole, 2 g PO once	Inform partners to be treated; patients should avoid alcohol and vinegar products to avoid nausea and vomiting, intestinal cramping, and headaches; not recommended during lactation; stop breastfeeding, treat; resume in 48 hr after last dose. Women may use breast pump and discard milk to prevent interruption of milk supply.
Candidiasis	Over-the-counter topical agents: butoconazole, clotrimazole, miconazole, or terconazole; use for 7 days	May be used during lactation.
Bacterial vaginosis	Metronidazole, 250 mg PO three times per day × 7 days	See *Trichomonas*; infection may increase risk of preterm labor; women are usually asymptomatic.

possible obstetric complications. HIV-positive women should be encouraged to seek prenatal care immediately if they suspect pregnancy to maximize chances for a positive outcome.

- Approximately 90% of all pediatric acquired immune deficiency syndrome (AIDS) cases are a result of transmission of the virus from mother to child during the perinatal period. Exposure may occur to the fetus through the maternal circulation as early as the first trimester of pregnancy, to the infant during labor and birth by inoculation or ingestion of maternal blood and other infected fluids, or to the infant through breast milk.

  –Treatment of HIV-infected women with the antiviral drug zidovudine (ZDV) during pregnancy and intrapartum, and treatment of their infants for the first 6 weeks of life with ZDV, decreases the rate of viral transmission to 8%. Use of combination ART or HAART reportedly reduces perinatal HIV transmission to 2%. All HIV-positive women also should be given the option of having a scheduled cesarean birth at 38 weeks to decrease the risk of transmission of HIV to the infant.

  –*Obstetric complications.* It is difficult to determine obstetric risk because many confounding variables are often present. Many HIV-positive women also have drug and alcohol addiction, poor nutrition, limited access to prenatal care, or concurrent STIs. HIV-positive women are probably at risk for preterm labor and birth, PROM, IUGR, perinatal mortality, and postpartum endometritis.

  –*Antepartum care.* HIV counseling and testing should be offered to all women at their initial entry into prenatal care. Universal testing is recommended versus selective testing for maternal HIV, because it results in a greater number of women being screened and treated. HIV-infected women should also be tested for other STIs, such as gonorrhea; syphilis; chlamydial infection; hepatitis B, C, and D; and herpes. Cytomegalovirus and toxoplasmosis antibody testing should be done because both infections can cause significant maternal and fetal complications and can be successfully treated with antimicrobial agents. Any history of vaccination and immune status should be documented, and chickenpox (varicella) and rubella titers should be determined. A tuberculin skin test should be performed; a positive test result necessitates the taking of a chest x-ray film to identify active pulmonary disease. A Papanicolaou (Pap) test should be done.

—All HIV-infected women should be treated with ZDV or other antiretroviral drugs during pregnancy, regardless of their CD_4 counts. ZDV, administered orally, is usually started after the first trimester and continued throughout pregnancy. The major side effect of this drug is bone marrow suppression; periodic hematocrit, WBC count, and platelet count assessments should be performed. Women with CD_4 counts less than 200 cells/mm^3 should receive prophylactic treatment for *Pneumocystis carinii* pneumonia with daily trimethoprim-sulfamethoxazole. Any other opportunistic infections should be treated with medications specific for the infection; often dosages must be higher for women with HIV infection or AIDS.

—Women who are HIV positive should also be vaccinated against hepatitis B, pneumococcal infection, *Haemophilus influenzae* type B, and viral influenza. To support any pregnant woman's immune system, appropriate counseling is provided about optimal nutrition, sleep, rest, exercise, and stress reduction. The HIV-infected woman needs nutritional support and counseling about diet choices, food preparation, and food handling. Weight gain or maintenance in pregnancy is a challenge with the HIV-infected patient. The infected patient is counseled regarding "safer sex" practices. Use of condoms is encouraged to minimize further exposure to HIV if her partner is the source. Orogenital sex is discouraged.

• *Intrapartum care.* Several therapy regimens are available. IV ZDV is administered to the HIV-positive woman during the intrapartum period. A loading dose is initiated on her admission in labor, followed by a continuous maintenance dose throughout labor.

—Every effort should be made during the birthing process to decrease the neonate's exposure to infected maternal blood and secretions. The membranes should be left intact until the birth if feasible.

—Women who give birth within 4 hours after membrane rupture are less likely to transmit the virus to their neonates than women who experience a longer interval between rupture and birth.

—Fetal scalp electrode and scalp pH sampling should be avoided, because these procedures may result in inoculation of the virus into the fetus. Likewise, the use of forceps or vacuum extractor should be avoided when possible.

—Women with intact membranes who give birth by cesarean before labor begins have decreased maternal-infant transmission.

• *Postpartum and newborn care.* Immediately after birth, infants should be wiped free of all body fluids and then bathed as soon as they are in stable condition. All staff members working with the mother or infant must adhere strictly to infection control techniques and observe Standard Precautions for blood and body fluids.

—Women who have HIV but who are without symptoms may have an unremarkable postpartum course. Immuno-suppressed women with symptoms may be at increased risk for postpartum UTIs, vaginitis, postpartum endometritis, and poor wound healing.

—Breastfeeding is discouraged because of HIV vertical transmission in breast milk.

—In planning for discharge, comprehensive care and support services will need to be arranged.

—After discharge, the woman and her infant are referred to physicians who are experienced in the treatment of AIDS and associated conditions.

SUBSTANCE ABUSE

The term *substance abuse* refers to the continued use of substances (e.g., alcohol and drugs) despite related problems in physical, social, or interpersonal areas. This discussion focuses on care of the pregnant woman who is a substance abuser.

• The damaging effects of alcohol and illicit drugs on pregnant women and their unborn babies are well documented. Alcohol and other drugs easily pass from a mother to her baby through the placenta. Smoking during pregnancy has serious health risks, including bleeding complications, miscarriage, still-birth, prematurity, low birth weight, and sudden infant death syndrome. Congenital abnormalities have occurred in infants of mothers who have taken drugs.

Collaborative Care

- The care of the substance-dependent pregnant woman is based on historical data, symptoms, physical findings, and laboratory results. Screening questions for alcohol and drug abuse should be included in the overall assessment of the first prenatal visit of all women. Women who are heavily involved in substance abuse often receive no prenatal care or make only a limited number of visits beginning late in pregnancy.

- Because women frequently deny or greatly underreport usage when asked directly about drug or alcohol consumption, it is crucial that the nurse display a nonjudgmental and matter-of-fact attitude while taking the history in order to gain the woman's trust and elicit a reasonably accurate estimate. Information about drug use should be obtained by asking first about the woman's intake of over-the-counter (OTC) and prescribed medications. Next, her usage of "legal" drugs, such as caffeine, nicotine, and alcohol, should be ascertained. Finally, the woman should be questioned about her use of illicit drugs, such as cocaine, heroin, and marijuana.

- Urine toxicology testing is often performed to screen for illicit drug use although the test is unreliable for alcohol use. Drugs may be found in urine days to weeks after ingestion, depending on how quickly they are metabolized and excreted from the body. Meconium (from the neonate) and hair can also be analyzed to determine past drug use over a longer period of time. In addition to screening for alcohol and drug abuse, the nurse should also screen for physical and sexual abuse and history of psychiatric illness, factors frequently accompanying substance use.

- Although the ideal long-term outcome is total abstinence, it is not likely that the woman will either desire or be able to stop alcohol and drug use suddenly. Indeed, it may be harmful to the fetus for her to do so. A realistic goal may be to decrease substance use, and short-term outcomes will be necessary.

- Intervention with the pregnant substance abuser begins with education about specific effects on pregnancy, the fetus, and the newborn for each drug used. Consequences of perinatal drug use should be clearly communicated and abstinence recommended as the safest course of action. Treatment for the substance abuse will be individualized for each woman depending on the type of drug used and the frequency and amount of use. Detoxification, short-term in-patient or out-patient treatment, long-term residential treatment, aftercare services, and self-help support groups are all possible options for alcohol and drug abuse.

- Methadone treatment for pregnant women dependent on heroin or other narcotics is controversial. If women withdraw from heroin during pregnancy, blood flow to the placenta is impaired. The substitution of methadone for the heroin not only promotes withdrawal from heroin but also does not cause impaired blood flow to the placenta. However, methadone can cause detrimental fetal effects, and withdrawal from it after birth can be worse for the newborn than heroin withdrawal.

- Cocaine use during pregnancy has increased dramatically. Maternal and fetal complications accompany cocaine use, including placental abruption, stillbirth, prematurity, and SGA infants. Pregnant women who use cocaine should be advised to stop using immediately. Such women will need a great deal of assistance, such as an alcohol and drug treatment program, individual or group counseling, and participation in self-help support groups, to successfully accomplish this major lifestyle change.

- Initial and serial ultrasound studies are usually performed to determine gestational age, because the woman may have had amenorrhea as a result of her drug use or may not know when her last menstrual period occurred. Because of concerns about stillbirth, an increased frequency of the birth of infants who are SGA, and the potential for hypoxia, non-stress testing may be done in women who are known substance abusers.

- Although substance abusers may be difficult to care for at any time, they are often particularly challenging during the intra-partum and postpartum periods because of manipulative and demanding behavior. Typically, these women display poor control over their behavior and a low threshold for pain. Increased dependency needs and poor parenting skills may also be apparent.

- Nurses must understand that substance abuse is an illness and that these women deserve to be treated with patience, kindness, consistency, and firmness when necessary. Even women who are actively abusing drugs will experience pain during labor and after giving birth and may need pain medication, as well as nonpharmacologic interventions. Mother-infant attachment should be promoted by identifying the woman's strengths and reinforcing positive maternal feelings and behaviors. Staffing should be sufficient to ensure strict surveillance of visitors and prevent unsupervised drug use.

- Advice regarding breastfeeding must be individualized. Breastfeeding is contraindicated in women who use amphetamines, alcohol, cocaine, heroin, or marijuana. The baby's nutrition and safety needs are of primary importance in this consideration. For some women, a desire to breastfeed may provide strong motivation to achieve and maintain sobriety.

- Smoking can interfere with the let-down reflex. Women who smoke in the postpartum period and breastfeed should avoid smoking for 2 hours before a feeding to minimize the nicotine in the milk and improve the let-down reflex. Mothers should also be discouraged from smoking in the same room with the infant because exposure to secondhand smoke can increase the likelihood that the infant will experience behavioral and respiratory health problems.

- Before a known substance abuser is discharged with her baby, the home situation is assessed to determine that the environment is safe and that someone will be available to meet the infant's needs if the mother proves unable to do so. If serious questions about the infant's well-being exist, the case will probably be referred to the state's child protective services agency for further action.

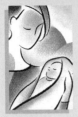

CHAPTER 9

Management of Discomfort

DISCOMFORT DURING LABOR AND BIRTH

Factors Influencing Pain Response

A woman's pain during childbirth is unique to her and is influenced by a variety of factors, including the following:

- Physiologic factors (e.g., endorphins level and maternal position)
- Cultural background (see Cultural Considerations box)
- Anxiety level
- Previous childbirth experience
- Childbirth preparation (e.g., gate control theory used for techniques to relieve pain)
- Comfort and support given by nurse and significant others
- Quality of the labor and birth environment

Neurologic Origins

- The pain from cervical changes, distention of the lower uterine segment, and uterine ischemia that predominates during the first stage of labor is visceral pain. It is located over the lower portion of the abdomen.
- During the second stage of labor the woman has somatic pain, which is often described as intense, sharp, burning, and well localized. Pain results from stretching and distention of perineal tissues and the pelvic floor to allow passage of the fetus, from distention and traction on the peritoneum and uterocervical supports during contractions, and from lacerations of soft tissue (e.g., cervix, vagina, and perineum).
- Pain experienced during the third stage of labor and the afterpains of the early postpartum period are uterine, similar to the pain experienced early in the first stage of labor.

Cultural Considerations

Some Cultural Beliefs about Pain

The following are examples of how women of different cultural backgrounds may react to pain. Because they are generalizations, the nurse must assess each woman experiencing pain related to childbirth.

- Chinese women may not exhibit reactions to pain, although it is acceptable to exhibit pain during childbirth. They consider it impolite to accept something when it is first offered; therefore pain interventions must be offered more than once. Acupuncture may be used for pain relief.
- Arab or Middle Eastern women may be vocal in response to labor pain. They may prefer medication for pain relief.
- Japanese women may be stoic in response to labor pain, but they may request medication when pain becomes severe.
- Southeast Asian women may endure severe pain before requesting relief.
- Hispanic women may be stoic until late in labor, when they may become vocal and request pain relief.
- Native American women may use medications or remedies made from indigenous plants. They are often stoic in response to labor pain.
- African-American women may express pain openly. Use of medication for pain relief varies.

NONPHARMACOLOGIC MANAGEMENT OF DISCOMFORT

Many of the nonpharmacologic methods for relief of discomfort require practice for best results (e.g., hypnosis, patterned breathing and controlled relaxation techniques, and biofeedback), although the nurse may use some of them successfully without the woman or couple having prior knowledge (e.g., slow paced breathing, massage and touch, effleurage, and counterpressure). Women should be encouraged to try a variety of methods and to seek alternatives, including pharmacologic methods, when the measure being used is no longer effective.

Childbirth Preparation Methods

All childbirth methods attempt to reduce fear, tension, and pain by increasing the woman's knowledge of the labor and birth process, enhancing her self-confidence and sense of control, preparing a support person, and training the woman in physical conditioning and relaxation breathing.

Specific Strategies

- *Focusing and relaxation techniques* may use a favorite object, such as a photograph or stuffed animal, or an object in the labor room during contractions as an object of attention.
  - With imagery, the woman focuses her attention on a pleasant scene, a place where she feels relaxed, or an activity she enjoys.
  - Support, feedback, and touch can be used to facilitate the woman's relaxation and thereby reduce tension and stress and enhance the progress of labor.
- *Breathing techniques* are emphasized by different approaches to childbirth preparation to provide distraction, thereby reducing the perception of pain and helping the woman maintain control throughout contractions (Box 9-1). For couples who have prepared for labor by practicing relaxing and breathing techniques, occasional reminders may be all that are necessary to help them along. For those who have had no preparation, instruction in simple breathing and relaxation can be given early in labor.
- *Effleurage* (light massage) is light stroking, usually of the abdomen, in rhythm with breathing during contractions. It is used to distract the woman from contraction pain. *Counterpressure* is steady pressure applied by a support person to the sacral area with the fist or heel of the hand. It is especially helpful when back pain is caused by pressure of the occiput against spinal nerves when the fetal head is in a posterior position.
- *Music,* either taped or live, enhances relaxation during labor, thereby reducing stress, anxiety, and the perception of pain.
- *Water therapy (hydrotherapy)* involves bathing, showering, or jet hydrotherapy (whirlpool baths) with warm water (e.g., at or below body temperature) to promote comfort and relaxation during labor. There is no limit to the time women can stay in the bath, and often women are encouraged to stay in it as long

BOX 9-1

Paced Breathing Techniques

CLEANSING BREATH
Relaxed breath in through nose and out mouth. Used at the beginning and end of each contraction.

SLOW-PACED BREATHING (APPROXIMATELY 6 TO 8 BREATHS/MIN)
Not less than half normal breathing rate (number of breaths per minute divided by 2)
IN-2-3-4/OUT-2-3-4/IN-2-3-4/OUT-2-3-4 . . .

MODIFIED-PACED BREATHING (APPROXIMATELY 32 TO 40 BREATHS/MIN)
Not more than twice normal breathing rate (number of breaths per minute multiplied by 2)

IN-OUT/IN-OUT/IN-OUT/IN-OUT . . .
For more flexibility and variety the woman may combine the slow and modified breathing by using the slow breathing for beginnings and ends of contractions and modified breathing for more intense peaks. This technique conserves energy, lessens fatigue, and reduces risk for hyperventilation.

PATTERNED-PACED BREATHING (SAME RATE AS MODIFIED)
Enhances concentration
a. 3:1 Patterned breathing: IN-OUT/IN-OUT/IN-OUT/IN-BLOW (repeat through contraction)
b. 4:1 Patterned breathing: IN-OUT/IN-OUT/IN-OUT/IN-OUT/IN-BLOW (repeat through contraction)

Source: Nichols, F. (2000). Paced breathing techniques. In F. Nichols & S. Humenick (Eds.), *Childbirth education: Practice, research, and theory* (2nd ed.). Philadelphia: Saunders; Perinatal Education Associates. (2003). *Breathing through labor and birth.* Internet document available at http://www.birthsource.com/articlefile/Article39.html (accessed March 23, 2006).

as desired. Fluids to maintain hydration and a cool face cloth for comfort are offered during the bath. The recommended temperature for the bath is between 36° and 38° C to avoid harmful effects.

- *Transcutaneous electrical nerve stimulation (TENS)* involves the placing of two pairs of flat electrodes on either side of the woman's thoracic and sacral areas of the spine that provide continuous low-intensity electrical impulses or stimuli from a battery-operated device. High intensity should be maintained for at least 1 minute to facilitate release of endorphins. TENS is most useful for lower back pain during the early first stage of labor.

- *Acupressure* and *acupuncture* techniques apply pressure, heat, or cold to acupuncture points called *tsubos*. Acupressure is best applied over the skin without using lubricants. Pressure is usually applied with the heel of the hand, fist, or pads of the thumbs and fingers. Tennis balls or other devices also may be used to apply pressure. Acupressure points are found on the neck, shoulders, wrists, lower back including sacral points, hips, area below the kneecaps, ankles, nails on the small toes, and soles of the feet. Acupuncture is the insertion of fine needles into specific areas of the body to restore the flow of qi (energy) and to decrease pain, which is thought to be obstructing the flow of energy. It should be done by a trained certified therapist.

- *Application of heat and cold* can involve warmed blankets, warm compresses, heated rice bags, a warm bath or shower, or a moist heating pad, all of which are effective for back pain. Also, cold application such as cool cloths or ice packs may be effective in increasing comfort when the woman feels warm and may be applied to areas of pain.

- *Touch* and *massage* have been an integral part of the traditional care process for women in labor. Touch can be as simple as holding the woman's hand, stroking her body, and embracing her. Therapeutic touch (TT) uses the concept of energy fields within the body called *prana*. Prana are thought to be deficient in some people who are in pain. TT uses laying-on of hands by a specially trained person to redirect energy fields associated with pain. Healing touch (HT) is another energy-based healing modality, combining a variety of techniques to align and balance the human energy field, thereby enhancing the body's ability to heal itself. Head, hand, back, and foot massage may be very effective in reducing tension and enhancing comfort.

- *Hypnosis* techniques used for labor and birth place an emphasis on enhancing relaxation and diminishing fear, anxiety, and perception of pain. The woman may be given direct suggestions about pain relief or indirect suggestions that she is experiencing diminished sensations. To be successful, the woman must learn and practice the techniques during the prenatal period.

- *Biofeedback* is based on the theory that if a person can recognize physical signals, certain internal physiologic events can be changed (i.e., whatever physical signs the woman has that are associated with her pain). During the prenatal period, the woman must learn how to use thinking and mental processes (e.g., focusing) to control body responses and functions. Formal biofeedback, which uses machines to detect skin temperature, blood flow, or muscle tension, also can prepare women to intensify their relaxation responses.

- *Aromatherapy* uses oils distilled from plants, flowers, herbs, and trees to promote health and well-being and treat illnesses. Lavender, clary sage, and bergamot promote relaxation and can be used by adding a few drops to a warm bath, to warm water used for soaking compresses that can be applied to the body, to an aromatherapy lamp to vaporize a room, or to oil for a back massage.

- An *intradermal water block* involves the injection of small amounts of sterile water (e.g., 0.05 to 0.1 ml) by using a fine needle (e.g., 25 gauge) into four locations on the lower back to relieve back pain for approximately 45 minutes to 2 hours.

PHARMACOLOGIC MANAGEMENT OF DISCOMFORT

Pharmacologic measures for pain management should be implemented before pain becomes so severe that catecholamines increase and labor is prolonged.

Sedatives

- Sedatives relieve anxiety and induce sleep and may be given to a woman experiencing a prolonged latent phase of labor and when there is a need to decrease anxiety or promote sleep. Barbiturates can cause undesirable side effects, including respiratory and vasomotor depression affecting the woman and newborn, and are seldom used.

- Phenothiazines (e.g., promethazine [Phenergan] and hydroxyzine [Vistaril]) do not relieve pain but decrease anxiety and apprehension, increase sedation, and may potentiate opioid analgesic effects. Metoclopramide (Reglan) is an antiemetic that also can be used for this purpose.

- Benzodiazepines (e.g., diazepam [Valium] and lorazepam [Ativan]), when given with an opioid analgesic, seem to enhance pain relief and reduce nausea and vomiting.

Analgesia and Anesthesia

Systemic analgesia

- Systemic analgesics cross the maternal blood-brain barrier to provide central analgesic effects. They also cross through the placenta to the fetus.
- Intravenous (IV) administration is preferred to intramuscular (IM) administration because the medication's onset of action is faster and more predictable; as a result, a higher level of pain relief usually occurs.
- An agonist is an agent that activates or stimulates a receptor to act; an antagonist is an agent that blocks a receptor or a medication designed to activate a receptor.
- *Opioid agonist analgesics,* such as meperidine (Demerol) and fentanyl (Sublimaze), are effective for relieving severe, persistent, or recurrent pain (see Medication Guide in Appendix B–Opioid Analgesics for Labor and Medication Guide–Fentanyl).
- *Opioid agonist-antagonist analgesics,* such as butorphanol (Stadol) and nalbuphine (Nubain), in the doses used during labor, provide adequate analgesia without causing significant respiratory depression in the mother or neonate. These opioid analgesics are not suitable for women with an opioid dependence because the antagonist activity could precipitate withdrawal symptoms (abstinence syndrome) in both the mother and her newborn (see Appendix B-Medication Guide–Opioid Analgesics for Labor.
- *Opioid (narcotic) antagonists,* such as naloxone (Narcan), can promptly reverse the central nervous system (CNS) depressant effects, especially respiratory depression (see Appendix B-Medication Guide–Naloxone). An opioid antagonist can be given to the newborn as one part of the treatment for neonatal narcosis, which is a state of CNS depression in the newborn produced by an opioid.

Nerve block analgesia and anesthesia

The principal pharmacologic effect of local anesthetics is the temporary interruption of the conduction of nerve impulses, notably pain. Examples of common agents are bupivacaine, lidocaine, mepivacaine, ropivacaine, and chloroprocaine. The solution strength of the local anesthetic agent and the amount used will depend on the type of nerve block being performed.

- *Local perineal infiltration* anesthesia may be used when an episiotomy is to be performed or when lacerations need to be sutured after the birth in a woman who does not have regional anesthesia.

- *Pudendal nerve block* is useful for the second stage of labor, episiotomy, and birth. Although it does not relieve the pain from uterine contractions, it does relieve pain in the lower vagina, vulva, and perineum.

- *Spinal anesthesia (block)* is an anesthetic solution containing a local anesthetic alone or in combination with fentanyl that is injected through the third, fourth, or fifth lumbar interspace into the subarachnoid space. This technique is commonly used for cesarean births and may be used for vaginal birth, but it is not suitable for labor. Marked hypotension, impaired placental perfusion, and an ineffective breathing pattern may occur during spinal anesthesia. After induction of the anesthetic, maternal blood pressure, pulse, and respirations and fetal heart rate (FHR) and fetal heart pattern must be checked and documented every 5 to 10 minutes. If signs of serious maternal hypotension or fetal distress develop, emergency care must be given (see Emergency box).

  -Advantages of spinal anesthesia include ease of administration and absence of fetal hypoxia with maintenance of normotension. Maternal consciousness is maintained, excellent muscular relaxation is achieved, and blood loss is not excessive.

  -Disadvantages of spinal anesthesia include medication reactions (e.g., allergy), hypotension, and an ineffective breathing pattern; cardiopulmonary resuscitation may be needed. When a spinal anesthetic is given, the need for operative birth (e.g., episiotomy, forceps-assisted birth, or vacuum-assisted birth) tends to increase because voluntary expulsive

EMERGENCY

Maternal Hypotension with Decreased Placental Perfusion

SIGNS AND SYMPTOMS
- Maternal hypotension (20% decrease from preblock baseline level or 100 mm Hg systolic)
- Fetal bradycardia
- Decreased beat-to-beat FHR variability

INTERVENTIONS
- Turn woman to lateral position or place pillow or wedge under hip to deflect uterus.
- Maintain IV infusion at rate specified, or increase "as needed" administration per hospital protocol.
- Administer oxygen by face mask at 10 to 12 L/min or per protocol.
- Elevate the woman's legs.
- Notify the primary health care provider, anesthesiologist, or nurse anesthetist.
- Administer IV vasopressor (e.g., ephedrine, 5 to 10 mg) per protocol if previous measures are ineffective.
- Remain with woman; continue to monitor maternal blood pressure and FHR every 5 minutes until her condition is stable or per primary health care provider's order.

FHR, Fetal heart rate; *IV,* intravenous.

efforts are reduced or eliminated. After birth the incidence of bladder and uterine atony, as well as postspinal headache, is higher.

—Leakage of cerebrospinal fluid (CSF) from the site of puncture of the dura mater (membranous covering of the spinal cord) is thought to be the major causative factor in *postdural puncture headache (PDPH)*. Initial treatment for a postdural puncture headache usually includes oral analgesics, bed rest in a quiet dimly lit or dark room, caffeine, and increased fluid intake.

—An autologous *epidural blood patch* is the most rapid, reliable, and beneficial relief measure for PDPH. The woman's blood (i.e., 10 to 20 ml) is injected slowly into the lumbar epidural space, creating a clot that patches the tear or hole in the dura mater around the spinal cord. Postprocedure instructions include resting in bed for 24 to 48 hours, applying cold packs to the site as needed for comfort, avoiding analgesics that affect platelet aggregation (e.g., nonsteroidal antiinflammatory drugs [NSAIDs]) for 2 days, drinking plenty of fluids, and observing for signs of infection at the site and for neurologic symptoms such as pain, numbness and tingling in legs, and difficulty with walking or elimination. The woman should be cautioned to avoid lifting, straining at stool, coughing, or tub bathing, for at least 2 days.

Epidural Anesthesia or Analgesia (Block)

- Relief from the pain of uterine contractions and birth (vaginal and cesarean) can be relieved by injecting a suitable local anesthetic agent (e.g., bupivacaine or ropivacaine), an opioid analgesic (e.g., fentanyl or sufentanil), or both into the epidural (peridural) space. Injection is made between the fourth and fifth lumbar vertebrae for a lumbar epidural block.

- For the induction of a lumbar epidural block, the woman is positioned sitting with her back curved or she may assume a modified Sims position with her shoulders parallel, legs slightly flexed, and back arched.

- After the epidural has been started, the woman is positioned preferably on her side so that the uterus does not compress the ascending vena cava and descending aorta, which can impair venous return, reduce cardiac output and blood pressure, and decrease placental perfusion.

- Oxygen should be available if hypotension occurs despite maintenance of hydration with IV fluid and displacement of the uterus to the side.

- Ephedrine (a vasopressor used to increase maternal blood pressure) and increased IV fluid infusion may be needed (see Emergency box).

- The FHR, fetal heart pattern, and progress in labor must be monitored carefully because the woman in labor may not be aware of changes in the strength of the uterine contractions or the descent of the presenting part.

- The advantages of an epidural block are numerous: the woman remains alert and able to participate, good relaxation is achieved, airway reflexes remain intact, only partial motor paralysis develops, gastric emptying is not delayed, and blood loss is not excessive. Fetal complications are rare but may occur in the event of rapid absorption of the medication or marked maternal hypotension. The dose, volume, and type of medication or medications used can be modified to allow the woman to push and to assume upright positions and even walk, to produce perineal anesthesia, and to permit forceps-assisted, vacuum-assisted, or cesarean birth if required.

- The disadvantages of epidural block also are numerous. The woman's ability to move freely is limited, related to the use of an IV infusion and electronic monitoring, orthostatic hypotension and dizziness, sedation, and weakness of the legs. CNS effects, such as excitation, bizarre behavior, tinnitus, disorientation, paresthesia, and convulsions, can occur if a solution containing a local anesthetic agent is accidentally injected into a blood vessel. Respiratory arrest can occur if the relatively high dosage used with an epidural block is accidentally injected into the subarachnoid space. Women who receive an epidural have a higher rate of fever (i.e., intrapartum temperature of 38° C or higher). Hypotension as a result of sympathetic blockade can be an outcome of an epidural block (see Emergency box). Urinary retention can occur. Pruritus (itching) is a side effect associated with the use of an opioid, especially fentanyl. A relation between epidural analgesia and longer second-stage labor, increased incidence of fetal malposition, use of oxytocin, and forceps-assisted or vacuum-assisted birth has been documented. Current research findings have been unable to demonstrate a significant increase in cesarean birth associated with epidural analgesia.

Combined Spinal-Epidural Analgesia. Using opioids such as fentanyl and sufentanil to potentiate the effects of local anesthetic agents has resulted in the reduction of the amount of the local anesthetic used, thereby reducing motor blockade. The opioid is injected into the subarachnoid space for rapid activation of the opioid receptors. Combined spinal-epidural analgesia may be associated with fetal bradycardia, necessitating close assessment of FHR and fetal heart pattern.

Epidural and Intrathecal Opioids. Opioids also can be used alone, eliminating the effect of a local anesthetic altogether. The use of epidural or intrathecal (spinal) opioids without the addition of a local anesthetic agent does not cause maternal hypotension or affect vital signs. The woman feels contractions but not pain. Her ability to bear down during the second stage of labor is preserved because the pushing reflex is not lost, and her motor power remains intact. Fentanyl, sufentanil, or preservative-free morphine may be used. For most women, intrathecal opioids do not provide adequate analgesia for second-stage labor pain, episiotomy, or birth.

- A more common indication for the administration of epidural or intrathecal analgesics is the relief of postoperative pain. For example, women who give birth by cesarean can receive fentanyl or morphine through a catheter. The catheter may then be removed, and the women are usually free of pain for 24 hours.

- Side effects of opioids administered by the epidural and intrathecal routes include nausea, vomiting, pruritus, urinary retention, and delayed respiratory depression. Antiemetics, antipruritics, and opioid antagonists are used to relieve these symptoms.

- Respiratory depression is a serious concern; for this reason the woman's respiratory rate should be assessed and documented every hour for 24 hours or as designated by hospital protocol. Naloxone should be readily available for use if the respiratory rate decreases to less than 10 breaths/min or if the oxygen saturation rate decreases to less than 89%. Administration of oxygen by face mask also may be initiated, and the anesthesiologist should be notified.

Nitrous Oxide for Analgesia. Nitrous oxide mixed with oxygen can be inhaled in a low concentration (50% or less) to reduce but not eliminate pain during the first and second stages of labor. A face mask or mouthpiece is used to self-administer the gas. At the lower doses used for analgesia, the woman remains awake, and the danger of aspiration is avoided because the laryngeal reflexes are unaffected.

General Anesthesia. If general anesthesia is being considered, the nurse gives the woman nothing by mouth and ensures that an IV infusion is in place. If time allows, the nurse premedicates the woman with a nonparticulate (clear) oral antacid (e.g., sodium citrate, Bicitra, or Alka-Seltzer) to neutralize the acidic contents of the stomach. Aspiration of highly acidic gastric contents will damage lung tissue. Some anesthesiologists and physicians also order the administration of a histamine (H_2)–receptor blocker, such as cimetidine (Tagamet), to decrease the production of gastric acid and metoclopramide (Reglan) to increase gastric emptying. Before the anesthesia is given, a wedge should be placed under one of the woman's hips to displace the uterus to prevent aortocaval compression, which interferes with placental perfusion.

CARE MANAGEMENT

Assessment

Because pain is a subjective phenomenon, the nurse must listen to the woman's description of her pain. One self-assessment tool that can be used is a visual analog scale (VAS). The VAS allows the woman to indicate on a line how severe or intense she perceives her pain to be from "no pain" to "pain as bad as it could possibly be." Other scales are available. Self-assessment is recommended to ensure that pain management is based on the subjective nature of the woman's pain rather than just on the nurse's judgment.

The nurse also must be alert for changes in fetal well-being; nonreassuring changes in FHR and fetal heart pattern should be noted and reported to the primary health care provider.

Interventions

Informed consent. The woman receives (in an understandable manner) the following:

- Explanation of alternative methods of anesthesia and analgesia available
- Description of anesthetic and procedure for administration
- Description of the benefits, discomforts, risks, and consequences for the mother and the fetus
- Explanation of how complications can be treated
- Information that the anesthetic is not always effective
- Indication that the woman may withdraw consent at any time
- Opportunity to have any questions answered

- Opportunity to have components of the consent explained in the woman's own words

The consent form will fulfill the following:

- Be written or explained in the woman's primary language
- Have the woman's signature
- Have the date of consent
- Carry the signature of anesthetic care provider, certifying that the woman has received and appears to understand the explanation

- *Preparation for procedures.* The methods of pain relief available to the woman are reviewed, and information is clarified as necessary. The procedure and what will be asked of the woman (e.g., to maintain flexed position during insertion of epidural needle) must be explained.

- *Administration of medication*
  - The preferred route of administration of medications such as meperidine, fentanyl, or nalbuphine is through IV tubing, administered into the port nearest the woman while the infusion of the IV solution is stopped. The medication is given slowly in small doses during a contraction. It may be given over the period of three to five consecutive contractions if needed to complete the dose. It is given during contractions to decrease fetal exposure to the medication because uterine blood vessels are constricted during contractions, and the medication stays within the maternal vascular system for several seconds before the uterine blood vessels reopen. When the medication is infused, the IV infusion is then restarted slowly to prevent a bolus of medication from being administered. With this method of injection, along with smaller but more frequent dosing, the amount of medication crossing the placenta to the fetus is reduced while the woman's degree of pain relief is maximized.
  - IM injections given in the upper arm (deltoid muscle) seem to result in more rapid absorption and higher blood levels of the medication than injections in other intramuscular sites.
  - An IV infusion is usually established before the induction of nerve blocks (e.g., epidural or subarachnoid). Anesthesia protocols often include the prophylactic administration

of IV fluid before epidural and spinal anesthesia for blood volume expansion to prevent maternal hypotension.

–Because nerve blocks can reduce bladder sensation, resulting in difficulty voiding, the woman should empty her bladder before the induction of the block and should be encouraged to void at least every 2 hours thereafter.

- *Safety and general care*
  –After a nerve block is administered, the woman is protected from injury by raising the side rails and placing a call bell within easy reach when the nurse is not in attendance. Oxygen and suction should be readily available at the bedside. The nurse must make sure there is no prolonged pressure on an anesthetized part (e.g., lying on one side with weight on one leg or tight linen on feet). If stirrups are used for birth, the nurse should pad them, adjust both stirrups to the same level and angle, place both of the woman's legs into them simultaneously while avoiding putting pressure on the popliteal angle, and apply restraints (if used) without restricting circulation.
  –Depending on the level of motor blockade, the woman should be assisted to remain as mobile as possible.
  –The second stage of labor is often prolonged in women who use epidural analgesia for pain management. Research evidence indicates that as long as the well-being of the maternal-fetal unit is established, a period of "laboring down" to allow the fetus to descend and rotate with uterine contractions and the use of open-glottis pushing techniques when the fetus has reached a +1 station and is rotating to an anterior position are the best approaches to use for the management of second-stage labor. Use of upright positions for second-stage labor can be encouraged, including squatting and sitting upright.

Nursing considerations

The nurse monitors and records the woman's response to nonpharmacologic pain relief methods and to medication or medications given. This includes the degree of pain relief, the level of apprehension, the return of sensations and perception of pain, and allergic or adverse reactions (e.g., hypotension, respiratory depression, hypothermia, fever, pruritus, nausea, and vomiting).

- The nurse continues to monitor maternal vital signs, blood pressure, the strength and frequency of uterine contractions, changes in the cervix and station of the presenting part, the presence and quality of the bearing-down reflex, bladder filling, and state of hydration.
- Determining the fetal response after administration of analgesia or anesthesia is vital.
- The woman is asked if she (or the family) has any questions. The nurse also assesses the woman's and her family's understanding of the need for ensuring her safety (e.g., keeping side rails up, calling for assistance as needed).
- Both the nurse and the anesthesia provider are responsible for documenting assessments and care in relation to the epidural.

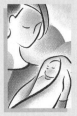

C H A P T E R *10*

Fetal Assessment during Labor

BASIS FOR MONITORING

- Fetal well-being during labor can be measured by the response of the fetal heart rate (FHR) to uterine contractions. In general, reassuring FHR patterns are characterized by the following:
  - A baseline FHR in the normal range of 110 to 160 beats per minute (beats/min) with no periodic changes and a moderate baseline variability (see later discussion on p. 264).
  - Accelerations with fetal movement
- A normal uterine activity pattern in labor is characterized by the following:
  - Contractions occurring every 2 to 5 minutes and lasting less than 90 seconds
  - Contractions moderate to strong in intensity, as evidenced by palpation, or intensity is less than 80 mm Hg, as measured by an intrauterine pressure catheter (IUPC)
  - 30 seconds or more elapsing between the end of one contraction and the beginning of the next contraction
- Uterine relaxation should be detected by palpation or by an average intrauterine pressure of 20 mm Hg or less
- Nonreassuring FHR patterns are those associated with fetal hypoxemia, which is a deficiency of oxygen in the arterial blood. If uncorrected, hypoxemia can deteriorate to severe fetal hypoxia, which is an inadequate supply of oxygen at the cellular level. Nonreassuring FHR patterns include the following:
  - Progressive increase or decrease in baseline rate
  - Tachycardia of 160 beats/min or more
  - Progressive decrease in baseline variability

—Severe variable decelerations (FHR less than 60 beats/min lasting longer than 30 to 60 seconds, with rising baseline, decreasing variability, or slow return to baseline)

—Late decelerations of any magnitude, especially those that are repetitive and uncorrectable

—Absent or undetected FHR variability

—Prolonged deceleration (greater than 60 to 90 seconds)

—Severe bradycardia (less than 70 beats/min)

MONITORING TECHNIQUES

Intermittent Auscultation

- Intermittent auscultation (IA) uses listening to fetal heart sounds at periodic intervals to assess the FHR. IA of the fetal heart can be performed with a Leff scope, a DeLee-Hillis fetoscope, or an ultrasound device.
- One procedure for performing auscultation is as follows:
  —Perform Leopold maneuvers (see p. 298) by palpating the maternal abdomen to identify fetal presentation and position.
  —Place the listening device over the area of maximal intensity and clarity of the fetal heart sounds to obtain the clearest and loudest sound, which is easiest to count. Apply ultrasound gel to Doppler ultrasound device if used.
  —Palpate the abdomen for the absence of uterine activity to be able to count the FHR between contractions.
  —Count the maternal radial pulse while listening to the FHR to differentiate it from the fetal rate.
  —Count the FHR for 30 to 60 seconds between contractions to identify the baseline rate. This rate can be assessed only during the absence of uterine activity.
  —Auscultate the FHR during a contraction and for 30 seconds after the end of the contraction to identify any increases or decreases in FHR in response to the contraction.
- In the absence of risk factors, one recommended practice is to auscultate the FHR as follows:
  —*First stage* (active phase): every 30 minutes
  —*Second stage:* every 15 minutes
- If risk factors are present, the FHR is auscultated as follows:
  —*First stage* (active phase): every 15 minutes
  —*Second stage:* every 5 minutes

- The FHR also is assessed before and after ambulation, rupture of membranes, and administration of medications and anesthesia, and it is assessed more frequently when a nonreassuring fetal heart rate is detected.
- When used as the primary method of fetal assessment, auscultation requires a 1:1 nurse-to-patient staffing ratio. If acuity and census change so that auscultation standards are no longer met, the nurse must inform the physician or nurse-midwife that continuous EFM will be used until staffing can be arranged to meet the standards.
- When using IA, uterine activity is assessed by palpation.

Electronic Fetal Monitoring

The two modes of electronic fetal monitoring (EFM) include the external mode, which uses external transducers placed on the maternal abdomen to assess FHR and uterine activity, and the internal mode, which uses a spiral electrode applied to the fetal presenting part to assess the FHR and an intra-uterine pressure catheter (IUPC) to assess uterine activity and pressure.

FETAL HEART RATE PATTERNS

Baseline Fetal Heart Rate

- *Baseline FHR* is the average rate during a 10-minute segment that excludes periodic or episodic changes, periods of marked variability, and segments of the baseline that differ by more than 25 beats/min. The normal range at term is 110 to 160 beats/min.
- *Variability* of the FHR can be described as irregular fluctuations in the baseline FHR of two cycles per minute or greater. It is a characteristic of baseline FHR and does not include accelerations or decelerations of the FHR. Variability has been described as short term (beat to beat) or long term (rhythmic waves or cycles from baseline). The current definition for research does not distinguish between short-term and long-term variability because in actual practice they are viewed together; however, this definition does identify four ranges of variability as seen in Fig. 10-1. These are based on visualization of the amplitude of the FHR in the peak-to-trough segment in beats per minute and include the following:

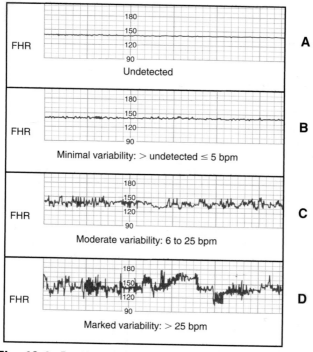

Fig. 10-1   Fetal heart rate variability. **A,** Absent or undetected. **B,** Minimal. **C,** Moderate. **D,** Marked. (Modified from Tucker, S. [2004]. *Pocket guide to fetal monitoring and assessment* [5th ed.]. St. Louis: Mosby.)

–Absent or undetected variability
–Minimal variability (greater than undetected variability but not more than 5 beats/min)
–Moderate variability (6 to 25 beats/min)
–Marked variability (greater than 25 beats/min)
• Table 10-1 contrasts key differences between increased and decreased variability.
• Tachycardia is a baseline FHR greater than 160 beats/min for a duration of 10 minutes or longer. Bradycardia is a baseline FHR less than 110 beats/min for a duration of 10 minutes or longer. Table 10-2 contrasts tachycardia with bradycardia.

Text continued on p. 272.

TABLE 10-1

Increased and Decreased Variability

INCREASED VARIABILITY	DECREASED VARIABILITY
CAUSE	Hypoxia or acidosis
Early mild hypoxemia	CNS depressants
Fetal stimulation by the following:	Analgesics or narcotics
—Uterine palpation	—Meperidine (Demerol)
—Uterine contractions	—Alphaprodine (Nisentil)
—Fetal activity	—Morphine
—Maternal activity	—Pentazocine (Talwin)
Drugs	Barbiturates
—Illicit drugs (e.g., cocaine and methamphetamines)	—Secobarbital (Seconal)
—Sympathomimetics (e.g., terbutaline and asthma drugs)	—Pentobarbital (Nembutal)
	—Amobarbital (Amytal)
	Tranquilizers
	—Diazepam (Valium)
	Ataractics
	—Promethazine (Phenergan)
	—Propiomazine (Largon)
	—Hydroxyzine (Vistaril)
	—Promazine (Sparine)

Parasympatholytics
—Atropine
General anesthetics
Prematurity: <24 wk
Fetal sleep cycles
Congenital abnormalities
Fetal cardiac arrhythmias

Benign when associated with periodic fetal sleep states, which last 20-30 min; if caused by drugs, variability usually increases as drugs are excreted

Decreased variability is not reassuring and is considered a sign of fetal stress *unless* it has an identifiable temporary (e.g., fetal sleep) or correctable cause

Decreased variability associated with uncorrectable late decelerations indicates presence of fetal acidosis and can result in low Apgar scores

CLINICAL SIGNIFICANCE

Significance of marked variability not known; increased variability from a previous average variability is earliest FHR sign of mild hypoxemia

Continued

CNS, Central nervous system; *FHR,* fetal heart rate.

Source: Tucker, S. 2004. *Pocket guide to fetal monitoring and assessment* (5th ed.). St. Louis: Mosby.

TABLE 10-1

Increased and Decreased Variability—cont'd

INCREASED VARIABILITY	DECREASED VARIABILITY
NURSING INTERVENTION Priority depends on cause: observe FHR tracing carefully for any nonreassuring patterns, including decreasing variability and late decelerations; if using external mode of monitoring, consider using internal mode (spiral electrode) for a more accurate tracing; intervention usually not required unless nonreassuring FHR pattern develops	Dependent on cause; intervention not warranted if associated with fetal sleep states or temporarily associated with CNS depressants; consider performing external stimulation or scalp stimulation during a vaginal examination to elicit an acceleration of FHR or return to moderate variability; consider application of spiral electrode; assist health care provider with fetal oxygen saturation monitoring if ordered; prepare for birth if so indicated by the primary health care provider

TABLE 10-2

Tachycardia and Bradycardia

TACHYCARDIA	BRADYCARDIA
DEFINITION	
FHR >160 beats/min lasting >10 min	FHR <110 beats/min lasting >10 min
CAUSE	
Early fetal hypoxemia	Late fetal hypoxemia or hypoxia
Maternal fever	Beta-adrenergic blocking drugs (propranolol;
Parasympatholytic drugs (atropine, hydroxyzine)	anesthetics for epidural, spinal, caudal, and
Beta-sympathomimetic drugs (ritodrine,	pudendal blocks)
isoxsuprine)	Maternal hypotension
Intraamniotic infection	Prolonged umbilical cord compression
Maternal hyperthyroidism	Fetal congenital heart block
Fetal anemia	Maternal hypothermia
Fetal heart failure	Prolonged maternal hypoglycemia
Fetal cardiac arrhythmias	
Illicit drugs (cocaine, methamphetamines)	

Continued

TABLE 10-2

Tachycardia and Bradycardia—cont'd

TACHYCARDIA	BRADYCARDIA
CLINICAL SIGNIFICANCE	
Persistent tachycardia in absence of periodic changes does not appear serious in terms of neonatal outcome (especially true if tachycardia is associated with maternal fever); tachycardia is a nonreassuring sign when associated with late decelerations, severe variable decelerations, or absence of variability	Bradycardia with moderate variability and absence of periodic changes is not a sign of fetal compromise if FHR remains >80 beats/min; bradycardia caused by hypoxia is a nonreassuring sign when associated with loss of variability and late decelerations
NURSING INTERVENTION	
Priority dependent on cause	Priority dependent on cause and based on stage of labor, fetal position and station, and fetal status
—Reduce maternal fever with antipyretics as ordered, hydration, and cooling measures	

—Oxygen at 8-10 L/min by face mask may be of some value
—Carry out health care provider's orders based on alleviating cause (e.g., assist with fetal pulse oximetry if performed to collect more data about cause)

—Intervention not warranted in fetus with heart block diagnosed by ECG scalp stimulation may be performed to determine whether the fetus has the ability to compensate physiologically for stress (FHR will accelerate)
—All interventions to improve fetal oxygenation (i.e., lateral maternal positioning, hydration, correction of maternal hypotension, maternal oxygenation, and discontinuing oxytocin) may be implemented
—carry out health care provider's orders based on alleviating cause

ECG, Electrocardiography; *FHR*, fetal heart rate.
Source : Tucker, S. 2004. *Pocket guide to fetal monitoring and assessment* (5th ed.). St. Louis: Mosby.

Changes in Fetal Heart Rate

- Changes in FHR from the baseline are categorized as periodic or episodic. Periodic changes are those that occur with uterine contractions. Episodic changes are those that are not associated with uterine contractions. These patterns include accelerations and decelerations.
- *Acceleration* of the FHR is defined as a visually apparent abrupt increase in FHR above the baseline rate. The increase is 15 beats/min or greater and lasts 15 seconds or more, with the return to baseline less than 2 minutes from the beginning of the acceleration (Fig. 10-2).
- *Deceleration* (caused by dominance of parasympathetic response) may be benign or nonreassuring. Three types of decelerations are encountered during labor: early, late, and variable. FHR decelerations are described by their visual relation to the onset and end of a contraction and by their shape.
- *Early deceleration* of the FHR is a visually apparent gradual decrease and return to baseline FHR in response to fetal head compression. It is a normal and benign finding (Fig. 10-3, *A*).
- The different characteristics of accelerations of the FHR and early decelerations are contrasted in Table 10-3.
- *Late deceleration* of the FHR is a visually apparent gradual decrease in and return to baseline FHR associated with uteroplacental insufficiency. The deceleration begins after the contraction has started, and the lowest point of the deceleration occurs after the peak of the contraction. The deceleration usually does not return to baseline until after the contraction is over (see Fig. 10-3, *B*).
- *Variable deceleration* is defined as a visually abrupt decrease in FHR below the baseline. The decrease is 15 beats/min or more, lasts at least 15 seconds, and returns to baseline in less than 2 minutes from the time of onset (see Fig. 10-3, *C*). Variable decelerations occur any time during the uterine contracting phase and are caused by compression of the umbilical cord. Table 10-4 contrasts late deceleration with variable deceleration.
- A prolonged deceleration is a visually apparent decrease in FHR below the baseline of 15 beats/min or more and lasting more than 2 minutes but less than 10 minutes.

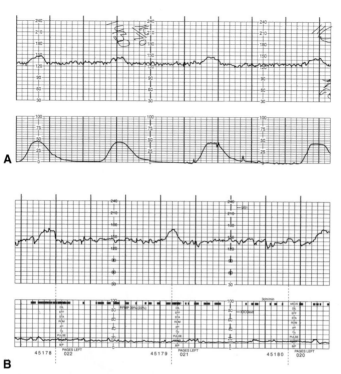

Fig. 10-2 **A,** Acceleration of fetal heart rate (FHR) with uterine contractions. **B,** Acceleration of FHR with movement. (From Tucker, S. [2004]. *Pocket guide to fetal monitoring and assessment* [5th ed.]. St. Louis: Mosby.)

CARE MANAGEMENT

Assessment and nursing diagnoses

Assess using agency's form. All the assessment information must be documented in the woman's medical record.

Interventions

It is the responsibility of the nurse providing care to women in labor to assess FHR patterns, implement independent nursing
Text continued on p. 284.

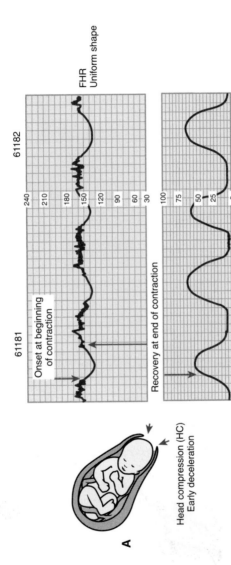

Fig. 10-3 Deceleration patterns. **A,** Early decelerations caused by head compression.

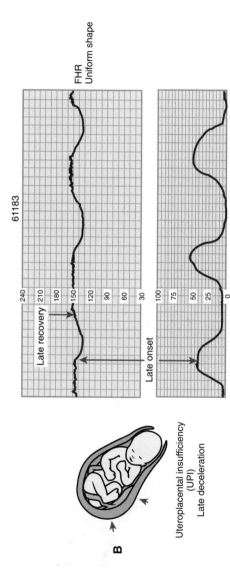

FHR
Uniform shape

61183

Late recovery

Late onset

Continued

Uteroplacental insufficiency
(UPI)
Late deceleration

B

Fig. 10-3, cont'd B, Late decelerations caused by uteroplacental insufficiency.

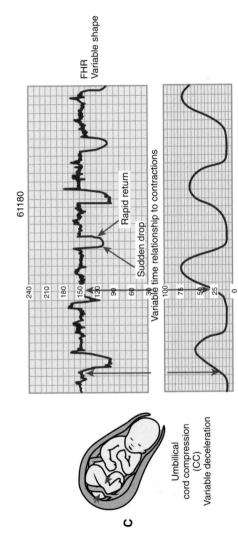

Fig. 10-3, cont'd C, Variable decelerations caused by cord compression. *FHR,* Fetal heart rate. (From Tucker, S. [2004]. *Pocket guide to fetal monitoring and assessment* [5th ed.]. St. Louis: Mosby.)

TABLE 10-3

Accelerations and Early Decelerations

	ACCELERATION	EARLY DECELERATION
Description	Transitory increase of fetal heart rate (FHR) above baseline (see Fig. 10-2)	Transitory decrease of FHR below baseline concurrent with uterine contractions (see Fig. 10-3, A)
Shape	May resemble shape of uterine contraction or be spikelike	Uniform shape; mirror image of uterine contraction
Onset	Onset to peak (30 sec; often precedes or occurs simultaneously with uterine contraction)	Early in contraction phase before peak of contraction
Recovery	Less than 2 min from onset	By end of contraction as uterine pressure returns to its resting tone
Amplitude	Usually 15 beats/min above baseline	Usually proportional to amplitude of contraction; rarely decelerates below 100 beats/min
Baseline	Usually associated with average baseline variability	Usually associated with average baseline variability

Continued

Source: Tucker, S. 2004. *Pocket guide to fetal monitoring and assessment* (5th ed.). St. Louis: Mosby.

TABLE 10-3

Accelerations and Early Decelerations – cont'd

	ACCELERATION	EARLY DECELERATION
Occurrence	Variable; may be repetitive with each contraction	Repetitious (occurs with each contraction); usually occurs between 4- and 7-cm dilation and in second stage of labor
Cause	Spontaneous fetal movement Vaginal examination Electrode application Scalp stimulation Reaction to external sounds Breech presentation Occiput posterior position Uterine contractions Fundal pressure Abdominal palpation	Head compression resulting from the following: —Uterine contractions —Vaginal examination —Fundal pressure —Placement of internal mode of monitoring
Clinical significance	Acceleration with fetal movement signifies fetal well-being, representing fetal alertness or arousal states	Reassuring pattern not associated with fetal hypoxemia, acidemia, or low Apgar scores
Nursing intervention	None required	None required

TABLE 10-4

Late Decelerations and Variable Decelerations

	LATE DECELERATION	VARIABLE DECELERATION
Description	Transitory gradual decrease in fetal heart rate (FHR) below baseline rate in contracting phase (see Fig. 10-3, *B*)	Abrupt decrease in FHR that is variable in duration, intensity, and timing related to onset of contractions (see Fig. 10-3, *C*)
Shape	Uniform; mirror images of uterine contraction; may be deep or shallow	Variable; characterized by sudden decrease in FHR in V, U, or W shape
Onset	Late in contraction phase; after peak of contraction; nadir of deceleration occurs after peak of contraction	Onset of deceleration to the beginning of nadir, 30 sec; decrease in FHR baseline is ≥15 beats/min, lasting ≥15 sec; variable times in contracting phase; often preceded by transitory acceleration

Continued

IV, Intravenous.
Source: Tucker, S. 2004. *Pocket guide to fetal monitoring and assessment* (5th ed.). St. Louis: Mosby.

TABLE 10-4

Late Decelerations and Variable Decelerations—cont'd

	LATE DECELERATION	VARIABLE DECELERATION
Recovery	Well after end of contraction	Return to baseline is rapid and <2 min from onset, sometimes with transitory acceleration or acceleration immediately before and after deceleration (shouldering or "overshoot"); slow return to baseline with severe variable decelerations
Deceleration	Usually proportional to amplitude of contraction; rarely decelerates to <100 beats/min; however, shallow late decelerations have the same significance	*Mild:* decelerates to any level, <30 sec with abrupt return to baseline *Moderate:* decelerates to <70 beats/min for 30-60 sec or <70 to 80 beats/min for 60 sec *Severe:* decelerates to <70 beats/min for >60 sec, with slow return to baseline
Baseline	Often associated with loss of variability and increasing baseline rate	Mild variables usually associated with average baseline variability; moderate and severe variables often associated with decreasing variability and increasing baseline rate

Continued

Occurrence	Occurs with each contraction; may be observed at any time during labor	Variable; commonly observed late in labor with fetal descent and pushing
Cause	Uteroplacental insufficiency caused by the following: —Uterine hyperactivity or hypertonicity —Maternal supine hypotension —Epidural or spinal anesthesia —Placenta previa —Abruptio placentae —Hypertensive disorders —Postmaturity —Intrauterine growth restriction —Diabetes mellitus —Intraamniotic infection	Umbilical cord compression caused by the following: —Maternal position with cord between fetus and maternal pelvis —Cord around fetal neck, arm, leg, or other body part —Short cord —Knot in cord —Prolapsed cord
Clinical significance	Nonreassuring pattern associated with fetal hypoxemia, acidemia, and low Apgar scores; considered ominous if persistent and uncorrected, especially when associated with fetal tachycardia and loss of variability	Variable decelerations occur in ≈50% of all labors and usually are transient and correctable *Reassuring* variable decelerations last <45 sec and abruptly return to the FHR baseline; normal baseline rate continues; variability does not decrease

TABLE 10-4
Late Decelerations and Variable Decelerations—cont'd

	LATE DECELERATION	VARIABLE DECELERATION
		Nonreassuring variable decelerations decrease to ≤70 beats/min for ≥60 sec and have a prolonged return to baseline; baseline rate increases; variability is absent
		Nonreassuring variable decelerations are associated with fetal acidemia, hypoxemia, and low Apgar scores; severe variable decelerations with average baseline variability just before birth are usually well tolerated
Nursing interventions	The usual priority is as follows: —Change maternal position (lateral) —Correct maternal hypotension by elevating legs	The usual priority is as follows: —Change maternal position (side to side, knee chest) —if decelerations are severe, proceed with following measures:

—Increase rate of maintenance IV solution
—Palpate uterus to assess for hyperstimulation
—Discontinue oxytocin if infusing
—Administer oxygen at 8-10 L/min with tight face mask
—Consider internal monitoring for a more accurate fetal and uterine assessment
—Fetal scalp or acoustic stimulation
—Assist with fetal oxygen saturation monitoring if ordered
—Assist with birth (cesarean or vaginal assisted) if pattern cannot be corrected

a. Discontinue oxytocin if infusing
b. Administer oxygen at 8-10 L/min with tight face mask
c. Assist with vaginal or speculum examination to assess for cord prolapse
d. Assist with amnioinfusion if ordered
e. Assist with fetal oxygen saturation monitoring if ordered
f. Assist with birth (vaginal assisted or cesarean) if pattern cannot be corrected

interventions, document observations and actions according to the established standard of care, and report nonreassuring patterns to the primary care provider (e.g., physician or certified nurse-midwife). Box 10-1 is a suggested protocol for FHR monitoring by IA and EFM during labor.

LEGAL TIP Fetal Monitoring Standards

Nurses who care for women during childbirth are legally responsible for correctly interpreting FHR patterns, initiating appropriate nursing interventions based on those patterns, and documenting the outcomes of those interventions. Perinatal nurses are responsible for the timely notification of the physician or nurse-midwife in the event of nonreassuring FHR patterns. Perinatal nurses also are responsible for initiating the institutional chain of command should differences in opinion arise among health care providers concerning the interpretation of the FHR pattern and the intervention required.

Nursing management of nonreassuring patterns

The term *intrauterine resuscitation* is sometimes used to refer to those interventions initiated when a nonreassuring FHR pattern is noted; they are directed primarily toward improving uterine and intervillous space blood flow and secondarily toward increasing maternal oxygenation and cardiac output.

- Preventive interventions include avoiding the maternal supine position and encouraging maternal position changes, encouraging spontaneous short bursts of pushing in response to involuntary bearing-down urges, and encouraging pushing with mouth open and glottis open with vocalizing.
- Nurses must assign priorities to interventions to maximize the efficacy of the intrauterine resuscitation. The *first priority* is to open the maternal and fetal vascular systems, the *second priority* is to increase blood volume, and the *third priority* is to optimize oxygenation of the circulating blood volume. For example, to relieve an acute FHR deceleration, the nurse can do the following:
  - Assist the woman to the side-lying position if she is not already in a lateral position.

Text continued on p. 289.

BOX 10-1

Sample Protocol for Fetal Heart Rate Monitoring

MATERNAL AND FETAL ASSESSMENTS
- Obtain a 20-minute strip of electronic fetal monitoring (EFM) for all patients admitted to labor unit.

Low Risk Patient
- Auscultate or assess tracing every 30 minutes in active phase of first stage of labor.
- Auscultate or assess tracing every 15 minutes in second stage.

High Risk Patient
- Auscultate or assess tracing every 15 minutes in active phase and every 5 minutes in second stage.

Auscultation: All Patients
- Count baseline fetal heart rate (FHR) between contractions.
- Assess FHR during the contraction and for 30 seconds after the contraction.
- Note increases or decreases of FHR.
- Assess FHR before ambulation.
- Interpret FHR data, nursing interventions, and patient responses.
- Notify primary health care provider.

EFM: All Patients
- Assess and interpret baseline FHR, variability of FHR, and presence or absence of decelerations and accelerations.

Assessments: All Patients
- Assess uterine activity for frequency and duration, the intensity of contractions, and uterine resting tone.
- Assess FHR immediately after rupture of membranes, vaginal examinations, and any invasive procedure.

EXTERNAL MONITORING
Ultrasound Transducer
Function
- Monitors FHR with high-frequency sound waves

Nursing Care
- Tap transducer before use to ensure sound transmission.

Continued

BOX 10-1

Sample Protocol for Fetal Heart Rate Monitoring—cont'd

- Apply ultrasound transmission gel to transducer, clean abdomen and transducer, and reapply gel every 2 hours and as needed.
- Massage reddened skin areas gently, and reposition belt or adhesive device every 2 hours and as needed.
- Auscultate FHR with stethoscope or fetoscope if in doubt as to validity of tracing.
- Position and reposition transducer as needed to ensure receipt of clear, interpretable FHR data.

Tocotransducer
Function
- Monitors uterine activity by way of a pressure-sensing device placed on the maternal abdomen

Nursing Care
- Position and reposition every 2 hours and as needed on the fundus, where there is the least maternal tissue.
- Keep abdominal strap snug but comfortable for the laboring woman.
- Adjust baseline between contractions to print between 10 and 20 mm Hg on the monitor strip paper.
- Palpate fundus every 30 to 60 minutes to assess strength of contraction; only frequency and duration of contractions can be assessed with tocotransducer.
- Do not determine woman's need for analgesia based on uterine activity displayed on monitor strip.
- Gently massage reddened areas under transducer and belt every hour and as needed.

INTERNAL MONITORING
Spiral Electrode
Function
- Obtains fetal electrocardiogram (ECG) from presenting part and converts it into FHR

Nursing Care
- Ensure that the connector to the scalp electrode is appropriately attached to leg plate.
- Reapply electrode paste to leg plate if needed.
- Observe FHR tracing on monitor strip for variability.

BOX 10-1

Sample Protocol for Fetal Heart Rate Monitoring—cont'd

- Turn electrode counterclockwise to remove; never pull straight out from presenting part.
- Administer perineal care after the woman voids during labor and as needed.

Intrauterine Catheter
Function
- Catheter (solid or fluid filled) that monitors intraamniotic pressure internally

Nursing Care
- Ensure that the length line on catheter is visible at introitus.
- For closed-system catheters, set baseline rate between uterine contractions when uterus is relaxed.
- Flush open-system catheter with sterile water before insertion and as needed.
- For open-system catheters, turn off stopcock to woman; then with pressure valve of strain gauge released, flush strain gauge, remove syringe, and set stylus to 0 lines of chart paper; test further according to manufacturer's instructions every 3 to 4 hours and as needed.
- Check proper functioning by tapping catheter, asking woman to cough, or applying fundal pressure; observe appropriate inflection on strip chart.
- Keep catheter or cable secured to woman's leg to prevent dislodgment.

REPORTABLE CONDITIONS
- Presence of nonreassuring patterns
  —Severe variable decelerations
  —Late decelerations
  —Absence of variability
  —Prolonged deceleration
  —Severe bradycardia
- Worsening of any pattern
- Presence of identifiable fetal arrhythmias
- Difficulty in obtaining adequate FHR tracing or inadequate audible FHR

Continued

BOX 10-1

Sample Protocol for Fetal Heart Rate Monitoring—cont'd

EMERGENCY MEASURES
- Implement the following measures immediately in the event of nonreassuring patterns. The priority will depend on the type of nonreassuring FHR pattern that is present (refer to Tables 10-1 to 10-3):
  —Reposition patient in lateral position to increase uteroplacental perfusion or relieve cord compression.
  —Administer oxygen at 8 to 10 L/min or per hospital protocol by face mask.
  —Discontinue oxytocin if infusing.
  —Correct maternal hypovolemia by increasing intravenous (IV) rate per protocol or as ordered.
  —Assess for bleeding or other cause of pattern change, such as maternal hypotension.
  —Notify primary health care provider.
  —Assist with other methods of assessment, such as fetal oxygen saturation monitoring or interventions such as amnioinfusion.
  —Anticipate emergency preparation for surgical intervention if nonreassuring pattern continues despite interventions.

DOCUMENTATION*
Patient Record: Auscultation
- FHR baseline, rate and rhythm, increases or decreases
Patient Record: EFM
- Method of monitoring, change in method, and adjustments to equipment
- FHR range, variability, and presence of decelerations or accelerations
- Uterine activity as determined by palpation or by external or internal monitoring
- Interpretation of FHR data, nursing interventions, and patient responses
- Notification of primary health care provider
Monitor Strip
- Patient identification data
- Assessments, procedures, and interventions (medications, etc.)

BOX 10-1

Sample Protocol for Fetal Heart Rate Monitoring—cont'd

- Notification of primary health care provider
- Significant occurrences (sterile vaginal examination, rupture of membranes, etc.)
- Adjustments of the monitor equipment

*If computer charting system is used, follow institutional policies and system guidelines and protocols.

—Increase the maternal blood volume by increasing the rate of the primary intravenous (IV) infusion or by raising the woman's legs.
—Provide oxygen by face mask.
- Some interventions are specific to the FHR pattern. Nursing interventions appropriate for the management of tachycardia and bradycardia are given in Table 10-2, and those appropriate for the management of increased or decreased variability are given in Table 10-1. No specific nursing interventions are required for the management of FHR acceleration or early deceleration (see Table 10-3). However, late and some types of variable FHR decelerations require aggressive intervention (see Table 10-4).

Other methods of assessment and intervention

Other methods of assessment and intervention are designed to be used in conjunction with EFM in an effort to identify and intervene in the presence of a nonreassuring FHR. These methods include FHR response to stimulation, fetal oxygen saturation monitoring, fetal blood sampling, amnioinfusion, and tocolysis. Umbilical cord acid-base determination is an assessment technique that is a useful adjunct to the Apgar score in assessing the immediate condition of the newborn. If acidosis is present (e.g., pH 7.10 to 7.18) the type of acidosis is deter-

TABLE 10-5

Types of Acidosis

BLOOD GASES*	RESPIRATORY	METABOLIC	MIXED
pH	↓	↓	↓
	(<7.1)	(<7.1)	(<7.1)
P_{CO_2} (mm Hg)	↑	Normal	↑
	(>60)	(<60)	(>60)
HCO_3^- (mEq/L)	Normal	↓	↓
	(16-24)	(<16)	(<16)
Base	Normal	↑	↑
	(<12)	(>12)	(>12)

Sources: Gilstrap, L. (2004). Fetal acid-base balance. In R. Creasy, R. Resnik, & J. Iams (Eds.), *Maternal-fetal medicine: Principles and practice* (5th ed.). Philadelphia: Saunders; Pagana, K., & Pagana, T. (2002). *Mosby's manual of diagnostic and laboratory tests* (2nd ed.). St. Louis: Mosby; Tucker, S. (2004). *Pocket guide to fetal monitoring and assessment* (5th ed.). St. Louis: Mosby.
*Arterial values.

mined (respiratory, metabolic, or mixed) by analyzing the blood gas values (Table 10-5). The nursing role is usually to assist the primary health care provider with these procedures.

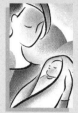

Nursing Care during Labor and Birth

PROCESS OF LABOR AND BIRTH

Signs Preceding Labor

- Box 11-1 lists signs that may precede labor.

Stages of Labor

- The first stage of labor is considered to last from the onset of regular uterine contractions to full dilation of the cervix. The first stage is much longer than the second and third combined.
- The first stage of labor has been divided into three phases: latent, active, and transition. During the latent phase, there is more progress in effacement of the cervix and little increase in descent. During the active phase and the transition phase, there is more rapid dilation of the cervix and increased rate of descent of the presenting part.
- The second stage of labor lasts from the time the cervix is fully dilated to the birth of the fetus.
  - The latent phase is a period that begins about the time of complete dilation of the cervix, when the contractions are weak or not noticeable and the woman is not feeling the urge to push, is resting, or is exerting only small bearing-down efforts with contractions.
  - The active phase is a period when contractions resume, the woman is making strong bearing-down efforts, and the fetal station is advancing.
- The third stage of labor lasts from the birth of the fetus until the placenta is delivered.
- The fourth stage of labor arbitrarily lasts about 2 hours after delivery of the placenta. It is the period of immediate recovery, when homeostasis is reestablished.

Maternal Adaptation

As the woman progresses through the stages of labor, various body system adaptations cause her to exhibit both objective and subjective symptoms (Box 11-2).

BOX 11-1

Signs Preceding Labor

- Lightening
- Return of urinary frequency
- Backache
- Stronger Braxton Hicks contractions
- Weight loss of 0.5 to 1.5 kg
- Surge of energy
- Increased vaginal discharge; bloody show
- Cervical ripening
- Possible rupture of membranes

BOX 11-2

Maternal Physiologic Changes during Labor

- Cardiac output increases 10% to 15% in first stage and 30% to 50% in second stage.
- Heart rate increases slightly in first and second stages.
- Systolic blood pressure increases during uterine contractions in first stage; systolic and diastolic pressures increase during uterine contractions in second stage.
- White blood cell count increases.
- Respiratory rate increases.
- Temperature may be slightly elevated.
- Proteinuria may occur.
- Gastric motility and absorption of solid food decrease; nausea and vomiting may occur during transition to second-stage labor.
- Blood glucose level decreases.

References: Monga, M. (2004). Maternal cardiovascular and renal adaptations to pregnancy. In R. Creasy, R. Resnik, & J. Iams (Eds.), *Maternal-fetal medicine: Principles and practice* (5th ed.). Philadelphia: Saunders; Pagana, K., & Pagana, T. (2003). *Mosby's diagnostic and laboratory test reference* (6th ed.). St. Louis: Mosby.

FIRST STAGE OF LABOR
CARE MANAGEMENT
Assessment
Interview

- Assessment begins at the first contact with the woman, whether by telephone or in person. Certain factors are assessed initially to determine whether the woman is in true or false labor and whether she should come for further assessment or admission (see Teaching Guidelines box).

- Admission forms such as one that your clinical agency uses provide guidelines for the acquisition of important assessment information when a woman in labor is being evaluated or admitted. Additional sources of data include the prenatal record, the initial interview, physical examination to determine baseline physiologic parameters, laboratory and diagnostic test results, expressed psychosocial and cultural factors, and the clinical evaluation of labor status.

- The nurse reviews the prenatal record to identify the woman's individual needs and risks. It is important to know the woman's age so that the plan of care can be tailored to the needs of her age group. Other factors to consider are the woman's general health status, current medical conditions or allergies, respiratory status, and previous surgical procedures.

- Her obstetric and pregnancy history are carefully noted. These include gravidity, parity, and problems such as history of vaginal bleeding, gestational hypertension, anemia, gestational diabetes, infections (e.g., bacterial or sexually transmitted), and immunodeficiency.

- It is important to confirm the expected date of birth (EDB). Other data in the prenatal record include patterns of maternal weight gain, physiologic measurements such as maternal vital signs (blood pressure, temperature, pulse, and respirations), fundal height, baseline fetal heart rate (FHR), and laboratory and diagnostic test results.

- The woman's primary complaint or reason for coming to the hospital is determined in the interview. She may be asked to describe the following:
  - Time and onset of contractions and progress in terms of frequency and duration

TEACHING GUIDELINES

How to Distinguish True Labor from False Labor

TRUE LABOR

- Contractions
  - —Occur regularly, becoming stronger, lasting longer, and occurring more closely together
  - —Become more intense with walking
  - —Usually felt in lower back, radiating to lower portion of abdomen
  - —Continue despite use of comfort measures
- Cervix (by vaginal examination)
  - —Shows progressive change (softening, effacement, and dilation signaled by the appearance of bloody show)
  - —Moves to an increasingly anterior position
- Fetus
  - —Presenting part usually becomes engaged in the pelvis, which results in increased ease of breathing; at the same time, the presenting part presses downward and compresses the bladder, resulting in urinary frequency

FALSE LABOR

- Contractions
  - —Occur irregularly or become regular only temporarily
  - —Often stop with walking or position change
  - —Can be felt in the back or abdomen above the navel
  - —Often can be stopped through the use of comfort measures
- Cervix (by vaginal examination)
  - —May be soft, but there is no significant change in effacement or dilation or evidence of bloody show
  - —Is often in a posterior position
- Fetus
  - —Presenting part usually not engaged in the pelvis

—Location and character of discomfort from contractions (e.g., back pain or suprapubic discomfort)

—Persistence of contractions despite changes in maternal position and activity (e.g., walking or lying down)

—Presence and character of vaginal discharge or show

—The status of amniotic membranes, such as a gush or seepage of fluid (rupture of membranes [ROM]); if there has been a discharge that may be amniotic fluid, she is asked the date and time the fluid was first noted and the fluid's characteristics (e.g., amount, color, and unusual odor); in many instances, a sterile speculum examination and a Nitrazine (pH) or fern test can confirm that the membranes are ruptured

- In case general anesthesia may be required in an emergency, it is important to assess the woman's respiratory status. The status of allergies is checked and the time and type of the woman's last solid and liquid intake is assessed because these can cause problems if general anesthesia is needed.

- Other pertinent data include the birth plan, the choice of infant feeding method, the type of pain management, the name of the pediatric health care provider, the woman's preparation for childbirth, the support person or family members desired during childbirth and their availability, and ethnic or cultural expectations and needs. The woman's use of alcohol, drugs, and tobacco before or during pregnancy should be determined.

- The woman's general appearance and behavior (and those of her partner) provide valuable clues to the type of supportive care she will need. However, the nurse should keep in mind that general appearance and behavior may vary, depending on the stage and phase of labor and sociocultural factors (Table 11-1).

Physical examination

- The initial physical examination encompasses a general systems assessment, including vital signs; performance of Leopold maneuvers to determine fetal presentation and position and the point of maximal intensity (PMI) for auscultating the FHR (see Procedure box); assessment of fetal status; assessment of uterine contractions; and vaginal examination to

Text continued on p. 299.

TABLE 11-1

Woman's Responses and Support Person's Actions during First Stage of Labor

WOMAN'S RESPONSES	NURSE'S OR SUPPORT PERSON'S ACTIONS*
DILATION OF CERVIX 0-3 CM (LATENT) **(contractions 30-45 sec long, 5-30 min apart, mild to moderate)**	
Mood: alert, happy, excited, mild anxiety	Provides encouragement, feedback for relaxation, and companionship
Settles into labor room; selects focal point	Assists woman to cope with contractions
Rests or sleeps if possible	Encourages use of focusing techniques
Uses breathing techniques	Helps to concentrate on breathing techniques
Uses effleurage, focusing, and relaxation techniques	Uses comfort measures
	Assists woman into comfortable position
	Informs woman of progress; explains procedures and routines
	Gives praise
	Offer fluids, food, and ice chips as ordered
DILATION OF CERVIX 4-7 CM (ACTIVE) (contractions 40-70 sec long, 3-5 min apart, moderate to strong)	
Mood: seriously labor oriented, concentration and energy needed for contractions, alert, more demanding	Acts as buffer; limits assessment techniques to between contractions
Continues relaxation and focusing techniques	Assists woman to cope with contractions
Uses breathing techniques	Encourages woman as needed to help her maintain breathing techniques
	Uses comfort measures
	Assists with frequent position changes, emphasizing side-lying and upright positions
	Encourages voluntary relaxation of muscles of back, buttocks, thighs, and perineum; performs effleurage
	Applies counterpressure to sacrococcygeal area

*Provided by nurses and support persons in collaboration with the nurse.

TABLE 11-1

Woman's Responses and Support Person's Actions during First Stage of Labor—cont'd

WOMAN'S RESPONSES	NURSE'S OR SUPPORT PERSON'S ACTIONS*
	Encourages and praises
	Keeps woman aware of progress
	Offers analgesics as ordered
	Checks bladder; encourages her to void
	Gives oral care; offers fluids, food, and ice chips as ordered

DILATION OF CERVIX 8-10 CM (TRANSITION)
(contractions 45-90 sec long, 2-3 min apart, strong)

Mood: irritable, intense concentration, symptoms of transition (e.g., nausea and vomiting)	Stays with woman; provides constant support
	Assists woman to cope with contractions
Continues relaxation, needs greater concentration to do this	Reminds, reassures, and encourages woman to reestablish breathing pattern and concentration as needed
Uses breathing techniques	Alerts woman to begin breathing pattern before contraction becomes too intense
—Uses patterned paced breathing (e.g., 4:1) if using psychoprophylactic techniques	Prompts panting respirations if woman begins to push prematurely
	Uses comfort measures
	Accepts woman's inability to comply with instructions
—Uses panting to overcome urge to push if appropriate	Accepts irritable response to helping, such as counterpressure
	Supports woman who has nausea and vomiting; gives oral care as needed; gives reassurance regarding signs of end of first stage
	Uses relaxation techniques (effleurage and voluntary relaxation)
	Keeps woman aware of progress

Procedure

Leopold Maneuvers

Wash hands.

Ask woman to empty bladder.

Position woman supine with one pillow under her head and with her knees slightly flexed.

Place small rolled towel under woman's right or left hip to displace uterus off major blood vessels (prevents supine hypotensive syndrome).

If right-handed, stand on woman's right, facing her:

1. Identify fetal part that occupies the fundus. The head feels round, firm, freely movable, and palpable by ballottement; the breech feels less regular and softer. This maneuver identifies fetal lie (longitudinal or transverse) and presentation (cephalic or breech) (Fig. A).

2. Using palmar surface of one hand, locate and palpate the smooth convex contour of the fetal back and the irregularities that identify the small parts (feet, hands, and elbows). This maneuver helps identify fetal presentation (Fig. B). With right hand, determine which fetal part is presenting over the inlet to the true pelvis. Gently grasp the lower pole of the uterus between the thumb and fingers, pressing in slightly (Fig. C). If the head is presenting and not engaged, determine the attitude of the head (flexed or extended).

3. Turn to face the woman's feet. Using both hands, outline the fetal head (Fig. D) with the palmar surface of the fingertips. When the presenting part has descended deeply, only a small portion of it may be outlined. Palpation of the cephalic prominence helps identify the attitude of the head. If the cephalic prominence is found on the same side as the small parts, this means that the head must be flexed and the vertex is presenting (see Fig. D). If the cephalic prominence is on the same side as the back, this indicates that the presenting head is extended and the face is presenting (see Fig. D).

4. Document fetal presentation, position, and lie and whether presenting part is flexed or extended, engaged or free floating. Use hospital's protocol for documentation (e.g., "Vertex, LOA, floating").

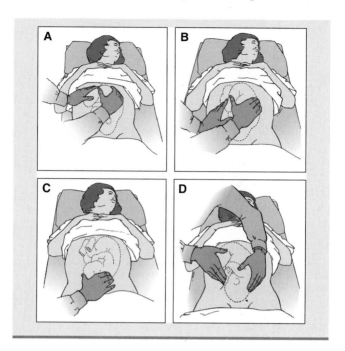

assess the status of cervical effacement and dilation, fetal descent, and amniotic membranes and fluid. The findings of the admission physical examination serve as a baseline for assessing the woman's progress from that point.

- Expected maternal progress and minimal assessment guidelines during the first stage of labor are presented in Table 11-2 and the Care Path for the Low Risk Woman in the First Stage of Labor.
- Standard Precautions should guide all assessment and care measures (Box 11-3 on p. 306).
- The FHR and pattern must be assessed (1) immediately after ROM, because this is the most common time for the umbilical cord to prolapse; (2) after any change in the contraction pattern or maternal status; and (3) before and after the woman receives medication or a procedure is performed.

Text continued on p. 306.

TABLE 11-2

Expected Maternal Progress in First Stage of Labor

CRITERION	PHASES MARKED BY CERVICAL DILATION*		
	LATENT (0-3 CM)	ACTIVE (4-7 CM)	TRANSITION (8-10 CM)
Duration†	About 6-8 hr	About 3-6 hr	About 20-40 min
Contractions			
—Strength	Mild to moderate	Moderate to strong	Strong to very strong
—Rhythm	Irregular	More regular	Regular
—Frequency	5-30 min apart	3-5 min apart	2-3 min apart
—Duration	30-45 sec	40-70 sec	45-90 sec
Descent			
—Station of presenting part	Nulliparous: 0	Varies: +1 to +2 cm	Varies: +2 to +3 cm
	Multiparous: −2 to 0 cm	Varies: +1 to +2 cm	Varies: +2 to +3 cm
Show			
—Color	Brownish discharge, mucous plug, or pale pink mucus	Pink to bloody mucus	Bloody mucus
—Amount	Scant	Scant to moderate	Copious
Behavior and appearance‡	Excited; thoughts center on self, labor, and baby; may be talkative or silent, calm or tense; some	Becomes more serious, doubtful of control of pain, more apprehensive; desires companionship	Pain described as severe; backache common; frustration, fear of loss of control, and irritability may

apprehension; pain controlled fairly well; alert, follows directions readily; open to instructions

and encouragement; attention more inwardly directed; fatigue evidenced; malar (cheeks) flush; has some difficulty following directions

be voiced; vague in communications; amnesia between contractions; writhing with contractions; nausea and vomiting, especially if hyperventilating; hyperesthesia; circumoral pallor, perspiration of forehead and upper lips; shaking tremor of thighs; feeling of need to defecate, pressure on anus

*In the nullipara, effacement is often complete before dilation begins; in the multipara, it occurs simultaneously with dilation.

†Duration of each phase is influenced by factors such as parity, maternal emotions, position, level of activity, and fetal size, and presentation and position. For example, the labor of a nullipara tends to last longer, on average, than the labor of a multipara. Women who ambulate and assume upright positions or change positions frequently during labor tend to experience a shorter first stage. Descent is often prolonged in breech presentations and occiput posterior positions.

‡Women who have epidural analgesia for pain relief may not demonstrate some of these behaviors.

CARE PATH Low Risk Woman in First Stage of Labor

CARE MANAGEMENT	0-3 CM (LATENT)	CERVICAL DILATION	
		4-7 CM (ACTIVE)	8-10 CM (TRANSITION)
	Frequency	Frequency	Frequency
I. ASSESSMENT MEASURES*			
• Blood pressure, pulse, respirations	• Every 30 to 60 minutes	• Every 30 minutes	• Every 15 to 30 minutes
• Temperature†	• Every 4 hours	• Every 4 hours	• Every 4 hours
• Uterine activity minutes	• Every 30 to 60 minutes	• Every 15 to 30 minutes	• Every 10 to 15 minutes
• Fetal heart rate (FHR)	• Every 30 to 60 minutes	• Every 15 to 30 minutes	• Every 15 to 30 minutes
• Vaginal show	• Every 30 to 60 minutes	• Every 30 minutes	• Every 15 minutes
• Behavior, appearance, mood, energy level of woman; condition of partner	• Every 30 minutes	• Every 15 minutes	• Every 5 minutes
• Vaginal examination‡	• As needed to identify progress	• As needed to identify progress	• As needed to identify progress

II. PHYSICAL CARE MEASURES§

- Stay at home for as long as possible
- Relaxation measures; rest and sleep if at night
- Activity—ambulation; emphasize upright positions
- Diversional activities
- Nourishment—light foods and full liquids
- Encourage voiding every 2 hours
- Perform basic hygiene measures

- Coach breathing techniques
- Encourage effleurage
- Assist in using relaxation techniques between contractions
- Encourage ambulation, upright positions
- Assist with position changes
- Use comfort measures desired by woman: massage, hot or cold packs, touch, etc.
- Initiate hydrotherapy (shower, bath, Jacuzzi)
- Provide nourishment as desired

- Coach breathing techniques
- Reduce touch if increased sensitivity is noted
- Help to relax between contractions
- Assist with position changes
- Use comfort measures according to acceptance level
- Continue hydrotherapy if effective
- Provide clear liquids: sips, ice chips
- Encourage voiding every 2 hours
- Provide hygiene measures, emphasizing mouth and perineal care

Continued

CARE PATH — Low Risk Woman in First Stage of Labor—cont'd

CARE MANAGEMENT	0-3 CM (LATENT)	CERVICAL DILATION		
		4-7 CM (ACTIVE)	8-10 CM (TRANSITION)	
		• Encourage voiding every 2 hours • Assist with hygiene, perineal care • Provide pharmacologic pain relief if requested by woman and ordered by primary health care provider • Provide relief for partner as needed	• Provide pharmacologic pain relief if requested by woman and ordered by primary health care provider • Prepare for birth	
III. EMOTIONAL SUPPORT	• Review birth plan • Review process of labor—what to expect, pain management techniques, available measures	• Provide feedback about performance • Reduce distractions during contractions • Role model comfort	• Provide continuous support • Reduce distractions	

- Redemonstrate breathing techniques as needed
- Keep informed: progress, procedures

- Reassure, encourage, and praise
- Take charge, talk through contraction until control regained
- Continue to keep informed

- Role model care measures to assist partner
- Continue reassurance, praise, and encouragement
- Keep informed
- Take charge as needed

*Full assessment using interview, physical examination, and laboratory testing is performed on admission. Subsequently, frequency of assessment is determined by the risk status of the maternal-fetal unit. More frequent assessment is required in high risk situations. Frequency of assessment and method of documentation are also determined by agency policy, which is usually based on the recommended care standards of medical and nursing organizations.

†If membranes have ruptured, the temperature should be assessed every 1 to 2 hours; assess orally or tympanically between contractions.

‡Perform vaginal examination at admission and thereafter only when signs indicate that progress has occurred (e.g., significant increase in frequency, duration, and intensity of contractions; rupture of membranes; perineal pressure); strict aseptic technique should be used. In the presence of vaginal bleeding, the primary health care provider performs the examination under a double setup in a delivery room, or an ultrasonography is performed to determine placental location.

§Physical care measures are performed by the nurse working together with the woman's partner and significant others. The woman is capable of greater independence in the latent phase but needs more assistance during the active and transition phases.

BOX 11-3

Standard Precautions during Childbirth

- Wash hands before and after putting on gloves and performing procedures.
- Wear gloves (clean or sterile, as appropriate) when performing procedures that require contact with the woman's genitalia and body fluids, including bloody show (e.g., during vaginal examination, amniotomy, hygienic care of the perineum, insertion of an internal scalp electrode and intrauterine pressure monitor, and catheterization).
- Wear a mask that has a shield or protective eyewear and a cover gown when assisting with the birth. Cap and shoe covers are worn for cesarean birth but are optional for vaginal birth in a birthing room. Gowns worn by the primary health care provider who is attending the birth should have a waterproof front and sleeves and should be sterile.
- Drape the woman with sterile towels and sheets as appropriate. Explain to the woman what can and cannot be touched.
- Help the woman's partner put on appropriate coverings for the type of birth, such as cap, mask, gown, and shoe covers. Show the partner where to stand and what can and cannot be touched.
- Wear gloves and gown when handling the newborn immediately after birth.
- Use an appropriate method to suction the newborn's airway, such as a bulb syringe, mechanical wall suction, or DeLee oral suction device, that prevents the newborn's mucus from getting into the user's mouth or airway.

- A uterine contraction is described in terms of the following characteristics:
  - *Frequency:* how often uterine contractions occur; the time that elapses from the beginning of one contraction to the beginning of the next
  - *Intensity:* the strength of a contraction at its peak
  - *Duration:* the time that elapses between the onset and the end of a contraction
  - *Resting tone:* the tension in the uterine muscle between contractions

- The following terms are used to describe what is felt on palpation:
  - *Mild:* slightly tense fundus that is easy to indent with fingertips (feels like touching finger to tip of nose)
  - *Moderate:* firm fundus that is difficult to indent with fingertips (feels like touching finger to chin)
  - *Strong:* rigid, boardlike fundus that is almost impossible to indent with fingertips (feels like touching finger to forehead)
- External electronic monitoring provides information about the relative strength of the uterine contractions. Internal electronic monitoring with an intrauterine pressure catheter is the most reliable way to assess the intensity of uterine contractions.
- The vaginal examination reveals whether the woman is in true labor (i.e., cervical dilation and effacement) and enables the examiner to determine whether the membranes have ruptured.

Laboratory and diagnostic tests

- A clean-catch urine specimen may be obtained to gather further data about the pregnant woman's health. It is a convenient and simple procedure that can provide information about her hydration status (e.g., specific gravity, color, and amount), nutritional status (e.g., ketones), infection status (e.g., leukocytes), and the status of possible complications, such as preeclampsia, shown by finding protein in the urine. The results can be obtained quickly and help the nurse determine appropriate interventions to implement.
- The blood tests performed vary with the hospital protocol and the woman's health status. If the woman's blood type has not been verified, blood is drawn for the purpose of determining the type and Rh factor.
- Assessment of amniotic membranes and fluid is done. The characteristics of the fluid are described in Table 11-3.

Signs of potential problems

Although some problems of labor are anticipated, others may appear unexpectedly during the clinical course of labor (see Signs of Potential Complications box).

TABLE 11-3

Assessment of Amniotic Fluid Characteristics

CHARACTERISTIC OF FLUID	NORMAL FINDING	DEVIATION FROM NORMAL FINDING	CAUSE OF DEVIATION FROM NORMAL
Color	Pale, straw colored; may contain white flecks of vernix caseosa, lanugo, and scalp hair	Greenish brown color Yellow-stained fluid Port wine colored	Hypoxic episode in fetus results in meconium passage into fluid May be normal finding in breech presentations related to pressure exerted on fetal abdominal wall during descent Fetal hypoxia ≥36 hr before ROM; fetal hemolytic disease; intrauterine infection Bleeding associated with premature separation of the placenta (abruptio placentae)

Viscosity and odor	Watery; no strong odor	Thick, cloudy, and foul smelling	Intrauterine infection Large amount of meconium can make fluid thick
Amount (normally varies with gestational age)	400 ml (20 wk of gestation) 1000 ml (36-38 wk of gestation)	≥2000 ml (32-36 wk of gestation) ≤500 ml (32-36 wk of gestation)	Hydramnios: associated with congenital anomalies of the fetus when fetus cannot drink or fluid is trapped in the body (e.g., fetal gastrointestinal obstruction or atresias); increased risk with maternal pregestational or gestational diabetes mellitus Oligohydramnios: associated with incomplete or absent kidney; obstruction of urethra; fetus cannot secrete or excrete urine

ROM, Rupture of membranes.

signs of
POTENTIAL COMPLICATIONS

Labor

- Intrauterine pressure of 80 mm Hg or higher (determined by intrauterine pressure catheter monitoring) or resting tone of 20 mm Hg or higher
- Contractions consistently lasting 90 seconds or longer
- Contractions consistently occurring 2 minutes or less apart
- Contraction pattern with less than a 30-second interval between the end of one contraction and the beginning of the next
- Fetal bradycardia, tachycardia, decreased variability not associated with fetal sleep cycles or temporary effects of CNS depressant drugs given to the woman, or late or severe variable deceleration
- Irregular fetal heart rate; suspected fetal arrhythmias
- Appearance of meconium-stained or bloody fluid from the vagina
- Arrest in progress of cervical dilation or effacement, descent of the fetus, or both
- Maternal temperature of 38°C or higher
- Foul-smelling vaginal discharge
- Persistent bright or dark red vaginal bleeding

Interventions

Standards of care

Standards of care guide the nurse in preparing for and implementing procedures with the expectant mother. These include the following tasks:

- Check the primary health care provider's orders.
- Review the primary health care provider's orders for completeness and correctness (e.g., the dose and route of the analgesic to be administered).
- Check labels on intravenous (IV) solutions, drugs, and other materials used for nursing care.
- Check the expiration date on any packs of supplies used for procedures.
- Ensure that information on the woman's identification band is accurate (e.g., the band is the appropriate color for allergies).

- Use an empathic approach when giving care.
- Use Standard Precautions, including precautions for invasive procedures.
- Document care according to hospital guidelines, and communicate information to the primary health care provider when indicated.

Physical nursing care during first stage of labor

The physical nursing care rendered to the woman in labor is an essential component of her care. The various physical needs, the requisite nursing actions, and the rationale for care are presented in Table 11-4 and the Care Path on p. 302-306.

Emergency interventions

Emergency conditions that require immediate nursing intervention can arise with startling speed. Interventions for a nonreassuring FHR, inadequate uterine relaxation, vaginal bleeding, infection, and prolapse of the cord are detailed in the Emergency box on p. 316-318.

SECOND STAGE OF LABOR

CARE MANAGEMENT

- Indicators for each phase of the second stage are given in Table 11-5.
- Assessment is continuous during the second stage of labor. Professional standards and agency policy determine the specific type and timing of assessments, as well as the way in which findings are documented. The Care Path for the Low Risk Woman in Second and Third Stages of Labor indicates typical assessments and the recommended frequency for their performance. Signs and symptoms of impending birth (see Table 11-5) may appear unexpectedly, requiring immediate action by the nurse (Box 11-4). The nurse continues to monitor maternal-fetal status and events of the second stage and provide comfort measures for the mother, such as helping her change position; providing mouth care; maintaining clean, dry bedding; and keeping extraneous noise, conversation, and other distractions to a

Text continued on p. 328.

TABLE 11-4

Physical Nursing Care during Labor

NEED	NURSING ACTIONS	RATIONALE
GENERAL HYGIENE		
Showers, bed baths, or Jacuzzi bath	Assess for progress in labor	Determines appropriateness of the activity
	Supervise showers closely if woman is in true labor	Prevents injury from fall; labor may be accelerated
	Suggest allowing warm water to flow over back	Aids relaxation; increases comfort
Perineum	Cleanse frequently, especially after rupture of membranes and when show increases	Enhances comfort and reduces risk of infection
Oral hygiene	Offer toothbrush or mouthwash or wash the teeth with an ice-cold wet washcloth as needed	Refreshes mouth; helps counteract dry, thirsty feeling
Hair	Brush or braid per woman's wishes	Improves morale; increases comfort
Handwashing	Offer washcloths before and after voiding and as needed	Maintains cleanliness; prevents infection
Face	Offer cool washcloth	Provides relief from diaphoresis; cools and refreshes
Gowns and linens	Change as needed; fluff pillows	Improves comfort; enhances relaxation

NUTRIENT AND FLUID INTAKE

Oral

Offer fluids and solid foods, following orders of primary health care provider and desires of laboring woman

Provides hydration and calories; enhances positive emotional experience and maternal control

Intravenous (IV)

Establish and maintain IV line as ordered

Maintains hydration; provides venous access for medications

ELIMINATION

Voiding

Encourage voiding at least q2h

A full bladder may impede descent of presenting part; overdistention may cause bladder atony and injury, as well as postpartum voiding difficulty

Reinforces normal process of urination

—Ambulatory woman

Allow ambulation to bathroom according to orders of primary health care provider, if the following are true:

—The presenting part is engaged

Precautionary measure to protect against prolapse of umbilical cord

—The membranes are not ruptured

—The woman is not medicated

Precautionary measure to protect against injury

Continued

TABLE 11-4

Physical Nursing Care during Labor—cont'd

NEED	NURSING ACTIONS	RATIONALE
—Woman on bed rest	Offer bedpan	Prevents complications of bladder distention and ambulation
	Allow tap water to run; pour warm water over the vulva; give positive suggestion	Encourages voiding
	Provide privacy	Shows respect for woman
	Put up side rails on bed	Prevents injury from fall
	Place call bell within reach	Reinforces safe care
	Offer washcloth for hands	Maintains cleanliness; prevents infection
	Wash vulvar area	Maintains cleanliness; enhances comfort; prevents infection
—Catheterization	Catheterize according to orders of primary health care provider or hospital protocol if measures to facilitate voiding are ineffective	Prevents complications of bladder distention

	Insert catheter between contractions	Minimizes discomfort
	Avoid force if obstacle to insertion is noted	"Obstacle" may be caused by compression of urethra by presenting part
	Perform vaginal examination	Determines degree of descent of presenting part
Bowel elimination—sensation of rectal pressure		Prevents misinterpretation of rectal pressure from the presenting part as the need to defecate
	Help the woman ambulate to bathroom or offer bedpan if rectal pressure is not from presenting part	Reinforces safe care and normal process of bowel elimination
	Cleanse perineum immediately after passage of stool	Reduces risk of infection and sense of embarrassment

EMERGENCY

Interventions for Emergencies

SIGNS

NONREASSURING FETAL HEART RATE PATTERN

- Fetal bradycardia (FHR less than 110 beats/min for more than 10 minutes)[†]
- Fetal tachycardia (FHR more than 160 beats/min for more than 10 minutes in term pregnancy)[§]
- Irregular FHR, abnormal sinus rhythm shown by internal monitor
- Persistent decrease in baseline FHR variability without an identified cause
- Late, severe variable, and prolonged deceleration patterns
- Absence of FHTs

INADEQUATE UTERINE RELAXATION

- Intrauterine pressure more than 80 mmHg (shown by intrauterine pressure catheter monitoring)
- Contractions consistently lasting longer than 90 seconds

INTERVENTIONS*

PRIORITIES ARE BASED ON WHAT SIGN IS PRESENT

- Notify primary health care provider.[‡]
- Change maternal position.
- Discontinue oxytocin (Pitocin) infusion if being infused.
- Start an IV line if one is not in place.
- Increase IV fluid rate (if fluid being infused) per protocol order.
- Administer oxygen at 8 to 10 L/min by snug face mask.
- Check maternal temperature for elevation.
- Assist with amnioinfusion if ordered.
- Stimulate fetal scalp or use sound stimulation.

- Notify primary health care provider.[‡]
- Discontinue oxytocin infusion if being infused.
- Change woman to side-lying position.
- Start an IV line if one is not in place.
- Increase IV fluid rate if fluid is being infused.

- Contraction interval less than 2 minutes

- Administer oxygen at 8 to 10 L/min by snug face mask.
- Palpate and evaluate contractions.
- Give tocolytics (terbutaline) as ordered.

VAGINAL BLEEDING

- Vaginal bleeding (bright red, dark red, or in an amount in excess of that expected during normal cervical dilation)
- Continuous vaginal bleeding with FHR changes
- Pain; may or may not be present

- Notify primary health care provider.[‡]
- Start an IV line if one is not in place.
- Assist with ultrasound examination if performed
- Anticipate emergency (stat) cesarean birth.
- *Do NOT perform a vaginal examination.*

INFECTION

- Foul-smelling amniotic fluid
- Maternal temperature more than 38° C in presence of adequate hydration (straw-colored urine)
- Fetal tachycardia above 160 beats/min for more than 10 minutes

- Notify primary health care provider.[‡]
- Institute cooling measures for laboring woman.
- Start an IV line if one is not in place.
- Assist with or perform collection of catheterized urine specimen and amniotic fluid sample, and send to the laboratory for urinalysis and cultures.

PROLAPSE OF CORD

- Fetal bradycardia with variable deceleration during uterine contraction
- Woman reports feeling the cord after membranes rupture

- Call for assistance.
- Have someone notify the primary health care provider immediately.

Continued

EMERGENCY—cont'd

- Cord lies alongside or below the presenting part of the fetus; can be seen or felt in or protruding from the vagina
- Major predisposing factors
  —Rupture of membranes with a gush
  —Loose fit of presenting part in lower uterine segment
  —Presenting part not yet engaged
  —Breech presentation

- Glove the examining hand quickly, and insert two fingers into the vagina to the cervix; with one finger on either side of the cord or both fingers to one side, exert upward pressure against the presenting part to relieve compression of the cord.
- Place a rolled towel under the woman's hip.
- Place woman in extreme Trendelenburg, modified Sims, or knee-chest position.
- Wrap the cord loosely in a sterile towel saturated with warm sterile normal saline if the cord is protruding from the vagina.
- Administer oxygen at 8 to 10 L/min by face mask until birth is accomplished.
- Start IV fluids, or increase existing drip rate.
- Continue to monitor FHR by internal fetal scalp electrode if possible.
- Do not attempt to replace cord into cervix.
- Prepare for immediate birth (vaginal or cesarean).

FHR, Fetal heart rate; *FHTs,* fetal heart tones; *IV,* intravenous.

*Because emergency situations are often frightening events, it is important for the nurse to explain to the woman and her support person what is happening and how it is being managed.

†Practice is to intervene within 2 to 30 minutes of FHR below 110 beats/min.

‡In most emergency situations, nurses take immediate action, following a protocol and standards of nursing practice. Another person can notify the primary health care provider, or this can be done by the nurse as soon as possible.

§Nonreassuring sign when associated with late decelerations or absence of variability, especially of more than 180 beats/min.

TABLE 11-5

Expected Maternal Progress in Second Stage of Labor

CRITERION	LATENT PHASE (AVERAGE DURATION 10-30 MIN)	DESCENT PHASE (AVERAGE DURATION VARIES)*	TRANSITION PHASE (AVERAGE DURATION 5-15 MIN)
Contractions —Magnitude (intensity)	Period of physiologic lull for all criteria; period of peace and rest; "laboring down"	Significant increase	Overwhelmingly strong Expulsive
—Frequency		2-2.5 min	1-2 min
—Duration		90 sec	90 sec
Descent, station	0 to +2	Increases and Ferguson reflex† activated, +2 to +4	Rapid, +4 to birth Fetal head visible in introitus
Show: color and amount		Significant increase in dark red bloody show	Bloody show accompanies birth of head
Spontaneous bearing-down efforts	Slight to absent, except during acme of strongest contractions	Increased urge to bear down	Greatly increased

Continued

TABLE 11-5

Expected Maternal Progress in Second Stage of Labor—cont'd

CRITERION	LATENT PHASE (AVERAGE DURATION 10-30 MIN)	DESCENT PHASE (AVERAGE DURATION VARIES)*	TRANSITION PHASE (AVERAGE DURATION 5-15 MIN)
Vocalization	Quiet; concern over progress	Grunting sounds or expiratory vocalization; announces contractions	Grunting sounds and expiratory vocalizations continue; may scream or swear
Maternal behavior	Experiences sense of relief that transition to second stage is finished Feels fatigued and sleepy Feels a sense of accomplishment and optimism, because the "worst is over"	Senses increased urge to push Alters respiratory pattern: has short 4- to 5-sec breath holds with regular breaths in between, five to seven times per contraction Makes grunting sounds or expiratory vocalizations	Describes extreme pain Expresses feelings of powerlessness Shows decreased ability to listen or concentrate on anything but giving birth

Feels in control

Frequent repositioning

Describes *ring of fire* (burning sensation of acute pain as vagina stretches and fetal head crowns)

Often shows excitement immediately after birth of head

Sources: Roberts, J. (2002). The "push" for evidence: Management of the second stage. *Journal of Midwifery & Women's Health, 47*(1), 2-15; Simkin, P., & Ancheta, R. (2000). *The labor progress handbook*. Malden, MA: Blackwell Science.

*Duration of descent phase can vary depending on maternal parity, effectiveness of bearing-down effort, and presence of spinal anesthesia or epidural analgesia.

†Pressure of presenting part on stretch receptors of pelvic floor stimulates release of oxytocin from posterior pituitary, resulting in more intense uterine contractions.

CARE PATH | Low Risk Woman in Second and Third Stages of Labor

CARE MANAGEMENT	SECOND STAGE OF LABOR	THIRD STAGE OF LABOR
I. ASSESSMENT MEASURES*		
• Blood pressure, pulse, respirations	**Frequency** • Every 5 to 30 minutes	**Frequency** • Every 15 minutes
• Uterine activity	• Assess every contraction	• Assess for placental separation
• Bearing-down effort • Fetal heart rate (FHR)	• Assess each effort • Every 5 to 15 minutes	• Determine Apgar score at 1 and 5 minutes
• Vaginal show	• Every 15 minutes	• Assess bleeding until placental expulsion
• Signs of fetal descent: urge to bear down, perineal bulging, crowning	• Every 10 to 15 minutes	
• Behavior, appearance, mood, energy level of woman; condition of partner	• Every 10 to 15 minutes	• Assess response to completion of childbirth process, reaction to newborn

II. PHYSICAL CARE MEASURES†

Latent Phase
- Assist to rest in position of comfort
- Encourage relaxation to conserve energy
- Promote urge to push; if delayed: ambulation, shower, pelvic rock, position changes

Descent Phase
- Assist to bear down effectively
- Help to use recommended positions that facilitate descent
- Encourage correct breathing during bearing-down efforts
- Help to relax between contractions
- Provide comfort measures as needed
- Cleanse perineum immediately if fecal material is expelled

Transition Phase
- Assist to pant during contraction to avoid rapid birth of head
- Coach to gently bear down between contractions
- Assist to bear down to facilitate delivery of separated placenta
- Administer oxytocic as ordered
- Provide pain relief as needed
- Provide hygiene and comfort measures as needed

CARE PATH		Low Risk Woman in 2nd and 3rd Stages of Labor—cont'd

CARE MANAGEMENT	SECOND STAGE OF LABOR	THIRD STAGE OF LABOR
III. EMOTIONAL SUPPORT	• Keep informed of progress of fetal descent • Provide feedback for bearing-down efforts • Explain purpose if medications given • Role model comfort measures • Provide continuous nursing presence • Create a quiet, calm environment • Reassure, encourage, praise • Take charge as needed, until woman regains confidence in ability to birth her baby • Offer mirror to watch birth	• Keep informed about progress of placental separation • Explain purpose if medications given • Describe status of perineal tissue and inform if repair is needed • Introduce parents to their baby • Assess and care for newborn within view of parents; delay eye prophylaxis to facilitate eye contact • Provide private time for family to bond with their new baby and help them to create memories • Encourage breastfeeding if desired

*Frequency of assessment is determined by the risk status of the maternal-fetal unit. More frequent assessment is required in high risk situations. Frequency of assessment and method of documentation are also determined by agency policy, which is usually based on the recommended care standards of medical and nursing organizations.

†Physical care measures are performed by the nurse working together with the woman's partner and significant others.

BOX 11-4

Guidelines for Assistance at the Emergency Birth of a Fetus in the Vertex Presentation

1. The woman usually assumes the position most comfortable for her. A lateral position is often recommended.
2. Reassure the woman that birth is usually uncomplicated and easy in these situations. Use eye-to-eye contact and a calm, relaxed manner. If there is someone else available, such as the partner, that person could help support the woman in the position, assist with coaching, and compliment her on her efforts.
3. Wash your hands, and put on gloves if available.
4. Place under woman's buttocks whatever clean material is available.
5. Avoid touching the vaginal area to decrease the possibility of infection.
6. As the head begins to crown, you should do the following:
   a. Tear the amniotic membrane if it is still intact.
   b. Instruct the woman to pant or pant-blow, thus minimizing the urge to push.
   c. Place the flat side of your hand on the exposed fetal head and apply *gentle* pressure toward the vagina to prevent the head from "popping out." The mother may participate by placing her hand under yours on the emerging head. NOTE: Rapid delivery of the fetal head must be prevented because a rapid change of pressure within the molded fetal skull follows, which may result in dural or subdural tears and may cause vaginal or perineal lacerations.
7. After the birth of the head, check for the umbilical cord. If the cord is around the baby's neck, try to slip it over the baby's head or pull it *gently* to get some slack so that you can slip it over the shoulders.
8. Support the fetal head as restitution (external rotation) occurs. After restitution, with one hand on each side of the baby's head, exert *gentle* pressure downward so that the anterior shoulder emerges under the symphysis pubis and acts as a fulcrum;

Continued

BOX 11-4

*Guidelines for Assistance
at the Emergency Birth of a Fetus
in the Vertex Presentation—cont'd*

then, as *gentle* pressure is exerted in the opposite direction, the posterior shoulder, which has passed over the sacrum and coccyx, emerges.

9. Be alert! Hold the baby securely because the rest of the body may emerge quickly. The baby will be slippery!

10. Cradle the baby's head and back in one hand and the buttocks in the other. Keep the head down to drain away the mucus. Use a bulb syringe, if one is available, to remove mucus from the baby's mouth.

11. Dry the baby quickly to prevent rapid heat loss. Keep the baby at the same level as the mother's uterus until the end of the cord stops pulsating. NOTE: It is important to keep the baby at the same level as the mother's uterus to prevent the baby's blood from flowing to or from the placenta and the resultant hypovolemia or hypervolemia. Also, do not "milk" the cord.

12. Place the baby on the mother's abdomen, cover the baby (remember to keep the head warm, too) with the mother's clothing, and have her cuddle the baby. Compliment her (them) on a job well done and on the baby, if appropriate.

13. Wait for the placenta to separate; *do not* tug on the cord. NOTE: Injudicious traction may tear the cord, separate the placenta, or invert the uterus. Signs of placental separation include a slight gush of dark blood from the introitus, lengthening of the cord, and change in the uterine contour from a discoid to globular shape.

14. Instruct the mother to push to deliver the separated placenta. Gently ease out the placental membranes using an up-and-down motion until the membranes are removed. If birth occurs outside a hospital setting, to minimize complications, do not cut the cord without proper clamps and a sterile cutting tool. Inspect the placenta for intactness. Place the baby on the placenta, and wrap the two together for additional warmth.

15. Check the firmness of the uterus. Gently massage the fundus and demonstrate to the mother how she can massage her own fundus properly.

BOX 11-4

Guidelines for Assistance at the Emergency Birth of a Fetus in the Vertex Presentation—cont'd

16. If supplies are available, clean the mother's perineal area and apply a perineal pad.

17. In addition to gentle massage of the fundus, the following measures can be taken to prevent or minimize hemorrhage:

   a. Put the baby to the mother's breast as soon as possible. Sucking or nuzzling and licking the nipple stimulate the release of oxytocin from the posterior pituitary. NOTE: If the baby does not or cannot nurse, manually stimulate the mother's nipples.

   b. Do not allow the mother's bladder to become distended. Assess the bladder for fullness and encourage her to void if fullness is found.

   c. Expel any clots from the mother's uterus.

18. Comfort or reassure the mother and her family or friends. Keep the mother and the baby warm. Give her fluids if available and tolerated.

19. If this is a multifetal birth, identify the infants in order of birth (using letters *A, B,* etc.).

20. Make notations regarding the following aspects of the birth:

   a. Fetal presentation and position

   b. Presence of cord around neck (nuchal cord) or other parts and number of times cord encircled part

   c. Color, character, and amount of amniotic fluid, if rupture of membranes occurs immediately before birth

   d. Time of birth

   e. Estimated time of determination of Apgar score (e.g., 1 and 5 minutes after birth), resuscitation efforts implemented, and ultimate condition of baby

   f. Sex of baby

   g. Time of placental expulsion, as well as the appearance and completeness of the placenta

   h. Maternal condition: affect, amount of bleeding, and status of uterine tonicity

   i. Any unusual occurrences during the birth (e.g., maternal or paternal response, verbalizations, or gestures in response to birth of baby)

minimum. The woman is encouraged to indicate other support measures she would like (Table 11-6).

Mechanism of birth: vertex presentation

The three phases of the spontaneous birth of a fetus in a vertex presentation are (1) birth of the head, (2) birth of the shoulders, and (3) birth of the body and extremities.

- Meconium aspiration should be prevented. If meconium has been present in the amniotic fluid during labor, preparations are made for wall suction, or in some cases a DeLee suction apparatus is placed on the sterile field for use. Fluids usually are withdrawn from the infant's mouth and nose before the first breath is taken. Use of the DeLee device with oral suction to withdraw fluid from the infant should be avoided unless the suction device is designed so that it can keep mucus from entering the user's airway.
- The time of birth is the precise time when the entire body is out of the mother. This time must be recorded on the record.
- Fundal pressure is the application of gentle, steady pressure against the fundus of the uterus to facilitate the vaginal birth. Use of fundal pressure by nurses is not advised because there is no standard technique available for this maneuver, and no current legal, professional, or regulatory standards exist for its use. In cases of shoulder dystocia, fundal pressure is not recommended: the all-fours position (Gaskin maneuver), suprapubic pressure, and maternal position changes are among the recommended interventions (see Chapter 12).

Immediate assessments and care of the newborn

The care given immediately after the birth focuses on assessing and stabilizing the newborn. A brief assessment of the newborn can be performed while the mother is holding the infant. This includes checking the infant's airway and Apgar score. Maintaining a patent airway, supporting respiratory effort, and preventing cold stress by drying the newborn and covering the newborn with a warmed blanket or placing him or her under a radiant warmer are the major priorities in terms of

Text continued on p. 331.

TABLE 11-6

Woman's Responses and Support Person's Actions during Second Stage of Labor

WOMAN'S RESPONSES*	NURSE'S OR SUPPORT PERSON'S ACTIONS†
LATENT PHASE	
Experiences a short period of peace and rest	Encourages woman to "listen" to her body
	Continues support measures allowing woman to rest
	Suggests an upright position to encourage progression of descent if descent phase does not begin after 20 min
DESCENT PHASE	
Senses increased urgency to bear down as Ferguson reflex is activated	Encourages respiratory pattern of short breath holds and open glottis pushing
Notes increase in intensity of uterine contractions; alters respiratory pattern: short 4-to 5-sec breath holds, five to seven times per contraction	Stresses normality and benefits of grunting sounds and expiratory vocalizations
Makes grunting sounds or expiratory vocalizations	Encourages bearing-down efforts with urge to push
	Encourages or suggests maternal movement and position changes (upright, if descent is not occurring)
	Encourages woman to "listen" to her body regarding movement and position change if descent is occurring
	Discourages long breath holds (no longer than 5-7 sec)

*Woman's responses will be altered if epidural analgesia is being administered.
†Provided by nurses and support persons in collaboration with the nurse.

TABLE 11-6

Woman's Responses and Support Person's Actions during Second Stage of Labor—cont'd

WOMAN'S RESPONSES	NURSE'S OR SUPPORT PERSON'S ACTIONS
	If birth is to occur in a delivery room, transfers woman to delivery room early to avoid rushing, or, if permitted, offers her option of walking to delivery room
	Places woman in lateral recumbent position to slow descent if descent is too fast
TRANSITIONAL PHASE	
Behaves in manner similar to behavior during transition in first stage (8-10 cm)	Encourages slow, gentle pushing
Experiences a sense of severe pain and powerlessness	Explains that "blowing away the contraction" facilitates a slower birth of the head
Shows decreased ability to listen	Provides mirror to help woman see or touch the emerging fetal head (best to extend over two or three contractions) to help her understand the perineal sensations
Concentrates on birth of baby until head is born	
Experiences contractions as overwhelming in intensity	
Reports feeling ring of fire as head crowns	Coaches woman to relax mouth, throat, and neck to promote relaxation of pelvic floor
Maintains respiratory pattern of three to five 7-sec breath holds per contraction, followed by forced expiration	Applies warm compress to perineum to promote relaxation
Eases head out with short expirations	
Responds with excitement and relief after head is born	

the newborn's immediate care. Further examination, identification procedures, and care can be postponed until later in the third stage of labor or early in the fourth stage.

Perineal lacerations

Perineal lacerations usually occur as the fetal head is being born. The extent of the laceration is defined in terms of its depth:

1. *First degree:* laceration that extends through the skin and structures superficial to muscles
2. *Second degree:* laceration that extends through muscles of the perineal body
3. *Third degree:* laceration that continues through the anal sphincter muscle
4. *Fourth degree:* laceration that also involves the anterior rectal wall

Episiotomy

- An episiotomy is an incision made in the perineum to enlarge the vaginal outlet. Clear evidence exists that routine performance of an episiotomy for birth is likely to be harmful or ineffective. The practice in many settings now is to support the perineum manually during birth and allow the perineum to tear rather than perform an episiotomy. Tears are often smaller than an episiotomy, are repaired easily or not at all, and heal quickly.
- Alternative measures for perineal management, such as warm compresses, manual support, and massage (e.g., prenatal and intrapartum), have been shown to reduce, to varying degrees, the incidence of episiotomies. Nurses acting as advocates can encourage women to use alternative birthing positions that reduce pressure on the perineum (e.g., lateral position) and to use spontaneous bearing-down efforts.

Emergency childbirth

Even under the best of circumstances, there probably will come a time when the perinatal nurse will be required to assist with the birth of an infant without medical assistance. Because it is neither possible nor desirable to prevent impending birth, the perinatal nurse must be able to function independently and be skilled in the safe birth of a vertex fetus (see Box 11-4).

THIRD STAGE OF LABOR

- The third stage of labor lasts from the birth of the baby until the placenta is expelled. The goal in the management of the third stage of labor is the prompt separation and expulsion of the placenta, achieved in the easiest, safest manner.
- To assist in the delivery of the placenta, the woman is instructed to push when signs of separation have occurred. Oxytocic agents may be administered after the placenta is removed because they stimulate the uterus to contract, thereby helping to prevent hemorrhage.
- Maternal physical status is assessed. The major risk for women during the third stage of labor is postpartum hemorrhage. When the primary health care provider completes the delivery of the placenta, the nurse observes the mother for signs of excessive blood loss, including alteration in vital signs, pallor, light-headedness, restlessness, decreased urinary output, and alteration in level of consciousness and orientation. Because of the rapid cardiovascular changes taking place (e.g., the increased intracranial pressure during pushing and the rapid increase in cardiac output), the risk of rupture of a preexisting cerebral aneurysm and the risk of formation of pulmonary emboli are greater than usual during this period. Another dangerous, unpredictable problem that may occur is the formation of an amniotic fluid embolism.
- When the third stage is complete and any lacerations are repaired or an episiotomy is sutured, the vulvar area is gently cleansed with warm water or normal saline, and a perineal pad or an ice pack is applied to the perineum. The birthing bed or table is repositioned, and the woman's legs are lowered simultaneously from the stirrups if she gave birth in a lithotomy position. Drapes are removed, and dry linen is placed under the woman's buttocks; she is provided with a clean gown and a warmed blanket if needed. Maternal and neonatal assessments for the fourth stage of labor are instituted.

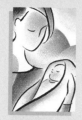

CHAPTER 12

Labor and Birth Complications

PRETERM LABOR AND BIRTH

Clinical Manifestations

- Preterm labor is defined as cervical changes and uterine contractions occurring between 20 and 37 weeks of pregnancy. Preterm birth is any birth that occurs before the completion of 37 weeks of pregnancy. The cause of preterm labor is unknown and is assumed to be multifactorial.
- The diagnosis of preterm labor is based on three major diagnostic criteria:
  - Gestational age between 20 and 37 weeks
  - Uterine activity (e.g., contractions)
  - Progressive cervical change (e.g., effacement of 80% or cervical dilation of 2 cm or greater)
- The known risk factors for preterm birth are shown in Box 12-1. However, at least 50% of all women who ultimately give birth prematurely have no identifiable risk factors.
- The two most common biochemical markers used in an effort to predict who might experience preterm labor are fetal fibronectin and salivary estriol.
  - Fetal fibronectins are glycoproteins found in plasma and produced during fetal life. They appear in the cervical canal early in pregnancy and then again in late pregnancy. Their appearance between 24 and 34 weeks of gestation predicts labor. The negative predictive value of fetal fibronectin is high (up to 94%). The positive predictive value is lower (46%). The test is done during a vaginal examination.
  - Salivary estriol is a form of estrogen produced by the fetus that is present in plasma at 9 weeks of gestation. Levels of salivary estriol have been shown to increase before preterm birth. Specimens of salivary estriol are collected by the

BOX 12-1

Risk Factors for Preterm Labor

DEMOGRAPHIC RISKS
- Nonwhite race
- Age (<15 years or >35 years)
- Low socioeconomic status
- Unmarried
- Less than high school education

BIOPHYSICAL RISKS
- Previous preterm labor or birth
- Second-trimester abortion (more than two spontaneous or therapeutic); stillbirths
- Grand multiparity; short interval between pregnancies (<1 year since last birth); family history of preterm labor and birth
- Progesterone deficiency
- Uterine anomalies or fibroids; uterine irritability
- Cervical incompetence, trauma, or shortened length
- Exposure to diethylstilbestrol (DES) or other toxic substances
- Medical diseases (e.g., diabetes, hypertension, or anemia)
- Small stature (<119 cm in height; <45.5 kg or underweight for height)
- Current pregnancy risks
  - Multifetal pregnancy
  - Hydramnios
  - Bleeding
  - Placental problems (e.g., placenta previa or abruptio placentae)
  - Infections (e.g., pyelonephritis, recurrent urinary tract infections, asymptomatic bacteriuria, bacterial vaginosis, or chorioamnionitis)
  - Gestational hypertension
  - Premature rupture of the membranes
  - Fetal anomalies
  - Inadequate plasma volume expansion; anemia

BEHAVIORAL-PSYCHOSOCIAL RISKS
- Poor nutrition; weight loss or low weight gain
- Smoking (>10 cigarettes per day)

BOX 12-1

Risk Factors for Preterm Labor—cont'd

- Substance abuse (e.g., alcohol or illicit drugs, especially cocaine)
- Inadequate prenatal care
- Commutes of more than 1½ hours each way
- Excessive physical activity (heavy physical work, prolonged standing, heavy lifting, or young child care)
- Excessive lifestyle stressors

From Cunningham, F. et al. (2005). *Williams Obstetrics* (22nd Ed). New York: McGraw-Hill; Gilbert, E., & Harmon, J. (2003). *Manual of high risk pregnancy and delivery* (3rd ed.). St. Louis: Mosby; Iams, J. (2002). Preterm birth. In S. Gabbe, J. Niebyl, & G. Simpson (Eds.), *Obstetrics: Normal and problem pregnancies* (4th ed.). New York: Churchill Livingstone; Martin, J. et al. (2003). Births: Final data for 2002. *National Vital Statistics Report, 52*(10), 1-113; Moore, M. (2003). Preterm labor and birth: What have we learned in the past two decades? *Journal of Obstetric, Gynecologic, and Neonatal Nursing 32*(5), 638-649.

woman in the home. The testing is done every 2 weeks for about 10 weeks. This marker also has a high negative predictive value (98%) and a lower positive predictive value (7% to 25%).

—Another possible predictor of imminent preterm labor is endocervical length determined by vaginal ultrasound. Women whose cervical length is 35 mm at 24 to 28 weeks of gestation are more likely to have a preterm birth than women whose cervical length exceeds 40 mm.

Care Management

- The onset of preterm labor is often insidious and can be easily mistaken for normal discomforts of pregnancy or Braxton Hicks contractions.

Interventions

- *Prevention.* One of the most important nursing interventions aimed at preventing preterm birth is the education of pregnant women about the early symptoms of preterm labor, so

BOX 12-2

Signs and Symptoms of Preterm Labor

UTERINE ACTIVITY
- Uterine contractions more frequent than every 10 minutes persisting for 1 hour or more
- Uterine contractions may be painful or painless

DISCOMFORT
- Lower abdominal cramping similar to gas pains; may be accompanied by diarrhea
- Dull, intermittent low back pain (below the waist)
- Painful, menstrual-like cramps
- Suprapubic pain or pressure
- Pelvic pressure or heaviness
- Urinary frequency

VAGINAL DISCHARGE
- Change in character and amount of usual discharge: thicker (mucoid) or thinner (watery), bloody, brown or colorless, increased amount, odor
- Rupture of amniotic membranes

that if symptoms occur the woman can be referred promptly to her care provider for more intensive care (Box 12-2).

- *Lifestyle modifications.* Nurses caring for women with symptoms of preterm labor should question the woman about whether she has symptoms when engaged in any of the following activities and to consider stopping those activities until 37 weeks of pregnancy when preterm birth is no longer a risk:
  - Sexual activity
  - Riding long distances in automobiles, trains, or buses
  - Carrying heavy loads, such as laundry, groceries, or a small child
  - Standing more than 50% of the time
  - Heavy housework
  - Climbing stairs
  - Hard physical work
  - Being unable to stop and rest when tired

- *Bed rest and home care.* Women who are at high risk for preterm birth commonly are told that it would be best if they were at home on bed rest for weeks or months.

  - The woman's environment can be modified for convenience by using tables and storage units around her bed to keep essential items within reach (e.g., telephone, television, radio, tape or CD player, computer with Internet access, snacks, books, magazines, newspapers, and items for hobbies).

  - Ensuring that the bed or couch is near a window and the bathroom is also helpful. Covering the bed with an egg crate mattress can relieve discomfort.

  - Women often find that a daily schedule of meals, activities, and hygiene and grooming (e.g., shower, dressing in street clothes, and applying make-up) that they create reduces boredom and helps them maintain control and normalcy.

  - Limiting naps, eating smaller but more frequent meals, and performing gentle range of motion exercises can help to reduce some of the detrimental effects of bed rest.

- *Tocolytic agents.* The use of tocolytic agents (medications that suppress uterine activity) may be considered in an attempt to prevent preterm birth. Once uterine contractions are suppressed, maintenance therapy may be implemented in an attempt to continue the suppression, or tocolytic treatment can be discontinued and resumed only if uterine contractions begin again.

  - It is now thought that the best reason to use tocolytic medications is that they afford the opportunity to begin administering antenatal glucocorticoids to accelerate fetal lung maturity and reduce the severity of sequelae in infants born preterm.

  - Medications used for this purpose include ritodrine (Yutopar), terbutaline (Brethine), magnesium sulfate (most commonly used), indomethacin (Indocin), and nifedipine (Procardia).

  - Because these medications have the potential for serious adverse reactions for mother and fetus, close nursing supervision during treatment is critical (Box 12-3 and see Medication Guide in Appendix B–Tocolytic Therapy).

> **BOX 12-3**
>
> ## Nursing Care for Women Receiving Tocolytic Therapy
>
> - Explain the purpose and side effects of tocolytic therapy to woman and her family.
> - Position woman on her side to enhance placental perfusion and reduce pressure on the cervix.
> - Monitor maternal vital signs, fetal heart rate (FHR), and labor status according to hospital protocol and professional standards.
> - Assess mother and fetus for signs of adverse reactions related to the tocolytic being administered.
> - Determine maternal fluid balance by measuring daily weight and intake and output (I&O).
> - Limit fluid intake to 2500 to 3000 ml/day, especially if a beta-adrenergic agonist is being administered.
> - Provide psychosocial support and opportunities for woman and family to express feelings and concerns.
> - Offer comfort measures as required.
> - Encourage diversional activities and relaxation techniques.

- *Promotion of fetal lung maturity.* Antenatal glucocorticoids given as intramuscular injections to the mother accelerate fetal lung maturity. All women between 24 and 34 weeks of gestation should be given antenatal glucocorticoids when preterm birth is threatened, unless there is a medical indication for immediate delivery such as cord prolapse, chorioamnionitis, or abruptio placentae. The regimen for administration of antenatal glucocorticoids is given in the Medication Guide in Appendix B—Betamethasone, Dexamethasone.

PRETERM PREMATURE RUPTURE OF MEMBRANES

Clinical Manifestations

Premature rupture of membranes (PROM) is the rupture of the amniotic sac and leakage of amniotic fluid beginning at least 1 hour before the onset of labor at any gestational age. Preterm premature rupture of the membranes (PPROM) (i.e., membranes rupture before 37 weeks of gestation) occurs in up to 25% of all cases of preterm labor. Infection often precedes PPROM, but the etiology of PPROM remains unknown. PPROM is diagnosed after the woman complains of either a sudden gush of fluid from the vagina or a slow leak of fluid from the vagina.

Infection is the serious side effect of PPROM that makes it a major complication of pregnancy. Chorioamnionitis is an intraamniotic infection of the chorion and amnion that is potentially life threatening for the fetus and the woman.

Care Management

Whenever PPROM is suspected, a Nitrazine or fern test is used to determine if the discharge is amniotic fluid or urine. Expectant management will continue as long as there are no signs of infection or fetal distress.

- Frequent biophysical profiles are performed to determine fetal health status and estimate amniotic fluid volume.
- The woman with PPROM also should be taught how to count fetal movements daily, because a slowing of fetal movement has been shown to be a precursor to severe fetal compromise.
- Signs of infection (e.g., fever, foul-smelling vaginal discharge, or rapid pulse) should be reported to the primary health care provider immediately.

DYSTOCIA

- Dystocia is defined as long, difficult, or abnormal labor; it is caused by any of the following:
  - Dysfunctional labor, resulting in ineffective uterine contractions or maternal bearing-down efforts (the powers): the most common cause of dystocia
  - Alterations in the pelvic structure (the passage)
  - Fetal causes, including abnormal presentation or position, anomalies, excessive size, and number of fetuses (the passenger)
  - Maternal position during labor and birth

—Psychologic responses of the mother to labor related to past experiences, preparation, culture and heritage, and support system
- Dystocia is suspected when there is an alteration in the characteristics of uterine contractions, a lack of progress in the rate of cervical dilation, or a lack of progress in fetal descent and expulsion.

Dysfunctional Labor

- A number of factors seem to increase a woman's risk for uterine dystocia, including the following:
  —Body build (e.g., 13.6 kg or more overweight or short stature)
  —Uterine abnormalities (e.g., congenital malformations; overdistention, as with multiple gestation; or hydramnios)
  —Malpresentations and positions of the fetus
  —Cephalopelvic disproportion (CPD)
  —Overstimulation with oxytocin
  —Maternal fatigue, dehydration and electrolyte imbalance, and fear
  —Inappropriate timing of analgesic or anesthetic administration

CARE MANAGEMENT

Assessment

Risk assessment is a continuous process in the laboring woman. The initial physical assessment and ongoing assessments provide information about maternal well-being; status of labor in terms of the characteristics of uterine contractions and progress of cervical effacement and dilation; fetal well-being in terms of fetal heart rate (FHR) and pattern, presentation, station, and position; and status of the amniotic membranes.

Interventions

Interventions that the nurse may implement or assist with include external cephalic version (ECV), trial of labor, cervical ripening with prostaglandins, induction or augmentation with oxytocin, amniotomy, and operative procedures (e.g., forceps- or vacuum-assisted birth).

External cephalic version (ECV)

- ECV is used to attempt to turn the fetus from a breech or shoulder presentation to a vertex presentation for birth. It may be attempted in a labor and birth setting after 37 weeks of gestation.

- ECV is accomplished by the exertion of gentle, constant pressure on the abdomen. Before it is attempted, ultrasound scanning is done to determine the fetal position; locate the umbilical cord; rule out placenta previa; evaluate the adequacy of the maternal pelvis; and assess the amount of amniotic fluid, the fetal age, and the presence of any anomalies.

- A nonstress test (NST) is performed to confirm fetal well-being, or the FHR pattern is monitored for a period of time (i.e., 10 to 20 minutes). Informed consent is obtained.

- A tocolytic agent such as magnesium sulfate or terbutaline often is given to relax the uterus and to facilitate the maneuver.

- During an attempted ECV, the nurse continuously monitors the FHR and pattern, especially for bradycardia and variable decelerations; checks the maternal vital signs; and assesses the woman's level of comfort because the procedure may cause discomfort.

- After the procedure is completed, the nurse continues to monitor maternal vital signs, uterine activity, and FHR and pattern and assess for vaginal bleeding until the woman's condition is stable.

- Women who are Rh negative should receive Rh immune globulin because the manipulation can cause fetomaternal bleeding.

Trial of labor

- A trial of labor (TOL) is the observance of a woman and her fetus for a reasonable period (e.g., 4 to 6 hours) of spontaneous active labor to assess safety of vaginal birth for the mother and infant.

- It may be initiated if the mother's pelvis is of questionable size or shape, if the fetus is in an abnormal presentation, or if the mother wishes to have a vaginal birth after a previous cesarean birth.

- Fetal sonography, maternal pelvimetry, or both may be done before a TOL to rule out CPD. The cervix must be ripe (e.g., soft and dilatable).
- During a TOL, the woman is evaluated for the occurrence of active labor, including adequate contractions, engagement and descent of the presenting part, and effacement and dilation of the cervix.
- The nurse assesses maternal vital signs and FHR and pattern and is alert for signs of potential complications. If complications develop, the nurse is responsible for initiating appropriate actions, including notifying the primary health care provider, and for evaluating and documenting the maternal and fetal responses to the interventions.
- Supporting and encouraging the woman and her partner and providing information regarding progress can reduce stress and enhance the labor process and facilitate a successful outcome.

Induction of labor
- Induction of labor is the chemical or mechanical initiation of uterine contractions before their spontaneous onset for the purpose of bringing about the birth.
- Intravenous oxytocin and amniotomy are the most common methods used in the United States. Prostaglandins are increasingly used for inducing labor.
- Less commonly used methods include stripping of membranes, nipple stimulation (manual or with a breast pump), and acupuncture. The ingestion of a laxative (e.g., castor oil), herbal preparations (e.g., green, chamomile, or raspberry tea; blue or black cohosh), or spicy food and administration of a soapsuds enema are other methods.
- Success rates for induction of labor are higher when the condition of the cervix is favorable, or inducible. A rating system such as the Bishop score (Table 12-1) can be used to evaluate the ability to be induced. For example, a score of 9 or more on this 13-point scale indicates that the cervix is soft, anterior, 50% or more effaced, and dilated 2 cm or more and that the presenting part is engaged. Induction of labor is likely to be more successful if the score is 9 or more for nulliparas and 5 or more for multiparas.

TABLE 12-1

Bishop Score

	SCORE			
	0	**1**	**2**	**3**
Dilation (cm)	0	1-2	3-4	≥5
Effacement (%)	0-30	40-50	60-70	≥80
Station (cm)	−3	−2	−1	+1, +2
Cervical consistency		Firm	Medium	Soft
Cervix position	Posterior	Midposition	Anterior	Anterior

Cervical ripening methods. Preparations of prostaglandin E_1 and prostaglandin E_2 can be used before induction to "ripen" (soften and thin) the cervix (see Medication Guides in Appendix B–Cytotec, Prepidil). Mechanical dilators ripen the cervix by stimulating the release of endogenous prostaglandins. Balloon catheters (e.g., Foley catheter) can be inserted into the intracervical canal to ripen and dilate the cervix. Hydroscopic dilators (substances that absorb fluid from surrounding tissues and then enlarge) also can be used for cervical ripening. Laminaria tents (natural cervical dilators made from desiccated seaweed) and synthetic dilators containing magnesium sulfate (Lamicel) are inserted into the endocervix without rupturing the membranes. As they absorb fluid, they expand and cause cervical dilation. These dilators are left in place for 6 to 12 hours before being removed to assess cervical dilation.

Amniotomy. Amniotomy (i.e., artificial rupture of membranes [AROM]) can be used to induce labor when the condition of the cervix is favorable (ripe) or to augment labor if progress begins to slow. Labor usually begins within 12 hours of the rupture. Before the procedure, the woman should be told what to expect; she also should be assured that the actual rupture of the membranes is painless for her and the fetus, although she may experience some discomfort when the Amnihook or other sharp instrument is inserted through the vagina and cervix (see Procedure box).

Procedure

Assisting with Amniotomy

PROCEDURE

Explain to the woman what will be done.

Assess fetal heart rate (FHR) before procedure begins to obtain a baseline reading.

Place several underpads under the woman's buttocks to absorb the fluid.

Position the woman on a padded bedpan, fracture pan, or rolled-up towel to elevate her hips.

Assist the health care provider who is performing the procedure by providing sterile gloves and lubricant for the vaginal examination.

Unwrap sterile package containing Amnihook or Allis clamp, and pass instrument to the primary health care provider, who inserts it alongside the fingers and then hooks and tears the membranes.

Reassess the FHR.

Assess the color, consistency, and odor of the fluid.

Assess the woman's temperature every 2 hours or per protocol.

Evaluate the woman for signs and symptoms of infection.

DOCUMENTATION

Record the following:

Time of rupture

Color, odor, and consistency of the fluid

FHR before and after the procedure

Maternal status (how well procedure was tolerated)

Oxytocin. Oxytocin is a hormone normally produced by the posterior pituitary gland; it stimulates uterine contractions. It may be used either to induce labor or to augment a labor that is progressing slowly because of inadequate uterine contractions.

• The indications for oxytocin induction or augmentation of labor may include, but are not limited to, the following:

  —Suspected fetal jeopardy (e.g., intrauterine growth restriction [IUGR])

  —Inadequate uterine contractions; dystocia

  —PROM

  —Postterm pregnancy

−Chorioamnionitis
−Maternal medical problems (e.g., woman with severe Rh isoimmunization, inadequately controlled diabetes mellitus, chronic renal disease, or chronic pulmonary disease)
−Severe preeclampsia (eclampsia)
−Fetal death
−Multiparous women with a history of precipitate labor or who live far from the hospital
- Contraindications to oxytocin stimulation of labor include, but are not limited to, the following:
  −CPD, prolapsed cord, or transverse lie
  −Nonreassuring FHR
  −Placenta previa or vasa previa
  −Prior classic uterine incision or uterine surgery
  −Active genital herpes infection
  −Invasive cancer of the cervix
- The primary health care provider orders induction or augmentation of labor with oxytocin. The nurse implements the order by initiating the primary intravenous infusion and administering the oxytocin solution through a secondary line. The nurse's actions related to assessment and care of a woman whose labor is being induced are guided by hospital protocol and professional standards (Box 12-4).
  −A commonly recommended initial dosage is 0.5 to 1 milliunits/min with increments of 1 to 2 milliunits/min every 15 to 60 minutes because 30 to 40 minutes is required for a steady state of oxytocin to be reached and for the full effect of a dosage increment to be reflected in more intense, frequent, and longer contractions.

Augmentation of labor. Augmentation of labor is the stimulation of uterine contractions after labor has started spontaneously but progress is unsatisfactory. Common augmentation methods include oxytocin infusion, amniotomy, and nipple stimulation. Noninvasive methods such as emptying the bladder, ambulation and position changes, relaxation measures, nourishment and hydration, and hydrotherapy should be attempted before invasive interventions are initiated. The administration procedure and nursing assessment and care measures for augmentation of labor with oxytocin are similar to those used for induction of labor with oxytocin.

BOX 12-4

Protocol: Induction of Labor with Oxytocin

PATIENT/FAMILY TEACHING
- Explain technique, rationale, and reactions to expect
  —Route and rate for administration of medication
  —What "piggyback" is for
  —Reasons for use: induce or improve labor
  —Reactions to expect concerning the nature of contractions: the intensity of contraction increases more rapidly, holds the peak longer, and ends more quickly; contractions will come regularly and more often
- Monitoring to anticipate
  —Maternal: blood pressure, pulse, uterine contractions, and uterine tone
  —Fetal: heart rate and activity
- Success to expect: a favorable outcome will depend on whether the cervix can be induced (e.g., Bishop score of 9)
- Keep woman and support person informed of progress

ADMINISTRATION
- Position woman in side-lying or upright position
- Assess status of maternal-fetal unit
- Prepare solutions and administer with pump delivery system according to prescribed orders
  —Infusion pump and solution are set up (e.g., 10 units/1000 ml isotonic electrolyte solution)
  —Piggyback solution is connected to IV line at proximal port (port nearest point of venous insertion)
  —Solution with oxytocin is flagged with a medication label
  —Begin induction at 0.5 to 1 milliunits/min
  —Increase dose 1 to 2 milliunits/min at intervals of 15 to 60 minutes until a dose of up to 20 to 40 milliunits/min is reached

MAINTAIN DOSE IF:
- Intensity of contractions results in intrauterine pressures of 40 to 90 mm Hg (shown by internal monitor)
- Duration of contractions is 40 to 90 seconds

BOX 12-4

Protocol: Induction of Labor with Oxytocin—cont'd

- Frequency of contractions is 2- to 3-minute intervals
- Cervical dilation of 1 cm/hr in the active phase

MATERNAL-FETAL ASSESSMENTS

- Monitor blood pressure, pulse, and respirations every 30 to 60 minutes and with every increment in dose
- Monitor contraction pattern and uterine resting tone every 15 minutes and with every increment in dose
- Assess intake and output; limit IV intake to 1000 ml/8 hr; output should be 120 ml or more every 4 hours
- Perform vaginal examination as indicated
- Monitor for nausea, vomiting, headache, and hypotension
- Assess fetal status using electronic fetal monitoring; evaluate tracing every 15 minutes and with every increment in dose
- Observe emotional responses of woman and her partner

REPORTABLE CONDITIONS

- Uterine hyperstimulation
- Nonreassuring FHR pattern
- Suspected uterine rupture
- Inadequate uterine response at 20 milliunits/min

EMERGENCY MEASURES

- Discontinue use of oxytocin per hospital protocol
  —Turn woman on her side
  —Increase primary IV rate up to 200 ml/hr, unless patient has water intoxication, in which case, the rate is decreased to one that keeps the vein open
  —Give woman oxygen by face mask at 8 to 10 L/min or per protocol or physician's or nurse-midwife's order

DOCUMENTATION

- Medication: kind, amount, time of beginning, increasing dose, maintaining dose, and discontinuing medication in patient record and on monitor strip

Continued

BOX 12-4

Protocol: Induction of Labor with Oxytocin—cont'd

- Reactions of mother and fetus
  —Pattern of labor
  —Progress of labor
  —FHR and pattern
  —Maternal vital signs
- Nursing interventions and woman's response
- Notification of physician or nurse-midwife

From: Ruchata, P., Metheby, N., Essenpreis, H., & Borcherding, K. (2002). Current practices in oxytocin dilution and fluid administration for induction of labor. *Journal of Obstetric, Gynecologic, and Neonatal Nursing, 31*(5), 545-550; Simpson, K. (2002). *Cervical ripening and induction and augmentation of labor.* (2nd ed). Washington, DC: Association of Women's Health, Obstetric and Neonatal Nursing (AWHONN).
FHR, Fetal heart rate; *IV,* intravenous.

- Some physicians advocate active management of labor, that is, the augmentation of labor to establish efficient labor with the aggressive use of oxytocin so that the woman gives birth within 12 hours of admission to the labor unit. Advocates of active management believe that intervening early (as soon as a nulliparous labor is not progressing at least 1 cm/hr) with use of higher pharmacologic oxytocin doses administered at frequent increment intervals (e.g., a starting dose of 6 milliunits/min with increases of 6 milliunits/min every 15 minutes to a maximum dose of 40 milliunits/min) shortens labor and is associated with a lower incidence of cesarean birth.
  —Additional components of the active management of labor include strict criteria to diagnose that the woman is in active labor with 100% effacement, amniotomy within 1 hour of admission of a woman in labor if spontaneous rupture of the membranes has not occurred, and continuous presence of a personal nurse who provides one-on-one care for the woman while she is in labor.

Forceps-assisted birth

- A forceps-assisted birth is one in which an instrument with two curved blades is used to assist in the birth of the fetal head.

–Maternal indications for forceps-assisted birth include the need to shorten the second stage of labor in the event of dystocia or to compensate for the woman's deficient expulsive efforts (e.g., if she is tired or has been given spinal or epidural anesthesia) or to reverse a dangerous condition (e.g., cardiac decompensation).

–Fetal indications include birth of a fetus in distress or in certain abnormal presentations, arrest of rotation, or delivery of the head in a breech presentation. The use of forceps during childbirth has been decreasing.

–Certain conditions are required for a forceps-assisted birth to be successful. The woman's cervix must be fully dilated to avert lacerations and hemorrhage. The bladder should be empty. The presenting part must be engaged, and a vertex presentation is desired. Membranes must be ruptured so that the position of the fetal head can be determined and the forceps can firmly grasp the head during birth. If a decrease in FHR occurs, the primary health care provider removes and reapplies the forceps.

Nursing considerations. When a forceps-assisted birth is deemed necessary, the nurse obtains the type of forceps requested by the primary health care provider. The nurse usually coaches the woman not to push during contractions unless the primary health care provider instructs the woman to push as traction is being applied during contractions.

–After birth, the mother is assessed for vaginal and cervical lacerations (e.g., bleeding that occurs even with a contracted uterus); urine retention, which may result from bladder or urethral injuries; and hematoma formation in the pelvic soft tissues, which may result from blood vessel damage.

–The infant should be assessed for bruising or abrasions at the site of the blade applications, facial palsy resulting from pressure of the blades on the facial nerve (cranial nerve VII), and subdural hematoma. Newborn and postpartum caregivers should be told that a forceps-assisted birth was performed.

Vacuum-assisted birth

• Vacuum-assisted birth, or vacuum extraction, is a birth method involving the attachment of a vacuum cup to the fetal head, using negative pressure to assist in the birth of the head. Indications for its use are similar to those for outlet forceps.

- Prerequisites for use include a vertex presentation, ruptured membranes, and absence of CPD.
- The cup is applied to the fetal head, and a caput develops inside the cup as the pressure is initiated. Traction is applied to facilitate descent of the fetal head, and the woman is encouraged to push as suction is applied. As the head crowns, an episiotomy is performed if necessary. The vacuum cup is released and removed after birth of the head.
- Risks to the newborn include cephalhematoma, scalp lacerations, and subdural hematoma.
  - Fetal complications can be reduced by strict adherence to the manufacturer's recommendations for method of application, degree of suction, and duration of application.
- Maternal complications are uncommon but can include perineal, vaginal, or cervical lacerations and soft-tissue hematomas.

  Nursing considerations. The nurse can prepare the woman for birth and encourage her to remain active in the birth process by pushing during contractions.

- The FHR should be assessed frequently during the procedure.
- After birth, the newborn should be observed for signs of trauma and infection at the application site and for cerebral irritation (e.g., poor sucking or listlessness).
- The newborn may be at risk for cephalhematoma and neonatal jaundice as bruising resolves.
- The parents may need to be reassured that the caput succedaneum will begin to disappear in a few hours. Neonatal caregivers should be told that the birth was vacuum assisted.

Cesarean birth

- Cesarean birth is the birth of a fetus through a transabdominal incision of the uterus. Spinal, epidural, and general anesthetics are used for cesarean births.
- The labor management approach that most consistently reduces cesarean birth rates is one-to-one support of the laboring woman by another woman such as a nurse, nurse-midwife, or doula.

Indications. The most common indications for cesarean birth are related to labor and birth complications, including CPD, malpresentations such as breech and shoulder, placental abnormalities (e.g., previa or abruptio), dysfunctional labor pattern, umbilical cord prolapse, fetal distress, and multiple gestation. Medical risk factors most closely associated with cesarean birth include hypertensive disorders, active genital herpes, positive human immunodeficiency virus (HIV) status, and diabetes.

Complications and risks. Maternal complications include aspiration, pulmonary embolism, wound infection, wound dehiscence, thrombophlebitis, hemorrhage, urinary tract infection, injuries to the bladder or bowel, and complications related to anesthesia. The fetus may be born prematurely if the gestational age has not been accurately determined; fetal injuries can occur during the surgery.

Preoperative care. Family-centered care is the goal for the woman who is to undergo cesarean birth and for her family. The primary health care provider discusses with the woman and her family the need for the cesarean birth and the prognosis for the mother and infant. The anesthesiologist assesses the woman's cardiopulmonary system and describes the options for anesthesia. Informed consent is obtained for the procedure.

–Blood and urine tests are usually done 1 or 2 days before a planned cesarean birth or on admission to the labor unit. Laboratory tests, most commonly ordered to establish baseline data, include a complete blood cell count and chemistry, blood typing and crossmatching, and urinalysis.

–Maternal vital signs and blood pressure and FHR and pattern continue to be assessed per the hospital routine until the operation begins. Physical preoperative preparation usually includes inserting a retention catheter to keep the bladder empty and administering prescribed preoperative medications. The primary health care provider may order an abdominal-mons shave or a clipping of pubic hair, although this is uncommon. In the event that general anesthesia will be needed, an antacid may be administered orally to neutralize gastric secretions in case of aspiration. Intravenous fluids are started to maintain hydration and to provide an open line for the administration of blood or medications if needed.

—Removal of dentures, nail polish, and jewelry may be optional, depending on hospital policies and type of anesthesia used. If the woman wears glasses and is going to be awake, the nurse should make sure her glasses accompany her to the operating room so she can see her infant. If the woman wears contact lenses, the nurse can find out whether they can be worn for the birth.

—During the preoperative preparation, the support person is encouraged to remain with the woman to provide continuing emotional support.

—The nurse provides essential information about the preoperative procedures during this time. Although the nursing actions may be carried out quickly if a cesarean birth is unplanned, verbal communication, particularly explanations, is important. Silence can be frightening to the woman and her support person. The nurse's use of touch can communicate feelings of care and concern for the woman.

Intraoperative care. Cesarean births occur in operating rooms in the surgical suite or in the labor and birth unit. If possible, the partner accompanies the woman. If the partner is not allowed or chooses not to be present, the nurse can stay in communication with him or her and give progress reports whenever possible.

—The nurse who is circulating may assist with positioning the woman on the birth (surgical) table. It is important to position her so that the uterus is displaced laterally to prevent compression of the inferior vena cava, which causes decreased placental perfusion. This is usually accomplished by placing a wedge under the hip.

—Care of the infant usually is delegated to a pediatrician or a nurse team skilled in neonatal resuscitation because these infants are considered to be at risk until there is evidence of physiologic stability after the birth.

—After birth, if the infant's condition permits and the mother is awake, the baby may be placed skin-to-skin on the mother or can be given to the woman's partner to hold. The infant whose condition is compromised is transported after initial stabilization to the nursery for observation and the implementation of appropriate interventions.

Immediate postoperative care. Once surgery is completed, the mother is transferred to a recovery room or back to her labor room. Nursing assessments in this immediate post-birth period follow agency protocol and include degree of recovery from the effects of anesthesia, postoperative and post-birth status, and degree of pain. A patent airway is maintained, and the woman is positioned to prevent possible aspiration. Vital signs are taken every 15 minutes for 1 to 2 hours or until stable. The condition of the incisional dressing, the fundus, and the amount of lochia is assessed, as well as the intravenous intake and the urine output through the Foley catheter. The woman is helped to turn and do coughing, deep-breathing, and leg exercises. Medications to relieve pain may be administered.

–If the baby is present, the mother and her partner are given some time alone with him or her to facilitate bonding and attachment. Breastfeeding can be initiated if the mother feels like trying.

–If the woman is in a recovery area or in her labor room, she usually is transferred to the postpartum unit after 1 to 2 hours or once her condition is stable and the effects of anesthesia have worn off.

Postoperative/postpartum care. The women's physiologic concerns for the first few days may be dominated by pain at the incision site and pain resulting from intestinal gas, and hence the need for pain relief. If epidural anesthesia was used for the surgery, epidural opioids can be given in the immediate postoperative period to provide pain relief for approximately 24 hours. Otherwise, pain medications usually are given every 3 to 4 hours, or patient-controlled analgesia may be ordered instead. Other comfort measures such as position changes, splinting of the incision with pillows, and relaxation and breathing techniques (e.g., those learned in childbirth classes) may be implemented (see Teaching Guidelines box).

–Daily care includes perineal care, breast care, and routine hygienic care, including showering after the dressing has been removed. The nurse assesses the woman's vital signs, incision, fundus, and lochia according to hospital policies, procedures, or protocols. Breath sounds, bowel sounds, circulatory status of lower extremities, and urinary and bowel

TEACHING GUIDELINES

Postpartum Pain Relief after Cesarean Birth

INCISIONAL
- Splint incision with a pillow when moving or coughing.
- Use relaxation techniques such as music, breathing, and dim lights.
- Apply a heating pad to the abdomen.

GAS
- Walk as often as you can.
- Do not eat or drink gas-forming foods, carbonated beverages, or whole milk.
- Do not use straws for drinking fluids.
- Take antiflatulence medication if prescribed.
- Lie on your left side to expel gas.
- Rock in a rocking chair.

elimination also are assessed. It is important to note maternal emotional status.

- Discharge teaching and planning should include information about nutrition; measures to relieve pain and discomfort; exercise and specific activity restrictions; time management that includes periods of uninterrupted rest and sleep; hygiene, breast, and incision care; timing for resumption of sexual activity and contraception; signs of complications (see Patient Instructions for Self-Care: Signs of Postoperative Complications After Discharge box); and infant care. The nurse assesses the woman's need for continued support or counseling to facilitate her emotional recovery from the birth. Referral to support groups or to community agencies may be indicated to promote the recovery process further.

Vaginal birth after cesarean

- A woman who has had a cesarean birth may subsequently become pregnant and not have any contraindications to labor and vaginal birth in that pregnancy and may attempt a vaginal birth after cesarean (VBAC).

PATIENT INSTRUCTIONS FOR SELF-CARE

Signs of Postoperative Complications after Discharge

Report the following signs to your health care provider:
- Temperature exceeding 38° C
- Painful urination
- Lochia heavier than a normal period
- Wound separation
- Redness or oozing at the incision site
- Severe abdominal pain

- Vaginal birth is relatively safe, but there is risk for uterine rupture through a lower uterine segment scar. Labor and vaginal birth are not recommended if there are contraindications, such as a previous fundal classic cesarean scar, a scar from uterine surgery, or evidence of CPD. Women are strongly advised against attempting VBACs in birth centers because the health risks are too great.

- This labor should occur in a hospital facility that has the equipment and personnel available to begin the surgery within 30 minutes from the time a decision is made to perform cesarean birth. There is no evidence that administering oxytocin to induce or augment labor or the use of epidural anesthesia is contraindicated, although caution and close monitoring of the laboring woman are urged if these are used. However, use of prostaglandins, especially misoprostol (prostaglandin E$_1$), to ripen the cervix or induce labor is not recommended because they have been associated with an increased risk for uterine rupture.

POSTTERM PREGNANCY, LABOR, AND BIRTH

Clinical Manifestations

- A postterm or postdate pregnancy is one that extends beyond the end of week 42 of gestation, or 294 days from the first day of the last menstrual period.

–Clinical manifestations of postterm pregnancy include maternal weight loss (more than 1.4 kg/wk) and decreased uterine size (related to decreased amniotic fluid), meconium in the amniotic fluid, and advanced bone maturation of the fetal skeleton with an exceptionally hard fetal skull.

- Maternal risks often related to the birth of an excessively large infant include:
  –Dysfunctional labor
  –Birth canal trauma, including perineal lacerations and extension of episiotomy during vaginal birth
  –Postpartum hemorrhage
  –Infection
- Interventions such as induction of labor with prostaglandins or oxytocin, forceps- or vacuum-assisted birth, and cesarean birth are more likely to be necessary.
- Fetal risks appear to be twofold:
  –First is the possibility of prolonged labor, shoulder dystocia, birth trauma, and asphyxia from macrosomia
  –Second are the compromising effects on the fetus of an "aging" placenta. Placental function gradually decreases after 37 weeks of gestation, and amniotic fluid volume (AFV) declines to about 400 ml by 42 weeks of gestation. The resulting oligohydramnios can lead to fetal hypoxia related to cord compression.
- Neonatal problems may include asphyxia, meconium aspiration syndrome, dysmaturity syndrome, hypoglycemia, polycythemia, and respiratory distress. Whether an infant born after a postterm pregnancy has neurologic, behavioral, intellectual, or developmental problems must be investigated further.

Collaborative Care

- The management of postterm pregnancy is still controversial. The induction of labor at 41 to 42 weeks is suggested by some authorities as a means of reducing the rate of cesarean birth and stillbirth or neonatal death. Others follow a more individualized approach, allowing the pregnancy to proceed to 43 weeks of gestation as long as assessment of fetal well-being with a combination of tests is performed, and the results of the tests are normal. Tests are usually performed on a weekly or twice-weekly basis.

- Antepartum assessments for postterm pregnancy may include daily fetal movement counts, NSTs, amniotic fluid volume (AFV) assessments, contraction stress tests (CSTs), biophysical profiles (BPPs), and Doppler flow measurements.
- Cervical checks usually are performed weekly after 40 weeks of gestation to determine whether the condition of the cervix is favorable for induction (5 or greater on the Bishop score for multiparas and 9 or more for nulliparas) (see Table 12-1).
- During the postterm period, the woman is encouraged to assess fetal activity daily, assess for signs of labor, and keep appointments with her primary health care provider.
- If the woman's cervix is favorable, labor is usually induced with oxytocin. If not, continued fetal surveillance or a cervical ripening agent (e.g., prostaglandin insert or gel) may be administered, followed by oxytocin induction.
- The fetus of a woman with a postterm pregnancy should be monitored electronically for a more accurate assessment of the FHR and pattern. Fetal scalp pH sampling or fetal oxygen saturation monitoring may be done to determine whether acidosis is occurring. Inadequate fluid volume leads to compression of the cord, which results in fetal hypoxia that is reflected in variable or prolonged deceleration patterns and passage of meconium. If oligohydramnios is present, an amnioinfusion may be performed to restore AFV to maintain a cushioning of the cord.
- A vaginal birth is anticipated, but the couple should be prepared for a forceps-assisted, vacuum-assisted, or cesarean birth if complications arise.

OBSTETRIC EMERGENCIES

Shoulder Dystocia

Clinical manifestations

- Shoulder dystocia is a condition in which the head is born, but the anterior shoulder cannot pass under the pubic arch. Fetopelvic disproportion related to excessive fetal size (greater than 4000 g) or maternal pelvic abnormalities may be a cause of shoulder dystocia, although shoulder dystocia can occur in the absence of any known risk factors.
- The nurse should observe for signs that could indicate the presence of shoulder dystocia, including slowing of the

progress of labor and formation of a caput succedaneum that increases in size. When the head emerges, it retracts against the perineum (turtle sign), and external rotation does not occur.

- The fetus/newborn is more likely to experience birth injuries related to asphyxia, brachial plexus damage, and fracture, especially of the humerus or clavicle.
- The mother's primary risk stems from excessive blood loss as a result of uterine atony or rupture, lacerations, extension of the episiotomy, or endometritis.

Collaborative Care

- Many maneuvers, such as suprapubic pressure and maternal position changes, have been suggested and tried to free the anterior shoulder, although no one particular maneuver has been found to be most effective. Suprapubic pressure can be applied to the anterior shoulder by using the Mazzanti or Rubin technique (Fig. 12-1, *A* and *B*) in an attempt to push the shoulder under the symphysis pubis.
- In the McRoberts maneuver (see Fig. 12-1, *C*), the woman's legs are flexed apart, with her knees on her abdomen. This maneuver causes the sacrum to straighten, and the symphysis pubis rotates toward the mother's head; the angle of pelvic inclination is decreased, freeing the shoulder. Suprapubic pressure can be applied at this time. The McRoberts maneuver is the preferred method when a woman is receiving epidural anesthesia.
- Having the woman move to a hands-and-knees position (the Gaskin maneuver), a squatting position, or a lateral recumbent position also has been used to resolve cases of shoulder dystocia.
- Fundal pressure is usually not advised as a method of relieving shoulder dystocia.
- When shoulder dystocia is diagnosed, the nurse helps the woman to assume the position or positions that may facilitate birth of the shoulders, assists the primary health care provider with these maneuvers and techniques during birth, and documents the maneuvers. The nurse also provides encouragement and support to reduce anxiety and fear.

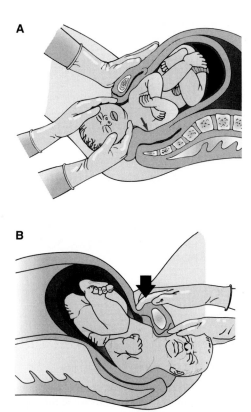

Fig. 12-1 Application of suprapubic pressure. **A,** Mazzanti technique. Pressure is applied directly posteriorly and laterally above the symphysis pubis. **B,** Rubin technique. Pressure is applied obliquely posteriorly against the anterior shoulder.

Continued

- Newborn assessment should include examination for fracture of the clavicle or humerus as well as brachial plexus injuries and asphyxia.
- Maternal assessment should focus on early detection of hemorrhage and trauma to the soft tissue of the birth canal.

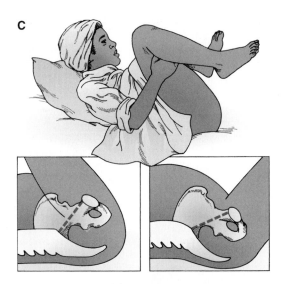

Fig. 12-1, *cont'd* **C,** McRoberts maneuver. (**C** modified from Gabbe, S., Niebyl, J., & Simpson, J. [2002]. *Obstetrics: Normal and problem pregnancies* [4th ed.]. New York: Churchill Livingstone.)

Prolapsed Umbilical Cord

Clinical manifestations

• Prolapse of the umbilical cord occurs when the cord lies below the presenting part of the fetus. Umbilical cord prolapse may be occult (hidden, not visible) at any time during labor whether or not the membranes are ruptured. It is most common to see frank (visible) prolapse directly after rupture of membranes, when gravity washes the cord in front of the presenting part. Contributing factors include a long cord (longer than 100 cm), malpresentation (breech), transverse lie, or unengaged presenting part.

Collaborative Care

• Prompt recognition of a prolapsed umbilical cord is important because fetal hypoxia resulting from prolonged cord compression (i.e., occlusion of blood flow to and from the fetus for more than 5 minutes) usually results in central nervous system damage or death of the fetus.

- Pressure on the cord may be relieved by the examiner putting a sterile gloved hand into the vagina and holding the presenting part off of the umbilical cord. The woman is assisted into a position such as a modified Sims, Trendelenburg, or knee-chest position, in which gravity keeps the pressure of the presenting part off the cord.

- If the cervix is fully dilated, a forceps- or vacuum-assisted birth can be performed for the fetus in a cephalic presentation; otherwise, a cesarean birth is likely to be performed. Nonreassuring FHR patterns, inadequate uterine relaxation, and bleeding also can occur as a result of a prolapsed umbilical cord.

- Indications for immediate interventions are presented in the Emergency box. Ongoing assessment of the woman and her fetus is critical to determine the effectiveness of each action taken.

Rupture of the Uterus
Clinical manifestations

- Rupture of the uterus is a rare but very serious obstetric injury. The most frequent causes of uterine rupture during pregnancy are separation of the scar of a previous classic cesarean birth, uterine trauma (e.g., accidents or surgery), and a congenital uterine anomaly. During labor and birth, uterine rupture may be caused by intense spontaneous uterine contractions, labor stimulation (e.g., oxytocin or prostaglandin), an overdistended uterus (e.g., multifetal gestation), malpresentation, external or internal version, or a difficult forceps-assisted birth. It occurs more commonly in multigravidas than in primigravidas.

- A uterine rupture is classified as either complete or incomplete. A complete rupture extends through the entire uterine wall into the peritoneal cavity or broad ligament. An incomplete rupture extends into the peritoneum but not into the peritoneal cavity or broad ligament. Bleeding is usually internal. An incomplete rupture also may be a partial separation at an old cesarean scar and may go unnoticed unless the woman undergoes a subsequent cesarean birth or other uterine surgery.

- Signs and symptoms vary with the extent of the rupture and may be silent or dramatic. In an incomplete rupture, pain may not be present.

EMERGENCY

Prolapsed Cord

SIGNS
- Fetal bradycardia with variable deceleration during uterine contraction signifies a prolapsed cord.
- Woman reports feeling the cord after membranes rupture.
- Cord is seen or felt in or protruding from the vagina.

INTERVENTIONS
- Call for assistance.
- Notify primary health care provider immediately.
- Glove the examining hand quickly and insert two fingers into the vagina to the cervix. With one finger on either side of the cord or both fingers to one side, exert upward pressure against the presenting part to relieve compression of the cord. Place a rolled towel under the woman's right or left hip.
- Place woman into the extreme Trendelenburg position, a modified Sims position, or a knee-chest position.
- If cord is protruding from vagina, wrap loosely in a sterile towel saturated with warm sterile normal saline solution.
- Administer oxygen to the woman by mask at 8 to 10 L/min until birth is accomplished.
- Start intravenous (IV) fluids or increase existing drip rate.
- Continue to monitor fetal heart rate (FHR) by internal fetal scalp electrode if possible.
- Explain to woman and support person what is happening and the way it is being managed.
- Prepare for immediate vaginal birth if cervix is fully dilated or cesarean birth if it is not.

–The fetus may or may not have late decelerations, decreased variability, an increased or decreased heart rate, or other nonreassuring signs.

–The woman may experience vomiting, faintness, increased abdominal tenderness, hypotonic uterine contractions, and lack of progress.

–Eventually, bleeding and the effects of blood loss will be noted.

—Fetal heart tones may be lost.

—In a complete rupture, the woman may complain of sudden, sharp, shooting abdominal pain and may state that "something gave way." If she is in labor, her contractions will cease, and pain is relieved.

—The woman may exhibit signs of hypovolemic shock caused by hemorrhage (i.e., hypotension; tachypnea; pallor; and cool, clammy skin).

—If the placenta separates, the FHR will be absent. Fetal parts may be palpable through the abdomen.

—The nurse should suspect pulmonary embolism if the woman complains of chest pain.

Collaborative Care

- Prevention is the best treatment. Women who have had a previous classic cesarean birth are advised not to attempt vaginal birth in subsequent pregnancies. Women at risk for uterine rupture are assessed closely during labor. Women whose labor is induced with oxytocin or prostaglandin (especially if their previous birth was cesarean) are monitored for signs of uterine hyperstimulation, because this can precipitate uterine rupture. If hyperstimulation occurs, the oxytocin infusion is discontinued or decreased, and a tocolytic medication may be given to decrease the intensity of the uterine contractions. After giving birth, women are assessed for excessive bleeding, especially if the fundus is firm and signs of hemorrhagic shock are present.

- If rupture occurs, the type of medical management depends on the severity. The nurse's role may include starting intravenous fluids, transfusing blood products, administering oxygen, and assisting with the preparation for immediate surgery. Supporting the woman's family and providing information about the treatment are important during this emergency.

Amniotic Fluid Embolism

Clinical manifestations

- Amniotic fluid embolism (AFE) occurs when amniotic fluid containing particles of debris (e.g., vernix, hair, skin cells, or meconium) enters the maternal circulation and obstructs pulmonary vessels, causing respiratory distress and circulatory collapse. Amniotic fluid is more damaging if it contains meconium and other particulate matter, such as mucus, fat globules, lanugo, and bacterial products. Maternal death occurs most often when thick meconium is present in the amniotic fluid. Even if death does not occur immediately, serious coagulation problems such as disseminated intravascular coagulopathy usually occur.

–Maternal factors (including multiparity, tumultuous labor, abruptio placentae, and oxytocin induction of labor) and fetal problems (including macrosomia, death, and meconium passage) have been associated with an increased risk for the development of AFE.

Collaborative Care

- The immediate interventions for AFE are summarized in the Emergency box. Such medical management must be instituted immediately. Cardiopulmonary resuscitation is often necessary. The woman is usually placed on mechanical ventilation, and blood replacement is initiated; coagulation defects are treated. Although the incidence of possible complications is small, their immediate recognition and prompt initiation of treatment are important.

- The nurse's immediate responsibility is to assist with the resuscitation efforts. If the woman survives, she is usually moved to a critical care unit, where hemodynamic monitoring and blood replacement and coagulopathy treatment are implemented. If cardiopulmonary arrest occurs, for optimal fetal survival, a perimortem cesarean birth should occur within 5 minutes.

- If the woman dies, emotional support and involvement of the perinatal loss support team or other resource for grief counseling are needed. Referral to grief and loss support groups would be appropriate.

EMERGENCY

Amniotic Fluid Embolism

SIGNS

Respiratory distress
- Restlessness
- Dyspnea
- Cyanosis
- Pulmonary edema
- Respiratory arrest

Circulatory collapse
- Hypotension
- Tachycardia
- Shock
- Cardiac arrest

Hemorrhage
- Coagulation failure: bleeding from incisions, venipuncture sites, trauma (lacerations); petechiae, ecchymoses, purpura
- Uterine atony

INTERVENTIONS

Oxygenate
- Administer oxygen by face mask (8 to 10 L/min) or resuscitation bag delivering 100% oxygen
- Prepare for intubation and mechanical ventilation
- Initiate or assist with cardiopulmonary resuscitation; tilt pregnant woman 30 degrees to side to displace uterus

Maintain cardiac output and replace fluid losses
- Position woman on her side
- Administer intravenous (IV) fluids
- Administer blood: packed cells, fresh frozen plasma
- Insert indwelling catheter, and measure hourly urine output

Correct coagulation failure

Monitor fetal and maternal status

Prepare for emergency birth once woman's condition is stabilized

Provide emotional support to woman, her partner, and family

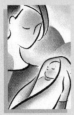

CHAPTER 13

Nursing Care of the Postpartum Woman

CARE MANAGEMENT—FOURTH STAGE OF LABOR

During the first 1 to 2 hours after birth, sometimes called the fourth stage of labor, maternal organs undergo their initial readjustment to the nonpregnant state and the functions of body systems begin to stabilize. Meanwhile, the newborn continues the transition from intrauterine to extrauterine existence.

Putting the infant to breast during this time is optimal because the infant is in an alert state and ready to nurse. Breast-feeding aids in the contraction of the uterus and the prevention of maternal hemorrhage.

Assessment

• Table 13-1 describes the physical assessment of the mother during the fourth stage of labor. The nurse should use the hospital/birth center forms to record the assessment. For healthy women, hemorrhage is probably the most dangerous potential complication during the fourth stage of labor.

• After birth, intense tremors that resemble shivering from a chill are commonly seen; they are not related to infection. The cause of these tremors is unknown; they may result from a sudden release of pressure on pelvic nerves after birth, a response to a fetus-to-mother transfusion that occurred during placental separation, a reaction to maternal adrenaline production during labor and birth, or a reaction to epidural anesthesia. Warm blankets and reassurance that the chills or tremors are common, are self-limiting, and last only a short while are useful interventions.

Text continued on p. 371.

TABLE 13-1

Assessment during the Fourth Stage of Labor

ASSESSMENT	SIGNS OF POTENTIAL COMPLICATIONS	RATIONALE
VITAL SIGNS		
Temperature	Temperature >38° C after the first 24 hr	Temperature may be elevated in first 24 hr because of dehydration
Pulse	Tachycardia or bradycardia	Bradycardia caused by decreased blood volume
Respiration	Dyspnea, rate <12 breaths/min	Magnesium sulfate; upper respiratory infection
Blood pressure	Hypotension Hypertension	Excessive blood loss Preeclampsia
Pain	Excessive pain	Vaginal hematoma
NEUROLOGIC		
Level of consciousness	Hard to arouse	Magnesium sulfate or medication may depress reflexes and make woman hard to arouse
Deep tendon reflexes	Hyperreflexia; hyporeflexia	Hyperreflexia associated with preeclampsia

Continued

TABLE 13-1

Assessment during the Fourth Stage of Labor—cont'd

ASSESSMENT	SIGNS OF POTENTIAL COMPLICATIONS	RATIONALE
NEUROLOGIC—cont'd		
Clonus (note number of beats)	+Clonus	Associated with preeclampsia
Homans sign	Homans sign positive; painful, reddened area; warmth on calf of leg	May indicate thrombophlebitis
CARDIOLOGIC		
Heart sounds	Murmurs, extra sounds	Some murmurs are innocuous and disappear after birth
Capillary refill time (CRT)	CRT ≥ 2 indicates poor perfusion	Decreased cardiac output, hypovolemia
Color	Circumoral, peripheral, or central cyanosis	Inadequate respiratory rate, anesthesia complication, cardiac problem
Edema	Edema of face and hands	Preeclampsia
Pedal pulses	Absent or diminished	Decreased cardiac output
RESPIRATORY		
Breath sounds	Crackles, rhonchi	Upper respiratory infection, inadequate chest excursion
Respiratory effort	Shallow respirations	Caused by anesthesia or magnesium sulfate or other medication
Secretions	Productive cough	Upper respiratory infection

GASTROINTESTINAL

Abdominal distention — Distention, peristaltic waves visible — Bowel obstruction

Bowel sounds — Diminished or no bowel sounds — Handling during cesarean birth

Flatus — No flatus — Normal in early postpartum; inactivity

Last bowel movement — Constipation, diarrhea — Normal at onset of labor

Appetite — Lack of appetite — Depression or having no culturally appropriate foods

Nutritional intake — Inadequate intake — Need to add about 300 calories per day to support milk production

GENITOURINARY

Fundus — Uterus deviated from the midline, boggy consistency, remains above the umbilicus after 24 hr — Full bladder

Lochia — Lochia heavy, foul odor, bright red bleeding that is not lochia; Clots — May have retained placenta, lacerations, or vaginal hematoma; infection

Perineum — Perineum has pronounced edema, not intact, signs of infection, marked discomfort — Infection, trauma, vaginal hematoma, hemorrhoids

Continued

TABLE 13-1

Assessment during the Fourth Stage of Labor—cont'd

ASSESSMENT	SIGNS OF POTENTIAL COMPLICATIONS	RATIONALE
Voiding	Unable to void, urgency, frequency, dysuria	Trauma to tissues urinary tract infection
SKIN		
Incision	Dehiscence	Obesity; staples removed too soon?
IV site	Red, warm, painful	Infection
Turgor	Poor	Dehydration
Striae	None	Normal finding
Linea nigra	None	Normal finding
Breasts	Breasts reddened, warm, painful	Engorgement, infection
	Palpable mass	
Nipples	Cracked and fissured nipples, inverted nipples	Improper latch on Plugged milk ducts
MUSCULOSKELETAL		
Mobility	Lethargy, extreme fatigue	Lack of sleep and long labor; depression
Level of activity	Hyperactivity	Anxiety
PSYCHOSOCIAL		
Affect	Flat	Depression
Depression	Inability to sleep or rest	Depression

Postanesthesia Recovery After Cesarean Birth or Regional Anesthesia for Vaginal Birth

- A postanesthesia recovery (PAR) score is determined for each patient on arrival and updated as part of every 15-minute assessment (Box 13-1).
- No woman should be discharged from the recovery area until she has completely recovered from the effects of anesthesia
- If the woman received general anesthesia:
  - She should be awake and alert.
  - She should be oriented to time, place, and person.
  - Respiratory rate should be within normal limits.
  - Oxygen saturation levels should be at least 95%, as measured by a pulse oximeter.
- If the woman received epidural or spinal anesthesia:
  - She should be able to raise her legs, extended at the knees, off the bed or to flex her knees.
  - She should be able to place her feet flat on the bed and raise her buttocks well off the bed.
  - The numb or tingling, prickly sensation should be entirely gone from her legs.
- Often, it takes several hours for these anesthetic effects to disappear.

Transfer from the Recovery Area

An oral report from the nurse who attended the woman during labor and birth should include conditions that could predispose the mother to hemorrhage, such as precipitous labor, large baby, grand multiparity (i.e., having given birth to six or more viable infants), or induced labor. The prenatal, labor, and birth records should be reviewed.

In preparing the transfer report, the recovery nurse uses information from the records of admission, birth, and recovery.

- Information that must be communicated to the postpartum nurse includes the following:
  - Identity of the health care provider
  - Gravidity and parity
  - Age
  - Anesthetic used

BOX 13-1

Postanesthesia Recovery (PAR) Score Form

PAR Score   ADMISSION: DISCHARGE:

Activity					
Respiration					
Blood pressure					
Conscious level					
Color					
TOTAL					

ACTIVITY

Able to move 4 extremities voluntarily or on command	2
Able to move 2 extremities voluntarily or on command	1
Able to move 0 extremities voluntarily or on command	0

RESPIRATION

Able to deep breathe and cough freely	2
Dyspnea or limited breathing	1
Apnea	0

BLOOD PRESSURE (BP)

BP ± mm Hg of preanesthetic level	2
BP ± 25-50 mm Hg of preanesthetic level	1
BP ≥ 50 mm Hg of preanesthetic level	0

CONSCIOUS LEVEL

Fully awake	2
Arousable on calling	1
Not responding	0

COLOR

Pink	2
Pale, dusky, blotchy, jaundiced, other	1
Cyanotic	0

—Any medications given
—Duration of labor and time of rupture of membranes
—Whether labor was induced or augmented
—Type of birth and repair
—Blood type and Rh status

−Group B streptococci status (if positive)
−Status of rubella immunity
−Syphilis and hepatitis B serology test results (if positive)
−Intravenous infusion of any fluids
−Physiologic status since birth
−Description of fundus, lochia, bladder, and perineum
−Sex and weight of infant
−Time of birth
−Name of pediatric care provider
−Chosen method of feeding
−Any abnormalities noted
−Assessment of initial parent-infant interaction

Most of this information is also documented for the nursing staff in the newborn nursery. In addition, specific information should be provided regarding the infant's Apgar scores, weight, voiding, and stooling and whether the infant was fed since birth. Nursing interventions that have been completed (e.g., eye prophylaxis or vitamin K injection) must also be recorded.

CARE MANAGEMENT—AFTER THE FIRST TWO HOURS

Initial Assessment

A complete physical assessment, including measurement of vital signs, is performed on admission to the postpartum unit. If the woman's vital signs are within normal limits, they are usually assessed every 4 to 8 hours for the remainder of her hospitalization. Other components of the initial assessment include the mother's emotional status, energy level, degree of physical discomfort, hunger, and thirst. Intake and output assessments should always be included if an intravenous infusion or a urinary catheter is in place. If the woman gave birth by cesarean, her incisional dressing should also be assessed.

Ongoing Physical Assessment

The new mother should be evaluated thoroughly during each shift throughout hospitalization. Physical assessments include evaluation of the breasts, uterine fundus, lochia, perineum, bladder and bowel function, vital signs, and legs. If a woman has an intravenous line in place, her fluid and hematologic status should be evaluated before it is removed. Table 13-1 lists signs of potential problems.

Routine Laboratory Tests

The following laboratory tests may be performed:
- Hemoglobin and hematocrit on the first postpartum day
- Urine specimen for routine urinalysis or culture and sensitivity, especially if an indwelling urinary catheter was inserted during the intrapartum period
- Rubella and Rh status if unknown

Newborn Safety

- Teach the mother to check the identity of any person who comes to remove the baby from her room. Hospital personnel usually wear picture identification badges. On some units, all staff members wear matching scrubs or special badges. Other units use closed-circuit television, computer monitoring systems, or fingerprint identification pads.
- As a rule, the baby is never carried in a staff member's arms between the mother's room and the nursery but is always wheeled in a bassinet, which also contains baby care supplies.

Prevention of Infection

- Maintain a clean environment.
- Change bed linens as needed.
- Disposable pads and draw sheets may need to be changed frequently.
- By not walking about barefoot, women avoid contaminating the linens when they return to bed.
- A sitz bath used in common must be scrubbed after each woman's use.
- Personnel must be conscientious about their handwashing techniques to prevent cross-infection.
- Standard Precautions must be practiced.
- Staff members with colds, coughs, or skin infections (e.g., a cold sore on the lips [herpes simplex virus type 1]) must follow hospital protocol when in contact with postpartum patients. In many hospitals, staff members with open herpetic lesions, strep throat, conjunctivitis, upper respiratory infections, or diarrhea are encouraged to avoid contact with mothers and infants by staying home until the condition is no longer contagious.

- Proper care of the episiotomy site and any perineal lacerations prevents infection in the genitourinary area and aids the healing process.
- Teach the woman to wipe from front to back (urethra to anus) after voiding or defecating.
- A squeeze bottle filled with warm water or an antiseptic solution is used after each voiding to cleanse the perineal area.
- Teach the woman to change her perineal pad from front to back each time she voids or defecates and wash her hands thoroughly before and after doing so.

Prevention of Excessive Bleeding

- A perineal pad saturated in 15 minutes or less and pooling of blood under the buttocks are indications of excessive blood loss, requiring immediate assessment, intervention, and notification of the physician or nurse-midwife.
- Blood loss is usually described subjectively as scant, light, moderate, or heavy (profuse). Fig. 13-1 shows examples of perineal pad saturation corresponding to each of these descriptions. Objective estimates of blood loss include measuring serial hemoglobin or hematocrit values, weighing blood clots and items saturated with blood (1 ml equals 1 g), and establishing how many milliliters it takes to saturate perineal pads being used. Different brands of perineal pads vary in their saturation volume and soaking appearance.

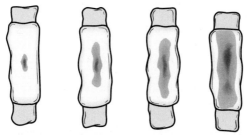

Fig. 13-1 Blood loss after birth is assessed by the extent of perineal pad saturation as (from left to right) scant (<2.5 cm), light (<10 cm), moderate (>10 cm), or heavy (one pad saturated within 2 hours).

- The nurse always checks under the mother's buttocks as well as on the perineal pad. Blood may flow between the buttocks onto the linens under the mother although the amount on the perineal pad is slight; thus excessive bleeding goes undetected.
- Blood pressure is not a reliable indicator of impending shock from early hemorrhage. More sensitive means of identifying shock are provided by respirations, pulse, skin condition, urinary output, and level of consciousness (see Emergency box).

Maintenance of Uterine Tone

Gentle massage of the uterine fundus helps to maintain firmness (Fig. 13-2). Fundal massage may cause a temporary increase in the amount of vaginal bleeding seen as pooled blood leaves the uterus. Clots may also be expelled. The uterus may remain boggy even after massage and expulsion of clots. See Appendix B for drugs used to manage postpartum hemorrhage for information about common oxytocic medications.

Promotion of Comfort, Rest, Ambulation, and Exercise

Comfort

- Afterbirth pains (afterpains), episiotomy or perineal lacerations, hemorrhoids, and breast engorgement may cause discomfort.
- Inspect and palpate areas of pain as appropriate for redness, swelling, discharge, and heat; and observe for body tension, guarded movements, and facial tension.
- Blood pressure, pulse, and respirations may be elevated in response to acute pain. Diaphoresis may accompany severe pain.
- A lack of objective signs does not necessarily mean there is no pain.
- Use both nonpharmacologic and pharmacologic interventions to promote comfort. Pain relief is enhanced by using more than one method or route.
- *Nonpharmacologic interventions.* Warmth, distraction, imagery, therapeutic touch, relaxation, and interaction with the infant may decrease the discomfort associated with afterbirth pain.

EMERGENCY

Hypovolemic Shock

SIGNS AND SYMPTOMS

Persistent significant bleeding—perineal pad soaked within 15 minutes; may not be accompanied by a change in vital signs or maternal color or behavior.

Woman states she feels weak, light-headed, "funny," "sick to my stomach," or "sees stars."

Woman begins to act anxious or exhibits air hunger.

Woman's skin turns ashen or grayish.

Skin feels cool and clammy.

Pulse rate increases.

Blood pressure declines.

INTERVENTIONS

Notify primary health care provider.

If uterus is atonic, massage gently and expel clots to cause uterus to contract; compress uterus manually, as needed, using two hands. Add oxytocic agent to IV drip, as ordered.

Give oxygen by face mask or nasal prongs at 8 to 10 L/min.

Tilt the woman to her side or elevate the right hip; elevate her legs to at least a 30-degree angle.

Provide additional IV infusion or maintain existing IV infusion of lactated Ringer's solution or normal saline solution to restore circulatory volume.

Administer blood or blood products as ordered.

Monitor vital signs.

Insert an indwelling urinary catheter to monitor perfusion of kidneys.

Administer emergency drugs as ordered.

Prepare for possible surgery or other emergency treatments or procedures.

Chart incident, medical and nursing interventions instituted, and results of treatments.

—To relieve discomfort of an episiotomy or perineal lacerations, encourage the woman to lie on her side and to use a pillow when sitting. Ice packs; topical application (if ordered); dry heat; cleansing with a squeeze bottle; and a cleansing shower, tub bath, or sitz bath are also effective. Many of these interventions are also effective for hemorrhoids,

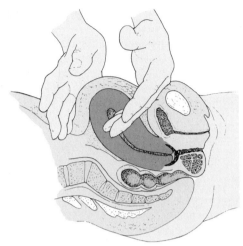

Fig. 13-2 Palpating fundus of uterus during the fourth stage of labor. Note that upper hand is cupped over fundus; lower hand dips in above symphysis pubis and supports uterus while it is massaged gently.

especially ice packs, sitz baths, and topical applications (e.g., witch hazel pads).

–The discomfort associated with engorged breasts may be lessened by applying ice, heat, or cabbage leaves to the breasts and wearing a well-fitted support bra.

• *Pharmacologic interventions.* Analgesics that are ordered are administered as needed. Topical application of antiseptic or anesthetic ointment or spray is effective for perineal pain. Patient-controlled analgesia pumps and epidural analgesia are technologies commonly used to provide pain relief after cesarean birth.

NURSE ALERT *The nurse should carefully monitor all women receiving opioids because respiratory depression and decreased intestinal motility are side effects.*

–Analgesics commonly used during the postpartum period are considered relatively safe for breastfeeding mothers. The timing of medications can be adjusted to minimize infant exposure. Pain medication may be given immediately after breastfeeding so that the interval between medication administration and the next nursing is as long as possible.

—If acceptable pain relief has not been obtained in 1 hour and there has been no change in the initial assessment, the nurse may need to obtain additional pain relief orders or further directions. Unrelieved pain might indicate the presence of a previously unidentified or untreated problem.

Rest

The excitement and exhilaration experienced after the birth of the infant may make rest difficult. The new mother may have difficulty sleeping. The demands of the infant, the hospital environment and routines, and the presence of frequent visitors contribute to alterations in her sleep pattern.

Fatigue

- Fatigue involves both physiologic components, associated with long labors, cesarean birth, anemia, and breastfeeding, and psychologic components, related to depression and anxiety. Infant behavior may also contribute to fatigue, particularly for mothers of more difficult infants.
- Back rubs, other comfort measures, and medication for sleep for the first few nights may be necessary. The side-lying position for breastfeeding minimizes fatigue in nursing mothers.

Ambulation

- Early ambulation is successful in reducing the incidence of thromboembolism and in promoting a rapid recovery of strength.

NURSE ALERT *Having a hospital staff or family member present the first time the woman gets out of bed after birth is wise because she may feel weak, dizzy, faint, or light-headed.*

- Women who must remain in bed after giving birth are at increased risk for the development of a thrombus. They may have antiembolic stockings (TED hose), a sequential compression device (SCD boots), or both ordered as prophylaxis. If a woman remains in bed longer than 8 hours (e.g., for postpartum magnesium sulfate therapy for preeclampsia), exercise to promote circulation in the legs is indicated using the following routine:

–Alternate flexion and extension of feet.
–Rotate ankle in circular motion.
–Alternate flexion and extension of legs.
–Press back of knee to bed surface; relax.

- If the woman is susceptible to thromboembolism, she is encouraged to walk about actively for true ambulation and is discouraged from sitting immobile in a chair. Women with varicosities are advised to wear support hose. If a thrombus is suspected, as evidenced by complaint of pain in calf muscles, or warmth, redness, or tenderness in the suspected leg (positive Homan's sign), the primary health care provider should be notified immediately; meanwhile the woman should be confined to bed, with the affected limb elevated on pillows.

Exercise

- Postpartum exercise can begin soon after birth, although the woman should be encouraged to start with simple exercises and gradually progress to more strenuous ones.
- Kegel exercises to strengthen pelvic muscle tone are extremely important, particularly after vaginal birth. Kegel exercises help women regain the muscle tone that is often lost as pelvic tissues are stretched and torn during pregnancy and birth. Women who maintain muscle strength may benefit years later by maintaining urinary continence.

Promotion of Nutrition

Restriction of food and fluid intake and the loss of fluids (blood, perspiration, or emesis) during labor cause many women to express a strong desire to eat or drink soon after birth. In the absence of complications, a woman who has given birth vaginally; has recovered from the effects of the anesthetic; and has stable vital signs, a firm uterus, and small to moderate lochial flow may have fluids and a regular diet as desired. Women may request that family members bring to the hospital favorite or culturally appropriate foods. Prenatal vitamins and iron supplements are often continued until 6 weeks postpartum or until the ordered supply has been used.

Promotion of Normal Bladder and Bowel Patterns

Bladder function

The mother should void spontaneously within 6 to 8 hours of giving birth. Measure the first several voidings to document adequate emptying of the bladder. A volume of at least 150 ml is expected for each voiding.

Bowel function

Teach the woman measures to avoid constipation, such as ensuring adequate roughage and fluid intake and promoting exercise. Narcotic analgesics contribute to decreased gastrointestinal tract motility. Stool softeners or laxatives may be necessary during the early postpartum period. Antigas medications may be ordered for women with gas pains. Ambulation or rocking in a rocking chair may stimulate passage of flatus and relief of discomfort.

Breastfeeding Promotion and Lactation Suppression

Breastfeeding promotion

During the first 2 hours after childbirth, the infant is in an alert state and ready to breastfeed. Breastfeeding aids in the contraction of the uterus and prevention of maternal hemorrhage.

Lactation suppression

- Suppression of lactation is necessary when the woman has decided not to breastfeed or in the case of neonatal death. Wearing a well-fitted support bra or breast binder continuously for at least the first 72 hours after giving birth is important. Women should avoid breast stimulation, including running warm water over the breasts, newborn suckling, or pumping of the breasts. A few nonbreastfeeding mothers experience severe breast engorgement (swelling of breast tissue caused by increased blood and lymph supply to the breasts preceding lactation). If breast engorgement occurs, it can usually be managed satisfactorily with nonpharmacologic interventions.

- Ice packs to the breasts can be used, with a 15 minutes on–45 minutes off schedule (to prevent the rebound swelling that can occur if ice is used continuously).
- Place cold fresh cabbage leaves inside the bra. Cabbage leaves have been used to treat swelling in other cultures for years. The exact mechanism of action is not known, but it is thought that naturally occurring plant estrogens or salicylates may be responsible for the effects. The leaves are replaced each time they wilt.
- A mild analgesic may also be necessary.
- Medications that were once prescribed for lactation suppression (e.g., estrogen, estrogen and testosterone, or bromocriptine) are no longer used.

Health Promotion for Future Pregnancies and Children

Rubella vaccination

For women who are not immune to rubella, a subcutaneous injection of rubella vaccine is recommended in the immediate postpartum period. The live attenuated rubella virus is not communicable in breast milk; therefore breastfeeding mothers can be vaccinated. However, because the virus is shed in urine and other body fluids, the vaccine should not be given if the mother or other household members are immunocompromised. Rubella vaccine is made from duck eggs, so women who have allergies to these eggs may develop a hypersensitivity reaction to the vaccine, for which they will need adrenaline. A transient arthralgia or rash is common in vaccinated women but is benign. Because the vaccine may be teratogenic, women who receive the vaccine must be informed about this fact.

LEGAL TIP Rubella Vaccination

Informed consent for rubella vaccination in the postpartum period includes information about possible side effects and the risk of teratogenic effects. Women must understand that they must practice contraception to avoid pregnancy for 2 months after being vaccinated.

Prevention of Rh isoimmunization

Injection of Rh immune globulin within 72 hours after birth prevents sensitization in the Rh-negative woman who has had a fetomaternal transfusion of Rh-positive fetal red blood cells (RBCs) (see Medication Guide in Appendix B—Rh Immune Globulin, RhoGAM, Gamulin Rh, HypRho-D, Rhophylac). Rh immune globulin promotes lysis of fetal Rh-positive blood cells before the mother forms her own antibodies against them.

NURSE ALERT *After birth, Rh immune globulin is administered to all Rh-negative, antibody (Coombs')–negative women who give birth to Rh-positive infants. Rh immune globulin is administered to the mother intramuscularly. It should never be given to an infant.*

The administration of 300 micrograms (one vial) of Rh immune globulin is usually sufficient to prevent maternal sensitization. If a large fetomaternal transfusion is suspected, however, the dosage needed should be determined by performing a Kleihauer-Betke test, which detects the amount of fetal blood in the maternal circulation. If more than 15 ml of fetal blood is present in maternal circulation, the dosage of Rh immune globulin must be increased.

There is some disagreement about whether Rh immune globulin should be considered a blood product. Health care providers need to discuss the most current information about this issue with women whose religious beliefs conflict with having blood products administered to them.

Psychosocial Needs

Meeting the psychosocial needs of new mothers involves assessing the parents' reactions to the birth experience, feelings about themselves, and interactions with the new baby and other family members. Sometimes the psychosocial assessment indicates serious actual or potential problems that must be addressed. The Signs of Potential Complications box lists several psychosocial needs that, at a minimum, warrant ongoing evaluation following hospital discharge. Patients exhibiting these needs should be referred to appropriate community resources for assessment and management.

PSYCHOSOCIAL NEEDS
Unable or unwilling to discuss labor and birth experience
Refers to self as ugly and useless
Excessively preoccupied with self (body image)
Markedly depressed
Lacks a support system
Partner and/or other family members react negatively to the baby
Refuses to interact with or care for baby (e.g., does not name baby, does not want to hold or feed baby, is upset by vomiting and wet or dirty diapers) (Cultural appropriateness of actions needs to be considered.)
Expresses disappointment over baby's sex
Sees baby as messy or unattractive
Baby reminds mother of family member or friend she does not like

Impact of the birth experience

Many women wish to review the birth process itself and look at their own intrapartal behavior in retrospect. Their partners may express similar desires. If their birth experience differed from that included in their birth plan (e.g., induction, epidural anesthesia, cesarean birth), the couple may need to mourn the loss of their expectations before they can adjust to the reality of their birth experience.

Maternal self-image

Assess the woman's self-concept, body image, and sexuality. How this new mother feels about herself and her body during the puerperium may affect her behavior and adaptation to parenting. The woman's self-concept and body image may also affect her sexuality.

Adaptation to parenthood/ parent-infant interactions

- The psychosocial assessment also includes evaluating adaptation to parenthood, as evidenced by the mother's and father's reactions to and interactions with the new baby. Parents are adapting well to their new role when they exhibit a realistic perception and acceptance of their newborn's needs and his or her limited abilities, immature social responses, and helplessness. Examples of positive parent-infant interactions include taking pleasure in their infant and in the tasks done for and with her or him, understanding their infant's emotional states and providing comfort, and reading their infant's cues for new experiences and sensing the infant's fatigue level.

- Should these indicators be missing, the nurse needs to investigate further what is hindering the normal adaptation process. There are several questions that the nurse can ask, such as "Do you feel sad often?" or "Are there concerns that you have regarding being a good parent?", which will help to determine if the woman is experiencing the normal "baby blues" or if there is another more serious underlying process taking place (i.e. postpartum depression).

Impact of cultural diversity

The final component of a complete psychosocial assessment is the woman's cultural beliefs and values. Much of a woman's behavior during the postpartum period is strongly influenced by her cultural background. Nurses are likely to come into contact with women from many different countries and cultures. All cultures have developed safe and satisfying methods of caring for new mothers and babies. Only by understanding and respecting the values and beliefs of each woman can the nurse design a plan of care to meet the woman's individual needs.

DISCHARGE

Early postpartum discharge, shortened hospital stay, and *1-day maternity stay* are all terms for the decreasing length of hospital stays of mothers and their babies after a low risk birth. Under the Newborns' and Mothers' Health Protection Act, all health plans are required to allow the new mother and newborn to remain in the hospital for a minimum of 48 hours after a normal vaginal birth and for 96 hours after a cesarean birth unless the attending provider, in consultation with the mother, decides on early discharge. Women who give birth in birthing centers may go home within a few hours, after the woman's and infant's conditions are stable.

Criteria for Discharge

Early discharge with postpartum home care is preferred by many women and their families. Hospital stays must be long enough to identify problems and to ensure that the woman has sufficiently recovered and is prepared to care for herself and the baby at home. Box 13-2 gives criteria for identifying low risk mothers and infants.

Content to be taught includes:
–Maternal and newborn care
–Recognition of the physical signs and symptoms that might indicate problems and how to obtain advice and assistance quickly if these signs appear
–Basic instruction regarding the resumption of sexual intercourse, prescribed medications, routine mother-baby checkups, and contraception (see Table 13-2)

Sexual Activity/Contraception

• Couples may safely resume sexual activity by approximately 2 weeks postpartum.
• Discuss the physical and psychologic effects that giving birth can have on sexual activity (see Patient Instructions for Self-Care box).
• Contraceptive options should also be discussed with women (and their partners, if present) before discharge.
• It is possible, particularly in women who bottle-feed, for ovulation to occur as soon as 1 month after birth.

Prescribed Medications

• Women continue to take their prenatal vitamins and iron during the postpartum period. It is especially important that women who are breastfeeding or who have a lower than normal hematocrit take these medications as prescribed.

Text continued on p. 391.

BOX 13-2

Criteria for Early Discharge

MOTHER

Uncomplicated pregnancy, labor, vaginal birth, and postpartum course

No evidence of premature rupture of membranes

Blood pressure and temperature stable and within normal limits

Ambulating unassisted

Voiding adequate amounts without difficulty

Hemoglobin >10 g

No significant vaginal bleeding; perineum intact or no more than second-degree episiotomy or laceration repair; uterus firm

Received instructions on postpartum self-care

INFANT

Term infant (38 to 42 weeks) with weight appropriate for gestational age

Normal findings on physical assessment

Temperature, respirations, and heart rate within normal limits and stable for the 12 hours preceding discharge

At least two successful feedings completed (normal sucking and swallowing)

Urination and stooling have occurred at least once

No evidence of significant jaundice in the first 24 hours after the birth

No excessive bleeding at the circumcision site for at least 2 hours

Screening tests performed according to state regulations; tests to be repeated at follow-up visit if done before the infant is 24 hours old

Initial hepatitis B vaccine given or scheduled for first follow-up visit

Laboratory data reviewed: maternal syphilis and hepatitis B status; infant or cord blood type and Coombs' test results if indicated

GENERAL

No social, family, or environmental risk factors identified

Family or support person available to assist mother and infant at home

Follow-up scheduled within 1 week if discharged before 48 hours after the birth

Documentation of skill of mother in feeding (breast or bottle), cord care, skin care, perineal care, infant safety (use of car seat, sleeping positions), and recognizing signs of illness and common infant problems

Sources: American Academy of Pediatrics. (1995). Hospital stay for healthy term infants, *Pediatrics, 96*(4), 788-790; Weekly, S.J., & Neumann, M.L. (1997). Speaking up for baby: The case for individualized neonatal discharge plans, *AWHONN Lifelines, 1*(1), 24-29.

PATIENT INSTRUCTIONS FOR SELF-CARE

Resumption of Sexual Intercourse

You can safely resume sexual intercourse by the second to fourth week after birth when bleeding has stopped and the episiotomy has healed. For the first 6 weeks to 6 months, the vagina does not lubricate well.

Your physiologic reactions to sexual stimulation for the first 3 months after birth will be slower and less intense. The strength of the orgasm is reduced.

A water-soluble gel, cocoa butter, or a contraceptive cream or jelly might be recommended for lubrication. If some vaginal tenderness is present, your partner can be instructed to insert one or more clean, lubricated fingers into the vagina and rotate them within the vagina to help relax it and to identify possible areas of discomfort. A position in which you have control of the depth of the insertion of the penis also is useful. The side-by-side or female-on-top position may be more comfortable.

The presence of the baby influences postbirth lovemaking. Parents hear every sound made by the baby; conversely, you may be concerned that the baby hears every sound you make. In either case, any phase of the sexual response cycle may be interrupted by hearing the baby cry or move, leaving both of you frustrated and unsatisfied. In addition, the amount of psychologic energy expended by you in child care activities may lead to fatigue. Newborns require a great deal of attention and time.

Some women have reported feeling sexual stimulation and orgasms when breastfeeding their babies. Breastfeeding mothers often are interested in returning to sexual activity before nonbreastfeeding mothers.

You should be instructed to correctly perform the Kegel exercises to strengthen your pubococcygeal muscle. This muscle is associated with bowel and bladder function and with vaginal feeling during intercourse.

TABLE 13-2

Maternal-Newborn Teaching Checklist

TOPICS FOR PATIENT TEACHING	I NEED INSTRUCTION	I ALREADY KNOW THIS
SELF-CARE		
Episiotomy and perineal care	_____	_____
Vaginal discharge	_____	_____
Hemorrhoids/ constipation	_____	_____
Breast care	_____	_____
Nutrition	_____	_____
Activity	_____	_____
Postpartal exercises	_____	_____
Return of menstruation	_____	_____
Family planning	_____	_____
Blood clots	_____	_____
Postpartum emotions	_____	_____
Postpartum warning signs	_____	_____
Incisional care (cesarean birth)	_____	_____
BABY CARE		
Diapering	_____	
Baby bath, skin and cord care	_____	_____
Circumcision care	_____	_____
Burping	_____	_____
Bowel movements, wet diapers	_____	_____
Sleeping habits	_____	_____
Newborn behavior	_____	_____
Jaundice	_____	_____
Use of pacifier	_____	_____
Signs of illness	_____	_____
Car seat safety	_____	_____
Taking temperature	_____	_____
General infant safety/poison control	_____	_____
Signs and symptoms of dehydration	_____	_____
Use of bulb syringe	_____	_____

Continued

TABLE 13-2

Maternal-Newborn Teaching Checklist—cont'd

TOPICS FOR PATIENT TEACHING	I NEED INSTRUCTION	I ALREADY KNOW THIS
BREASTFEEDING		
Latch on	_____	_____
Positioning		
Frequency of feeding	_____	_____
Sore nipples	_____	_____
Determining if baby is getting enough to eat	_____	_____
Engorgement	_____	_____
Feeding water	_____	_____
Nursing while working		
Weaning	_____	_____
BOTTLE-FEEDING		
Types of formula	_____	_____
Preparing formula	_____	_____
Frequency of feedings	_____	_____
AT HOME		
When to call health care provider	_____	_____
OTHER		
Working mothers	_____	_____
Day care	_____	_____
Sibling adjustment	_____	_____
Single parent support	_____	_____
Time out for parents	_____	_____
Infant safety and security	_____	_____
MEDICATIONS		
Dose, action, side effects	_____	_____

- Women with extensive episiotomies or vaginal lacerations (third or fourth degree) are usually prescribed stool softeners to take at home.
- Pain relief medications (analgesics or nonsteroidal antiinflammatory medications) may be prescribed, especially for women who had cesarean birth.
- The nurse should make certain that the woman knows the route, dosage, frequency, and common side effects of all ordered medications.

Routine Mother and Baby Checkups

- Women who have experienced uncomplicated vaginal births are commonly scheduled for the traditional 6-week postpartum examination. Women who have had a cesarean birth are often seen in the physician's or nursemidwife's office or clinic 2 weeks after hospital discharge. The date and time for the follow-up appointment should be included in the discharge instructions. If an appointment has not been made before the woman leaves the hospital, she should be encouraged to call the physician's or nurse-midwife's office or clinic to schedule an appointment.
- Parents who have not already done so need to make plans for newborn follow-up at the time of discharge. Most offices and clinics like to see newborns for an initial examination within the first week or by 2 weeks of age. If an appointment for a specific date and time was not made for the infant before leaving the hospital, the parents should be encouraged to call the office or clinic right away.

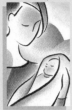

CHAPTER 14

Postpartum Complications

POSTPARTUM HEMORRHAGE

Postpartum hemorrhage (PPH) is a life-threatening event that can occur with little warning and is often unrecognized until the mother has profound symptoms. PPH is defined as follows:

- The loss of more than 500 ml of blood after vaginal birth
- The loss of more than 1000 ml of blood after cesarean birth
- A 10% change in hematocrit between admission for labor and postpartum or the need for erythrocyte transfusion
- Occurrence within 24 hours of the birth for early, acute, or primary PPH
- Occurrence more than 24 hours but less than 6 weeks postpartum for late or secondary PPH

Etiology and Risk Factors

Excessive bleeding may occur during the period from the separation of the placenta to its expulsion or removal.

- Commonly, such excessive bleeding is the result of incomplete placental separation, undue manipulation of the fundus, or excessive traction on the cord.
- After the placenta has been expelled or removed, persistent or excessive blood loss usually is the result of atony of the uterus or prolapse of the uterus into the vagina.
- Late PPH may be the result of subinvolution of the uterus, endometritis, or retained placental fragments. Box 14-1 lists risk factors for PPH.

BOX 14-1

Risk Factors for Postpartum Hemorrhage

Uterine atony
- Overdistended uterus
  —Large fetus
  —Multiple fetuses
  —Hydramnios
  —Distention with clots
- Anesthesia and analgesia
  —Conduction anesthesia
- Previous history of uterine atony
- High parity
- Prolonged labor or oxytocin-induced labor
- Trauma during labor and birth
  —Forceps-assisted birth
  —Vacuum-assisted birth
  —Cesarean birth

Lacerations of the birth canal
Retained placental fragments
Ruptured uterus
Inversion of the uterus
Placenta accreta
Coagulation disorders
Placental abruption
Placenta previa
Manual removal of a retained placenta
Magnesium sulfate administration during labor or postpartum period
Endometritis
Uterine subinvolution

Uterine Atony

- Uterine atony is marked hypotonia of the uterus.
- Uterine atony is the leading cause of PPH, complicating approximately 1 in 20 births.
- It is associated with high parity, hydramnios, a macrosomic fetus, and multifetal gestation. In such conditions, the uterus is "overstretched" and contracts poorly after the birth.
- Other causes of atony include traumatic birth, use of halogenated anesthesia (e.g., halothane) or magnesium sulfate, rapid

or prolonged labor, chorioamnionitis, and use of oxytocin for labor induction or augmentation.

Lacerations of the Genital Tract

- Lacerations of the cervix, vagina, and perineum also are causes of PPH.
- Hemorrhage related to lacerations should be suspected if bleeding continues despite a firm, contracted uterine fundus. This bleeding can be a slow trickle, an oozing, or frank hemorrhage.
- Factors associated with obstetric lacerations of the lower genital tract include the following:
  - Operative birth, precipitate birth, congenital abnormalities of the maternal soft parts, and contracted pelvis.
  - Size, abnormal presentation, and position of the fetus; relative size of the presenting part and the birth canal; previous scarring from infection, injury, or operation; and vulvar, perineal, and vaginal varicosities.
- Extreme vascularity in the labial and periclitoral areas often results in profuse bleeding if laceration occurs.
- Pelvic hematomas may be vulvar, vaginal, or retroperitoneal in origin.
  - Vulvar hematomas are the most common. Pain is the most common symptom, and most vulvar hematomas are visible.
  - Vaginal hematomas occur more commonly in association with a forceps-assisted birth, an episiotomy, or primigravidity. Symptoms include persistent perineal or rectal pain or a feeling of pressure in the vagina.
  - A retroperitoneal hematoma may cause minimal pain, and the initial symptoms may be signs of shock.
- Cervical lacerations usually occur at the lateral angles of the external os. Most are shallow, and bleeding is minimal. More extensive lacerations may extend into the vaginal vault or into the lower uterine segment.

Retained Placenta

- Nonadherent retained placenta may result from the following:

–Partial separation of a normal placenta

–Entrapment of the partially or completely separated placenta by an hourglass constriction ring of the uterus

–Mismanagement of the third stage of labor

–Abnormal adherence of the entire placenta or a portion of the placenta to the uterine wall

–Placental retention because of poor separation: common in very preterm births (20 to 24 weeks of gestation)

• Management of Nonadherent Retained Placenta

–Manual separation and removal are done by the primary health care provider.

–Supplementary anesthesia is not usually needed for women who have had regional anesthesia for birth.

–For other women, administration of light nitrous oxide and oxygen inhalation anesthesia or intravenous thiopental facilitates uterine exploration and placental removal.

–After this removal, the woman is at continued risk for PPH and for infection.

• Adherent retained placenta, or abnormal adherence of the placenta occurs for reasons unknown, but it is thought to result from zygotic implantation in an area of defective endometrium so that there is no zone of separation between the placenta and the decidua.

–Attempts to remove the placenta in the usual manner are unsuccessful, and laceration or perforation of the uterine wall may result, putting the woman at great risk for severe PPH and infection.

• Unusual placental adherence may be partial or complete. The following degrees of attachment are recognized:

–*Placenta accreta:* slight penetration of myometrium by placental trophoblast

–*Placenta increta:* deep penetration of myometrium by placenta

–*Placenta percreta:* perforation of uterus by placenta

• Bleeding with complete or total placenta accreta may not occur unless separation of the placenta is attempted.

• With more extensive involvement, bleeding will become profuse when removal of the placenta is attempted.

• Treatment includes blood component replacement therapy; hysterectomy may be indicated.

Inversion of the Uterus

Inversion of the uterus after birth is a potentially life-threatening complication. The primary presenting signs of uterine inversion are hemorrhage, shock, and pain.

- Uterine inversion may be partial or complete.
  - Complete inversion of the uterus is obvious; a large, red, rounded mass (perhaps with the placenta attached) protrudes 20 to 30 cm outside the introitus.
  - Incomplete inversion cannot be seen but must be felt; a smooth mass will be palpated through the dilated cervix.
- Contributing factors to uterine inversion include the following:
  - Fundal implantation of the placenta
  - Vigorous fundal pressure
  - Excessive traction applied to the cord; the umbilical cord should not be pulled on strongly unless the placenta has definitely separated
  - Uterine atony
  - Leiomyomas
  - Abnormally adherent placental tissue

Subinvolution of the Uterus

- Late postpartum bleeding may occur as a result of subinvolution of the uterus.
- Recognized causes of subinvolution include retained placental fragments and pelvic infection.
- Signs and symptoms include prolonged lochial discharge, irregular or excessive bleeding, and sometimes hemorrhage.
- A pelvic examination usually reveals a uterus that is larger than normal and may be boggy.

Collaborative Care
Assessment

PPH may be sudden and even exsanguinating. The nurse must therefore be alert to the symptoms of hemorrhage and hypovolemic shock and be prepared to act quickly to minimize blood loss (Fig. 14-1).

- The woman's history should be reviewed for factors that cause predisposition to PPH.
- The fundus is assessed to determine whether it is firmly contracted at or near the level of the umbilicus.
- Bleeding should be assessed for color and amount.
- The perineum is inspected for signs of lacerations or hematomas to determine the possible source of bleeding.
- Vital signs may not be reliable indicators of shock immediately postpartum because of the physiologic adaptations of this period. However, frequent vital sign measurements during the first 2 hours after birth may identify trends related to blood loss (e.g., tachycardia, tachypnea, or decreasing blood pressure).
- Assessment for bladder distention is important; a distended bladder can displace the uterus and prevent contraction.
- The skin is assessed for warmth and dryness; nail beds are checked for color and promptness of capillary refill.
- Laboratory studies include evaluation of hemoglobin and hematocrit levels.

Late PPH develops at least 24 hours after the birth or later in the postpartum period. The woman may be at home when the symptoms occur. Discharge teaching should emphasize the signs of normal involution, as well as potential complications.

Interventions
Medical Management
Hypotonic Uterus

- Evaluate the contractility of the uterus. If the uterus is hypotonic, massage the uterine fundus and express clots in the uterus.
- Eliminate bladder distention by having the woman void or by inserting a catheter.
- Infuse 10 to 40 units of oxytocin added to 1000 ml lactated Ringer's or normal saline solution.
  - If the uterus fails to respond to oxytocin, a 0.2-mg dose of ergonovine (Ergotrate) or methylergonovine (Methergine) may be given intramuscularly to produce sustained uterine contractions.
  - More commonly, a 0.25-mg dose of a derivative of prostaglandin $F_{2\alpha}$ (carboprost tromethamine) may be given intramuscularly. It also can be given intramyometrially at

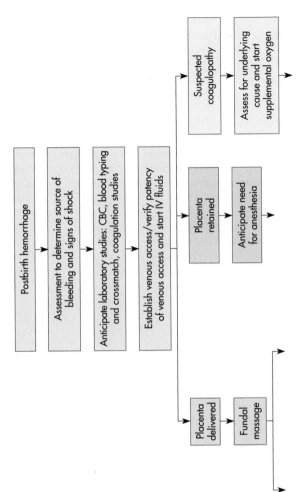

Postbirth hemorrhage

Assessment to determine source of bleeding and signs of shock

Anticipate laboratory studies: CBC, blood typing and crossmatch, coagulation studies

Establish venous access/verify patency of venous access and start IV fluids

Placenta delivered

Fundal massage

Placenta retained

Anticipate need for anesthesia

Suspected coagulopathy

Assess for underlying cause and start supplemental oxygen

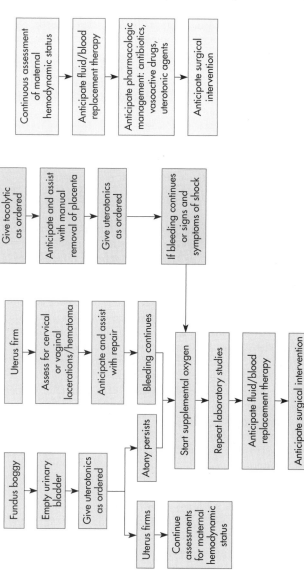

Fig. 14-1 Nursing assessments for postpartum bleeding. *CBC,* Complete blood count; *IV,* intravenous; *uterotonics,* medications to contract the uterus.

cesarean birth or intraabdominally after vaginal birth. See Appendix B for the table comparing drugs used to manage PPH.

—In addition to the medications used to contract the uterus, rapid administration of crystalloid solutions and/or blood or blood products will be needed to restore the woman's intravascular volume.

> **NURSE ALERT** *Use of ergonovine or methylergonovine is contraindicated in the presence of hypertension or cardiovascular disease. Prostaglandin $F_{2\alpha}$ should be used cautiously in women with cardiovascular disease or asthma.*

- Oxygen can be given to enhance oxygen delivery to the cells.
- Laboratory studies usually include a complete blood count with platelet count, fibrinogen, fibrin split products, prothrombin time, and partial thromboplastin time.
- Blood type and antibody screen are done if not previously performed.
- If bleeding persists, bimanual compression may be considered by the obstetrician or nurse-midwife. This procedure involves inserting a fist into the vagina and pressing the knuckles against the anterior side of the uterus and then placing the other hand on the abdomen and massaging the posterior aspect of the uterus with it.
- If the uterus still does not become firm, manual exploration of the uterine cavity for retained placental fragments is implemented.
- If the preceding procedures are ineffective, surgical management may be the only alternative. Surgical management options include vessel ligation (uteroovarian, uterine, or hypogastric), selective arterial embolization, and hysterectomy.

Bleeding with a Contracted Uterus

- If the uterus is firmly contracted and bleeding continues, the source of bleeding still must be identified and treated.
- Assessment may include visual or manual inspection of the perineum, vagina, uterus, cervix, or rectum and laboratory studies (e.g., hemoglobin, hematocrit, coagulation studies, or platelet count).

- Treatment depends on the source of the bleeding:
  - Lacerations are usually sutured.
  - Hematomas may be managed with observation, cold therapy, ligation of the bleeding vessel, or evacuation.
  - Fluids and blood replacement may be needed.

Uterine Inversion

- Uterine inversion is an emergency situation requiring immediate recognition, replacement of the uterus within the pelvic cavity, and correction of associated clinical conditions.
- Tocolytic agents or halogenated anesthetics may be given to relax the uterus before attempting replacement.
- Medical management of this condition includes treating shock, repositioning the uterus, giving oxytocic agents after the uterus is repositioned, and initiating broad-spectrum antibiotics.

Subinvolution

- Treatment of subinvolution depends on the cause.
- Ergonovine, 0.2 mg every 4 hours for 2 or 3 days, and antibiotic therapy are the most common medications used.
- Dilation and curettage (D&C) may be needed to remove retained placental fragments or to debride the placental site.

Nursing Interventions

Immediate nursing care of the woman with postpartum hemorrhage

- Vital signs and uterine consistency are assessed.
- Oxytocin or other drugs to stimulate uterine contraction are administered according to standing orders or protocols.
- The primary health care provider is notified if not present.
- The woman and her family will be anxious about her condition. The nurse can calmly provide explanations about interventions being performed and the need to act quickly.

Lacerations

- After the bleeding has been controlled, the care of the woman with lacerations of the perineum is similar to that for women with episiotomies (analgesia as needed for pain and hot or cold applications as necessary).

• The need for increased roughage in the diet and increased intake of fluids is emphasized.

• Stool softeners may be used to assist the woman in reestablishing bowel habits without straining and putting stress on the suture lines.

NURSE ALERT *To avoid injury to the suture line, a woman with third- or fourth-degree lacerations is not given rectal suppositories or enemas.*

Uterine Inversion. The care of the woman who has experienced an inversion of the uterus focuses on immediate stabilization of hemodynamic status:

• Her response to treatment to prevent shock or fluid overload is observed closely.

• If the uterus has been repositioned manually, care must be taken to avoid aggressive fundal massage.

Discharge Teaching. Discharge instructions for the woman who has had PPH are similar to those for any postpartum woman:

• She should be told that she will probably feel fatigue, even exhaustion, and will need to limit her physical activities to conserve her strength.

• She may need instructions in increasing her dietary iron and protein intake and iron supplementation to rebuild lost red cell (RBC) volume.

• She may need assistance with infant care and household activities until she has regained strength.

• Some women have problems with delayed or insufficient lactation and postpartum depression.

• Referrals for home care follow-up or to community resources may be needed.

THROMBOEMBOLIC DISEASE

A thrombosis results from the formation of a blood clot or clots inside a blood vessel and is caused by inflammation (thrombophlebitis) or partial obstruction of the vessel. Three thromboembolic conditions are of concern in the postpartum period:

- *Superficial venous thrombosis:* involvement of the superficial saphenous venous system
- *Deep venous thrombosis:* involvement varies but can extend from the foot to the iliofemoral region
- *Pulmonary embolism:* complication of deep venous thrombosis occurring when part of a blood clot dislodges and is carried to the pulmonary artery, where it occludes the vessel and obstructs blood flow to the lungs

Incidence and Etiology

- The major causes of thromboembolic disease are venous stasis and hypercoagulation, both of which are present in pregnancy and continue into the postpartum period.
- Other risk factors include cesarean birth, history of venous thrombosis or varicosities, obesity, maternal age older than 35 years, multiparity, and smoking.

Clinical Manifestations

- Superficial venous thrombosis is the most frequent form of postpartum thrombophlebitis. It is characterized by pain and tenderness in the lower extremity. Physical examination may reveal warmth, redness, and an enlarged, hardened vein over the site of the thrombosis.
- Deep vein thrombosis is more common in pregnancy and is characterized by unilateral leg pain, calf tenderness, and swelling.
  - Physical examination may reveal redness and warmth, but women also may have a large clot and have few symptoms.
  - Physical examination is not a sensitive diagnostic indicator for thrombosis.
  - A positive Homan's sign may be present, but further evaluation is needed because the calf pain may be attributed to other causes, such as a strained muscle resulting from the birthing position.
- Venography is the most accurate method for diagnosing deep venous thrombosis; however, it is an invasive procedure that

exposes the woman to ionizing radiation and is associated with serious complications.

- Pulmonary embolism is characterized by dyspnea and tachypnea. Other signs and symptoms frequently seen include apprehension, cough, tachycardia, hemoptysis, elevated temperature, and pleuritic chest pain.
- Noninvasive diagnostic methods are more commonly used; these include real-time and color Doppler ultrasound.
  - Cardiac auscultation may reveal murmurs with pulmonary embolism.
  - Electrocardiograms are usually normal.
  - Arterial PO_2 may be lower than normal.
  - A ventilation/perfusion scan, Doppler ultrasound, and pulmonary arteriogram may be used for diagnosis.

Medical Management

- Superficial venous thrombosis is treated with analgesia (nonsteroidal antiinflammatory agents), rest with elevation of the affected leg, and elastic stockings. Local application of heat also may be used.
- Deep venous thrombosis is initially treated with anticoagulant (usually continuous intravenous heparin) therapy, bed rest with the affected leg elevated, and analgesia.
  - After the symptoms have decreased, the woman may be fitted with elastic stockings to use when she is allowed to ambulate.
  - Intravenous heparin therapy continues for 5 to 7 days.
  - Oral anticoagulant therapy (warfarin) is started during this time and will be continued for about 3 months.
  - Continuous intravenous heparin therapy is used for pulmonary embolism until symptoms have resolved.
  - Intermittent subcutaneous heparin or oral anticoagulant therapy is usually continued for 6 months.

Nursing Interventions

Assessment

In the hospital setting, nursing care of the woman with a thrombosis consists of continued assessments:

- Inspection and palpation of the affected area
- Palpation of peripheral pulses

- Checking Homans sign
- Measurement and comparison of leg circumferences
- Inspection for signs of bleeding
- Monitoring for signs of pulmonary embolism, including chest pain, coughing, dyspnea, and tachypnea; and respiratory status for presence of crackles
- Monitoring of laboratory reports for prothrombin or partial thromboplastin times
- Assessment of the woman and her family for their level of understanding about the diagnosis and their ability to cope during the unexpected extended period of recovery

Interventions

- Give explanations and education about the diagnosis and the treatment.
- Assist with personal care as long as the woman is on bed rest.
- Encourage the family to participate in the care if that is what the woman and the family wish.
- While the woman is on bed rest, encourage her to change positions frequently but not to place the knees in a sharply flexed position that could cause pooling of blood in the lower extremities. Also, caution her not to rub the affected area because this action could cause the clot to dislodge.
- Once the woman is allowed to ambulate, teach her how to prevent venous congestion by putting on the elastic stockings before getting out of bed.
- Administer heparin and warfarin as ordered, and notify the physician if clotting times are outside the therapeutic level.
- If the woman is breastfeeding, assure her that neither heparin nor warfarin is excreted in significant quantities in breast milk. If the infant has been discharged, encourage the family to bring the infant for feedings as permitted by hospital policy; the mother also can express milk to be sent home.
- Pain can be managed with a variety of measures:
  - Position changes, elevating the leg, and application of moist warm heat may decrease discomfort.
  - Administration of analgesics and antiinflammatory medications may be needed.

> **NURSE ALERT** *Medications containing aspirin are not given to women receiving anticoagulant therapy because aspirin inhibits synthesis of clotting factors and can lead to prolonged clotting time and increased risk of bleeding.*

- The woman is usually discharged home with oral anticoagulants and will need explanations about the treatment schedule and possible side effects.
- If subcutaneous injections are to be given, teach the woman and family how to administer the medication and about site rotation.
- Also, give the woman and her family information about safe care practices to prevent bleeding and injury while she is receiving anticoagulant therapy, such as using a soft toothbrush and using an electric razor.
- Give the woman information about follow-up with her health care provider to monitor clotting times and to make sure the correct dose of anticoagulant therapy is maintained.
- Instruct the woman to use a reliable method of contraception if taking warfarin, because this medication is considered teratogenic.

POSTPARTUM INFECTIONS

Postpartum or puerperal infection is any clinical infection of the genital canal that occurs within 28 days after miscarriage, induced abortion, or childbirth.

- The definition used in the United States continues to be the presence of a fever of 38° C or more on 2 successive days of the first 10 postpartum days (not counting the first 24 hours after birth).
- Puerperal infection is probably the major cause of maternal morbidity and mortality throughout the world. It occurs after about 6% of births in the United States (5 to 10 times higher after cesarean births than after vaginal births).
- Common postpartum infections include endometritis, wound infections, mastitis, urinary tract infections (UTIs), and respiratory tract infections.
- The most common infecting organisms are the numerous streptococcal and anaerobic organisms. *Staphylococcus aureus*,

gonococci, coliform bacteria, and clostridia are less common but serious pathogenic organisms that also cause puerperal infection.

- Postpartum infections are more common in women who have concurrent medical or immunosuppressive conditions or who had a cesarean or other operative birth.
- Intrapartal factors, such as prolonged rupture of membranes, prolonged labor, and internal maternal or fetal monitoring, also increase the risk of infection. Factors that predispose the woman to postpartum infection are listed in Box 14-2.

Prevention

The most effective and least expensive treatment of postpartum infection is prevention:

- Preventive measures include good prenatal nutrition to control anemia and intrapartal hemorrhage.
- Good maternal perineal hygiene with thorough handwashing is emphasized.
- Strict adherence by all health care personnel to aseptic techniques during childbirth and the postpartum period is very important.

Endometritis

Endometritis is the most common type of postpartum infection.

- It usually begins as a localized infection at the placental site but can spread to involve the entire endometrium. Incidence is higher after cesarean birth.
- Assessment for signs of endometritis may reveal a fever (usually greater than 38° C); increased pulse; chills; anorexia; nausea; fatigue and lethargy; pelvic pain; uterine tenderness; or foul-smelling, profuse lochia. Leukocytosis and a markedly increased RBC sedimentation rate are typical laboratory findings of postpartum infections. Anemia also may be present. Blood cultures or intracervical or intrauterine bacterial cultures (aerobic and anaerobic) should reveal the offending pathogens within 36 to 48 hours.

BOX 14-2

Predisposing Factors for Postpartum Infection

PRECONCEPTION OR ANTEPARTAL FACTORS

History of previous venous thrombosis, urinary tract infection, mastitis, pneumonia
Diabetes mellitus
Alcoholism
Drug abuse
Immunosuppression
Anemia
Malnutrition

INTRAPARTAL FACTORS

Cesarean birth
Prolonged rupture of membranes
Chorioamnionitis
Prolonged labor
Bladder catheterization
Internal fetal or uterine pressure monitoring
Multiple vaginal examinations after rupture of membranes
Epidural anesthesia
Retained placental fragments
Postpartum hemorrhage
Episiotomy or lacerations
Hematomas

- Management of endometritis consists of intravenous broad-spectrum antibiotic therapy (cephalosporins, penicillins, or clindamycin and gentamicin) and supportive care, including hydration, rest, and pain relief.
- Antibiotic therapy is usually discontinued 24 hours after the woman is asymptomatic.
- Assessments of lochia, vital signs, and changes in the woman's condition continue during treatment.
- Comfort measures depend on the symptoms and may include cool compresses, warm blankets, perineal care, and sitz baths.
- Teaching should include side effects of therapy, prevention of spread of infection, signs and symptoms of worsening condi-

tion, and adherence to the treatment plan and the need for follow-up care.
- Women may need to be encouraged or assisted to maintain mother-infant interactions and breastfeeding (if allowed during treatment).

Wound Infections

- Wound infections also are common postpartum infections but often develop after the woman is at home. Sites of infection include the cesarean incision and the episiotomy or repaired laceration site. Predisposing factors are similar to those for endometritis.
  - Signs of wound infection include erythema, edema, warmth, tenderness, seropurulent drainage, and wound separation.
  - Fever and pain also may be present.
- Treatment of wound infections may combine antibiotic therapy with wound debridement.
  - Wounds may be opened and drained.
  - Nursing care includes frequent wound and vital sign assessments and wound care.
  - Comfort measures include sitz baths, warm compresses, and perineal care.
  - Teaching includes good hygiene techniques (i.e., changing perineal pads front to back, handwashing before and after perineal care), self-care measures, and signs of worsening conditions to report to the health care provider.
  - The woman is usually discharged to home for self-care or home nursing care after treatment is initiated in the inpatient setting.

Urinary Tract Infections

UTIs occur in 2% to 4% of postpartum women.
- Risk factors include urinary catheterization, frequent pelvic examinations, epidural anesthesia, genital tract injury, history of UTI, and cesarean birth.
- Signs and symptoms include dysuria, frequency and urgency, low-grade fever, urinary retention, hematuria, and pyuria. Costovertebral angle (CVA) tenderness or flank pain may indicate an upper UTI.

- Urinalysis results may reveal *Escherichia coli,* although other gram-negative aerobic bacilli also may cause UTIs.
- Medical management for UTIs consists of antibiotic therapy, analgesia, and hydration.
- Postpartum women are usually treated on an outpatient basis; therefore teaching should include instructions on how to monitor temperature, bladder function, and appearance of urine.
- The woman also should be taught about signs of potential complications and the importance of taking all antibiotics as prescribed.
- Other suggestions for prevention of UTIs include proper perineal care, wiping from front to back after urinating or having a bowel movement, and increasing fluid intake.

Mastitis

Mastitis affects about 1% of women soon after childbirth, most of whom are first-time mothers who are breastfeeding. Mastitis almost always is unilateral and develops well after the flow of milk has been established. The infecting organism generally is the hemolytic *S. aureus.*

- An infected nipple fissure usually is the initial lesion, but the ductal system is involved next.
- Inflammatory edema and engorgement of the breast soon obstruct the flow of milk in a lobe; regional mastitis and then generalized mastitis follow.
- If treatment is not prompt, mastitis may progress to a breast abscess.
- Symptoms rarely appear before the end of the first postpartum week and are more common in the second to fourth weeks.
  - Chills, fever, malaise, and local breast tenderness are noted first.
  - Localized breast tenderness, pain, swelling, redness, and axillary adenopathy also may occur.
  - Antibiotics are prescribed.
  - Lactation can be maintained by emptying the breasts every 2 to 4 hours by breastfeeding, manual expression, or breast pump.

- Because mastitis rarely occurs before the postpartum woman is discharged, teaching should include warning signs of mastitis and counseling about prevention of cracked nipples.
- Management includes intensive antibiotic therapy (e.g., cephalosporins and vancomycin, which are particularly useful in staphylococcal infections), support of breasts, local heat (or cold), adequate hydration, and analgesics.
- Almost all instances of acute mastitis can be avoided by proper breastfeeding technique to prevent cracked nipples.
  - Missed feedings, waiting too long between feedings, and abrupt weaning may lead to clogged nipples and mastitis.
  - Cleanliness practiced by all who have contact with the newborn and new mother also reduces the incidence of mastitis.

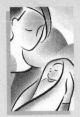

CHAPTER 15

Assessment and Care of the Newborn

CARE MANAGEMENT: FROM BIRTH THROUGH THE FIRST 2 HOURS

- Care begins immediately after birth and focuses on assessing and stabilizing the newborn's condition. As part of Standard Precautions, gloves should be worn when handling the newborn until blood and amniotic fluid are removed by bathing.
- The nurse verifies that respirations have been established, dries the infant, assesses temperature, and places identical identification bracelets on the infant and the mother. In some settings, the father or partner also wears an identification bracelet. Information on the bracelet includes name, sex, date and time of birth, and identification number. Infants also are foot-printed by using a form that includes the mother's fingerprints, name, and date and time of birth. These identification procedures must be performed before the mother and infant are separated after birth.
- The infant may be placed on the mother's abdomen to allow skin-to-skin contact, wrapped in a warm blanket and placed in the arms of the mother, given to the partner to hold, or kept partially undressed under a radiant warmer. The infant may be admitted to a nursery or remain with the parents throughout the hospital stay.
- The initial examination of the newborn can occur while the nurse is drying and wrapping the infant, or observations can be made while the infant is lying on the mother's abdomen or in her arms immediately after birth.

TABLE 15-1

Apgar Score

	SCORE		
SIGN	**0**	**1**	**2**
Heart rate	Absent	Slow (<100 beats/min)	>100 beats/min
Respiratory rate	Absent	Slow, weak cry	Good cry
Muscle tone	Flaccid	Some flexion of extremities	Well flexed
Reflex irritability	No response	Grimace	Cry
Color	Blue, pale	Body pink, extremities blue	Completely pink

Interference in the initial parent-infant acquaintance process should be minimized.

Apgar Score

The nurse usually assigns the Apgar score at 1 and 5 minutes after birth (Table 15-1). The Apgar score permits a rapid assessment of the need for resuscitation. Scores of 0 to 3 indicate severe distress; scores of 4 to 6 indicate moderate difficulty; and scores of 7 to 10 indicate that the infant is having no difficulty adjusting to extrauterine life. Apgar scores do not predict future neurologic outcome, but they are useful for describing the newborn's transition to extrauterine environment. If resuscitation is required, it should be initiated before the 1-minute Apgar score.

Initial Physical Assessment

If the infant is breathing effectively, is pink in color, and has no apparent life-threatening anomalies or risk factors requiring immediate attention (e.g., infant of a diabetic mother), further examination can be delayed until after the parents have had an opportunity to interact with the infant. Routine procedures and the admission process can be carried out in the mother's room or in a separate nursery.

The initial physical assessment includes a brief review of systems:

1. *External:* Note skin color, general activity, and position; assess nasal patency by covering one nostril at a time while observing respirations; assess skin: peeling, or lack of subcutaneous fat (dysmaturity or postterm); note meconium staining of cord, skin, fingernails, or amniotic fluid (staining may indicate fetal release of meconium, often related to hypoxia; offensive odor may indicate intrauterine infection); note length of nails and creases on soles of feet.

2. *Chest:* Auscultate apical heart for rate and rhythm, heart tones, and presence of abnormal sounds; note character of respirations and presence of crackles or other adventitious sounds; note equality of breath sounds by auscultation.

3. *Abdomen:* Observe characteristics of abdomen (rounded, flat, concave) and absence of anomalies; auscultate bowel sounds; note number of vessels in cord.

4. *Neurologic:* Check muscle tone; assess Moro and suck reflexes; palpate anterior fontanel; note by palpation the presence and size of the fontanels and sutures.

5. *Genitourinary:* Note external sex characteristics and any abnormality of genitalia; check anal patency and presence of meconium; note passage of urine.

6. *Other observations:* Note gross structural malformations obvious at birth that may require immediate medical attention.

A gestational age assessment is done within 2 hours of birth (Fig. 15-1). See later discussion on p. 461.

A more comprehensive physical assessment is completed within 24 hours of birth (Table 15-2).

Stabilization

Generally, the normal term infant born vaginally has little difficulty clearing the airway. Most secretions are moved by gravity and brought to the oropharynx by the cough reflex. The infant is often maintained in a side-lying position (head stabilized, not in Trendelenburg) with a rolled blanket at the back to facilitate drainage.

If the infant has excess mucus in the respiratory tract, the mouth and nasal passages may be suctioned with the bulb syringe.

Suctioning with a bulb syringe

- Suction the mouth first to prevent the infant from inhaling pharyngeal secretions by gasping as the nares are touched.
  - Compress the bulb, and insert into one side of the mouth.
  - Avoid the center of the infant's mouth because this could stimulate the gag reflex.
- Suction the nasal passages one nostril at a time.
- When the infant's cry sounds clear and not as though it is through mucus or a bubble, stop suctioning.
- Always keep the bulb syringe in the infant's crib.
- Demonstrate to the parents how to use the bulb syringe, and ask for a return demonstration.

Use of nasopharyngeal catheter with mechanical suction apparatus

Deeper suctioning may be needed to remove mucus from the newborn's nasopharynx or posterior oropharynx.

Wall suction: Adjust the pressure to <80 mm Hg. Proper tube insertion and suctioning for 5 seconds or less per tube insertion help prevent laryngospasms and oxygen depletion.

- Lubricate the catheter in sterile water and insert either orally along the base of the tongue or up and back into the nares.
- After the catheter is properly placed, create suction by placing your thumb over the control as the catheter is carefully rotated and gently withdrawn.
- Repeat the procedure until the infant's cry sounds clear and air entry into the lungs is heard by stethoscope.

Text continued on p. 454.

NEUROMUSCULAR MATURITY

	-1	0	1	2	3	4	5
Posture							
Square Window (wrist)	> 90°	90°	60°	45°	30°	0°	
Arm Recoil		180°	140° - 180°	110° - 140°	90° - 110°	< 90°	
Popliteal Angle	180°	160°	140°	120°	100°	90°	< 90°
Scarf Sign							
Heel to Ear							

A

PHYSICAL MATURITY

	-1	0	1	2	3	4	5
Skin	sticky friable transparent	gelatinous red, translucent	smooth pink, visible veins	superficial peeling or rash, few veins	cracking pale areas rare veins	parchment deep cracking no vessels	leathery cracked wrinkled
Lanugo	none	sparse	abundant	thinning	bald areas	mostly bald	
Plantar Surface	heel-toe 40-50 mm: -1; <40 mm: -2	>50 mm no crease	faint red marks	anterior transverse crease only	creases ant. 2/3	creases over entire sole	
Breast	imperceptible	barely perceptible	flat areola no bud	stippled areola 1-2 mm bud	raised areola 3-4 mm bud	full areola 5-10 mm bud	
Eye/Ear	lids fused loosely: -1; tightly: -2	lids open pinna flat stays folded	sl. curved pinna; soft; slow recoil	well-curved pinna; soft but ready recoil	formed & firm instant recoil	thick cartilage ear stiff	
Genitals (male)	scrotum flat, smooth	scrotum empty faint rugae	testes in upper canal rare rugae	testes descending few rugae	testes down good rugae	testes pendulous deep rugae	
Genitals (female)	clitoris prominent labia flat	prominent clitoris small labia minora	prominent clitoris enlarging minora	majora & minora equally prominent	majora large minora small	majora cover clitoris & minora	

MATURITY RATING

score	weeks
-10	20
-5	22
0	24
5	26
10	28
15	30
20	32
25	34
30	36
35	38
40	40
45	42
50	44

Fig. 15-1 Estimation of gestational age. **A,** New Ballard Scale for newborn maturity rating. *Continued*

CLASSIFICATION OF NEWBORNS—
BASED ON MATURITY AND INTRAUTERINE GROWTH
Symbols: X - 1st Examination O - 2nd Examination

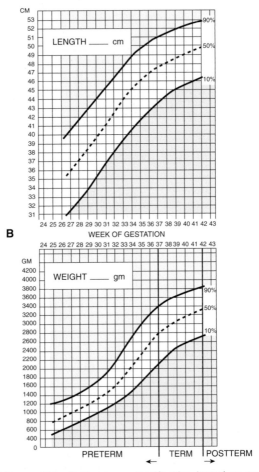

Fig. 15-1 cont'd B, Newborn classification based on maturity and intrauterine growth. (**A** from Ballard, J. et al. [1991]. New Ballard Score, expanded to include extremely premature infants. *Journal of Pediatrics, 119*[3], 417-423. **B** modified from Lubchenco, L., Hansman, C., & Boyd, E. [1966]. Intrauterine growth in length and head circumference as estimated from live births at gestational ages from 26 to 42 weeks. *Journal of Pediatrics, 37*[3], 403-408; Battaglia, F., & Lubchenco, L. [1967]. A practical classification of newborn infants by weight and gestational age. *Journal of Pediatrics, 71*[2], 159-167.)

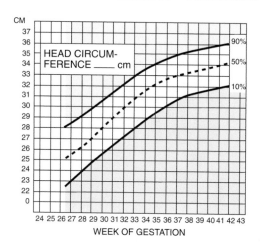

CM

	1st Examination (X)	2nd Examination (O)
LARGE FOR GESTATIONAL AGE (LGA)		
APPROPRIATE FOR GESTATIONAL AGE (AGA)		
SMALL FOR GESTATIONAL AGE (SGA)		
Age at Examination	hrs	hrs
Signature of Examiner		
	M.D.	M.D.

B

Fig. 15-1 cont'd

TABLE 15-2

Physical Assessment of Newborn

AREA ASSESSED	NORMAL FINDINGS	DEVIATIONS FROM NORMAL RANGE	ETIOLOGY
POSTURE Inspect newborn before disturbing	Arms, legs in moderate flexion; fists clenched Normal spontaneous movement bilaterally; asynchronous but equal extension in all extremities	Hypotonia	Prematurity or hypoxia in utero, maternal medications
		Hypertonia	Drug dependence, central nervous system [CNS] disorder
		Opisthotonos Limitation of motion in any of extremities	CNS disturbance
VITAL SIGNS Heart rate and pulses —Inspection —Palpation —Auscultation	Visible pulsations in left midclavicular line, fifth intercostal space Apical pulse, fourth intercostal space, 100-160 beats/min (listen for 1 full minute) 80-100 beats/min (sleeping) to 180 beats/min (crying)	Tachycardia: persistent, >180 beats/min Bradycardia: persistent, <80 beats/min Murmurs (if present, note other signs of cardiovascular dysfunction such as tachypnea, tachycardia,	Respiratory distress syndrome (RDS) Congenital heart block, maternal lupus Possibly functional

	Quality: *first sound* (closure of mitral and tricuspid valves) and *second sound* (closure of aortic and pulmonic valves) sharp and clear Possible murmur	pallor, cyanosis, absence of peripheral pulses, or poor perfusion)	
		Arrhythmias: irregular heart rate (irregular heart rate not attributed to changes in activity or respiratory pattern should be further evaluated)	
		Sounds: distant, poor quality, extra	Pneumomediastinum
		Heart on right side of chest	Dextrocardia, often accompanied by reversal of intestines
Peripheral pulses: femoral, brachial, popliteal, posterior tibial	Peripheral pulses equal and strong	Weak or absent peripheral pulses; unequal	Decreased cardiac output, thrombus
	Femoral pulses equal and strong	Weak or absent femoral pulses	Hip dysplasia, coarctation of aorta if weak on left and strong on right, thrombophlebitis

Continued

TABLE 15-2

Physical Assessment of Newborn—cont'd

AREA ASSESSED	NORMAL FINDINGS	DEVIATIONS FROM NORMAL RANGE	ETIOLOGY
VITAL SIGNS—cont'd			
Temperature Axillary method of choice	Axillary: 36.5°-37.2° C	Subnormal	Prematurity, infection, low environmental temperature, inadequate clothing, dehydration
		Increased	Infection, high environmental temperature, excessive clothing, proximity to heating unit or in direct sunshine, drug addiction, diarrhea and dehydration
	Temperature stabilized by 8-10 hr of age	Temperature not stabilized by 6-8 hr after birth	If mother received magnesium sulfate, maternal analgesics

Check respiratory rate and effort when infant is at rest	30-60 breaths/min	
Count respirations for full minute	Shallow and irregular in rate, rhythm, and depth when infant is awake	Apneic episodes: >15 sec	Preterm infant: "periodic breathing," rapid warming or cooling of infant
	Subnormal	Bradypnea: <25/min	Maternal narcosis from analgesics or anesthetics, birth trauma
	Breath sounds loud, clear, near	Tachypnea: >60/min	Narrowing of bronchi RDS, congenital, diaphragmatic hernia, transient tachypnea of the newborn
	Crackles may be heard after birth	Crackles, rhonchi, wheezes	Fluid in lungs
		Expiratory grunt	
		Distress evidenced by nasal flaring, retractions, chin tug, labored breathing	
Measure blood pressure (BP) using oscillometric monitor BP cuff,	80-90s/40s-50s (mmHg)	Difference between upper and lower extremity pressures	Coarctation of aorta
		Hypotension	Sepsis, hypovolemia

Continued

TABLE 15-2

Physical Assessment of Newborn—cont'd

AREA ASSESSED	NORMAL FINDINGS	DEVIATIONS FROM NORMAL RANGE	ETIOLOGY
VITAL SIGNS—cont'd palpate brachial, popliteal, or posterior tibial pulse (depending on measurement site) Check electronic monitor BP cuff: BP cuff width affects readings, use cuff 2.5cm wide and palpate radial pulse		Hypertension	Coarctation of aorta, renal involvement, thrombus
WEIGHT Weigh at same time each day	2500-4000 g Acceptable weight loss: ≤10% Second baby weighs more than first Birth weight regained within first 2 wk	Weight ≤2500 g	Prematurity, small for gestational age, rubella syndrome
		Weight ≥4000 g	Large for gestational age, maternal diabetes, heredity—normal for these parents
		Weight loss >10%-15%	Dehydration

Continued

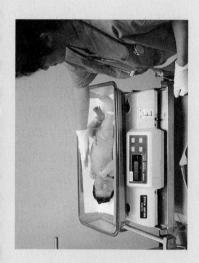

Weighing the infant. Note that a hand is held over the infant as a safety measure. The scale is covered to protect against cross-infection. (Courtesy Kim Molloy, Knoxville, IA.)

TABLE 15-2
Physical Assessment of Newborn—cont'd

AREA ASSESSED	NORMAL FINDINGS	DEVIATIONS FROM NORMAL RANGE	ETIOLOGY
LENGTH Length from top of head to heel	45-55 cm	<45 cm or >55 cm	Chromosomal abnormality, heredity—normal for these parents

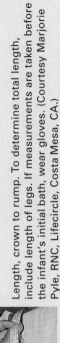

Length, crown to rump. To determine total length, include length of legs. If measurements are taken before the infant's initial bath, wear gloves. (Courtesy Marjorie Pyle, RNC, Lifecircle, Costa Mesa, CA.)

HEAD CIRCUMFERENCE

32-36.8 cm
Circumference of head and chest approximately the same for first 1 or 2 days after birth

Small head, ≤32 cm: microcephaly

Maternal rubella, toxoplasmosis, cytomegalic inclusion disease, fused cranial sutures (craniosynostosis)

Maldevelopment, infection

Hydrocephaly: sutures widely separated, circumference ≥4 cm more than chest circumference

Increased intracranial pressure

Hemorrhage, space-occupying lesion

Continued

TABLE 15-2

Physical Assessment of Newborn—cont'd

AREA ASSESSED	NORMAL FINDINGS	DEVIATIONS FROM NORMAL RANGE	ETIOLOGY
HEAD CIRCUMFERENCE—*cont'd*			

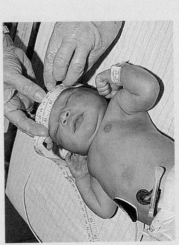

Circumference of head. (Courtesy Marjorie Pyle, RNC, Lifecircle, Costa Mesa, CA.)

CHEST CIRCUMFERENCE

Measure at nipple line

2-3 cm less than head circumference, averages between 30 and 33 cm

≤30 cm

Prematurity

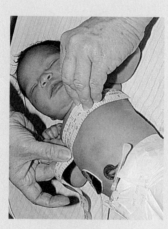

Circumference of chest. (Courtesy Marjorie Pyle, RNC, Lifecircle, Costa Mesa, CA.)

Continued

TABLE 15-2
Physical Assessment of Newborn—cont'd

AREA ASSESSED	NORMAL FINDINGS	DEVIATIONS FROM NORMAL RANGE	ETIOLOGY
ABDOMINAL CIRCUMFERENCE Measure above umbilicus Not usually measured unless specific indication	Same size as chest	Enlarging abdomen between feedings	Abdominal mass or blockage in intestinal tract

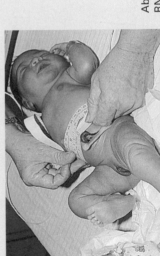

Abdominal circumference. (Courtesy Marjorie Pyle, RNC, Lifecircle, Costa Mesa, CA.)

SKIN		
Color	Generally pink	
	Varying with ethnic origin	
		Dark red	Prematurity, polycythemia
		Gray	Hypotension, poor perfusion
	Acrocyanosis, especially if chilled	Pallor	Cardiovascular problem, CNS damage, blood dyscrasia, blood loss, twin-to-twin transfusion, nosocomial infection
	Mottling		
	Harlequin sign		
	Plethora		
	Telangiectases ("stork bites" or capillary hemangiomas)	Cyanosis	Hypothermia; infection; hypoglycemia; cardiopulmonary diseases; cardiac, neurologic, or respiratory malformations
	Erythema toxicum or neonatorum ("newborn rash")		
	Milia		
	Petechiae over presenting part	Petechiae over any other area	Clotting factor deficiency, infection
	Ecchymoses from forceps in vertex births or over buttocks, genitalia, and legs in breech births	Ecchymoses in any other area	Hemorrhagic disease, traumatic birth

Continued

TABLE 15-2

Physical Assessment of Newborn—cont'd

AREA ASSESSED	NORMAL FINDINGS	DEVIATIONS FROM NORMAL RANGE	ETIOLOGY
SKIN—*cont'd*			
Jaundice	None at birth Physiologic jaundice in up to 50% of term infants in first week of life	Jaundice within first 24 hr	Increased hemolysis, Rh isoimmunization, ABO incompatibility
Birthmarks	Mongolian spot —Infants of African-American, Asian, and Native American origin: 70%-85% —Infants of Caucasian origin: 5%-13%	Hemangiomas Nevus flammeus: port-wine stain Nevus vasculosus: strawberry mark Cavernous hemangiomas	
Check condition	No skin edema Opacity: few large blood vessels visible indistinctly over abdomen	Edema on hands, feet; pitting over tibia Texture thin, smooth, or of medium thickness; rash or superficial peeling visible	Overhydration Prematurity, postmaturity

	Normal Findings	Deviations from Normal Range/Possible Causes
	Numerous vessels very visible over abdomen	Prematurity
	Texture thick, parchmentlike; cracking, peeling	Postmaturity
	Skin tags, webbing	
	Papules, pustules, vesicles, ulcers, maceration	Impetigo, candidiasis, herpes, diaper rash
Gently pinch skin between thumb and forefinger over abdomen and inner thigh to check for turgor	Dehydration: loss of weight best indicator After pinch released, skin returns to original state immediately Normal weight loss after birth: ≤10% of birth weight Possibly puffy	
	Loose, wrinkled skin	Prematurity, postmaturity, dehydration: fold of skin persisting after release of pinch
	Tense, tight, shiny skin	Edema, extreme cold, shock, infection
	Lack of subcutaneous fat, prominence of clavicle or ribs	Prematurity, malnutrition
Vernix caseosa: color and odor	Whitish, cheesy, odorless; usually more found in creases, folds	
	Absent or minimal	Postmaturity
	Excessive	Prematurity
	Green color	Possible in utero release of meconium or presence of bilirubin

Continued

TABLE 15-2

Physical Assessment of Newborn—cont'd

AREA ASSESSED	NORMAL FINDINGS	DEVIATIONS FROM NORMAL RANGE	ETIOLOGY
SKIN—*cont'd*			
Lanugo	Over shoulders, pinnae of ears, forehead	Odor	Possible intrauterine infection
		Absent	Postmaturity
		Excessive	Prematurity, especially if lanugo abundant and long and thick over back
	Making up one fourth of body length	Cephalhematoma	Birth trauma
	Molding	Indentation	Fracture from trauma
	Caput succedaneum, possibly showing some ecchymosis	Severe molding	
HEAD Fontanels: open versus closed	Anterior fontanel 5 cm diamond, increasing as molding resolves	Full, bulging	Tumor, hemorrhage, infection
	Posterior fontanel triangle, smaller than anterior	Large, flat, soft	Malnutrition, hydrocephaly, retarded bone age, hypothyroidism

Sutures	Palpable and unjoined sutures	Depressed	Dehydration
	Possible overlap of sutures with molding	Widely spaced	Hydrocephaly
		Premature closure	Craniosynostosis
Hair	Silky, single strands lying flat; growth pattern toward face and neck, variation in amount	Fine, woolly	Prematurity
		Unusual swirls, patterns or hairline, coarse, brittle	Endocrine or genetic disorders
EYES			
Eyeballs	Both present and of equal size, both round, firm	Agenesis or absence of one or both eyeballs	Chromosomal disorders, such as Down, cri-du-chat syndromes
	Eyes and space between eyes each one third the distance from outer-to-outer canthus	Epicanthal folds when present with other signs	
	Epicanthal folds: normal racial characteristic	Discharge: purulent	Infection
	Symmetric in size, shape		
	Blink reflex	Small eyeball	Rubella syndrome
		Lens opacity or absence of red reflex	Congenital cataracts, possibly from rubella
	No discharge	Discharge (purulent)	Infection
		Chemical conjunctivitis	Eye medication (requires no treatment)
	No tears	Lesions: coloboma, absence of part of iris	
	Subconjunctival hemorrhage		

Continued

TABLE 15-2
Physical Assessment of Newborn—cont'd

AREA ASSESSED	NORMAL FINDINGS	DEVIATIONS FROM NORMAL RANGE	ETIOLOGY
		Pink color of iris	Albinism
		Jaundiced sclera	Hyperbilirubinemia

Eyes. In pseudostrabismus, inner epicanthal folds cause the eyes to appear misaligned; however, corneal light reflexes are perfectly symmetric. Eyes are symmetric in size and shape and are well placed.

Pupils	Present, equal in size, reactive to light	Pupils: unequal, constricted, dilated, fixed	Intracranial pressure, medications, tumors
Eyeball movement	Random, jerky, uneven, focus possible briefly, following to midline	Persistent strabismus Doll's eyes	Increased intracranial pressure
	Transient strabismus or nystagmus until third or fourth month	Sunset	Increased intracranial pressure
Eyebrows	Distinct (not connected in midline)	Connection in midline	Cornelia de Lange syndrome
NOSE			
—Shape	Midline		
—Placement	Some mucus but no drainage	Copious drainage, with or without regular periods of cyanosis at rest and return of pink color with crying	Choanal atresia, congenital syphilis, chromosomal disorder
—Patency	Preferential nose breather	Malformed	
	Sneezing to clear nose		
	Slight deformity (flat or deviated to one side) from passage through birth canal	Flaring of nares	Respiratory distress

Continued

TABLE 15-2

Physical Assessment of Newborn—cont'd

AREA ASSESSED	NORMAL FINDINGS	DEVIATIONS FROM NORMAL RANGE	ETIOLOGY
EARS Pinna	Correct placement: line drawn through inner and outer canthi of eyes reaching to top notch of ears (at junction with scalp)	Agenesis Lack of cartilage Low placement	Prematurity Chromosomal disorder, mental retardation, kidney disorder
	Well-formed, firm cartilage	Preauricular tags Size: possibly overly prominent or protruding ears	
Hearing	Responds to voice and other sounds State (e.g., alert, asleep) influences response	No response to sound	Deaf, rubella syndrome

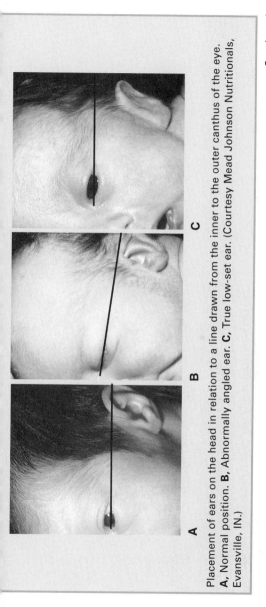

A **B** C

Placement of ears on the head in relation to a line drawn from the inner to the outer canthus of the eye.
A, Normal position. **B,** Abnormally angled ear. **C,** True low-set ear. (Courtesy Mead Johnson Nutritionals, Evansville, IN.)

Continued

TABLE 15-2
Physical Assessment of Newborn—cont'd

AREA ASSESSED	NORMAL FINDINGS	DEVIATIONS FROM NORMAL RANGE	ETIOLOGY
FACIES Observe overall appearance of face	"Normal" appearance; well-placed, proportionate, symmetric features Positional deformities	Infant appearance "odd" or "funny" Usually accompanied by other features, such as low-set ears, other structural disorders	Hereditary, chromosomal aberration
MOUTH Lips	Symmetry of lip movement	Gross anomalies in placement, size, shape Cyanosis, circumoral pallor Asymmetry in movement of lips	Cleft lip and/or palate, gums Respiratory distress, hypothermia Cranial nerve VII paralysis
Buccal mucosa	Dry or moist Pink Transient circumoral cyanosis		

Gums	Pink gums Inclusion cysts (Epstein pearls—Bohn nodules, whitish, hard nodules on gums or roof of mouth)	Teeth: predeciduous or deciduous
Tongue	Tongue not protruding, freely movable, symmetric in shape, movement Sucking pads inside cheeks	Macroglossia Short lingual frenulum Thrush: white plaques on cheeks or tongue that bleed if touched
Palate (soft, hard) —Arch —Uvula —Chin	Soft and hard palates intact Uvula in midline Epstein pearls Distinct chin	Cleft, hard or soft palate Micrognathia
—Saliva	Mouth moist	Excessive saliva

Hereditary

Prematurity, chromosomal disorder
Candida albicans

Pierre Robin or other syndrome
Esophageal atresia, tracheoesophageal fistula

Continued

TABLE 15-2

Physical Assessment of Newborn—cont'd

AREA ASSESSED	NORMAL FINDINGS	DEVIATIONS FROM NORMAL RANGE	ETIOLOGY
Reflexes —Rooting —Sucking —Extrusion	Reflexes present Reflex response dependent on state of wakefulness and hunger	Absent	Prematurity
NECK Sternocleidomastoid muscles	Short, thick, surrounded by skin folds; no webbing Head held in midline (sternocleidomastoid muscles equal), no masses Transient positional deformity Freedom of movement from side to side and flexion and extension, no movement of chin past shoulder	Webbing Restricted movement, holding of head at angle Absence of head control	Turner syndrome Torticollis (wryneck), opisthotonos Prematurity, Down syndrome

	Thyroid not palpable	Masses; Distended veins	Enlarged thyroid; Cardiopulmonary disorder
Thyroid gland	Thyroid not palpable	Masses Distended veins	Enlarged thyroid Cardiopulmonary disorder
CHEST			
Thorax	Almost circular, barrel shaped Tip of sternum possibly prominent	Bulging of chest, unequal movement Malformation	Pneumothorax, pneumomediastinum Funnel chest—pectus excavatum
Respiratory movements	Symmetric chest movements, chest and abdominal movements synchronized during respirations Occasional retractions, especially when crying	Retractions with or without respiratory distress, see saw respirations	Prematurity, RDS
Clavicles	Clavicles intact	Fracture of clavicle; crepitus	Trauma
Ribs	Rib cage symmetric, intact; moves with respirations	Poor development of rib cage and musculature	Prematurity
Nipples	Prominent, well formed; symmetrically placed	Supernumerary, along nipple line Malpositioned or widely spaced	

Continued

TABLE 15-2

Physical Assessment of Newborn—cont'd

AREA ASSESSED	NORMAL FINDINGS	DEVIATIONS FROM NORMAL RANGE	ETIOLOGY
CHEST—cont'd			
Breast tissue	Breast nodule: approximately 3-10 mm in term infant		Prematurity
	Secretion of witch's milk	Lack of breast tissue	Maternal hormones
ABDOMEN			
Umbilical cord	Two arteries, one vein	One artery	Renal anomalies
	Whitish gray	Meconium stained	Intrauterine distress
	Definite demarcation between cord and skin, no intestinal structures within cord	Bleeding or oozing around cord	Hemorrhagic disease
	Dry around base, drying	Redness or drainage around cord	Infection, possible persistence of urachus
	Odorless	Herniation of abdominal contents into area of cord (e.g., omphalocele); defect covered with thin, friable membrane, possibly extensive	
	Cord clamp in place for 24 hr		
	Reducible umbilical hernia		

Abdomen	Rounded, prominent, dome-shaped because abdominal musculature not fully developed	Gastroschisis: fissure of abdominal cavity	
	Some diastasis of abdominal musculature		
	Liver possibly palpable 1-2 cm below right costal margin		
	No other masses palpable	Distention at birth	Ruptured viscus, genitourinary masses or malformations: hydronephrosis, teratomas, abdominal tumors
		—Mild	Overfeeding, high gastrointestinal tract obstruction
		—Marked	Lower gastrointestinal tract obstruction, imperforate anus
		—Intermittent or transient	Overfeeding
		Partial intestinal obstruction	Stenosis of bowel
		Visible peristalsis	Obstruction

Continued

TABLE 15-2

Physical Assessment of Newborn—cont'd

AREA ASSESSED	NORMAL FINDINGS	DEVIATIONS FROM NORMAL RANGE	ETIOLOGY
		Malrotation of bowel or adhesions	
Bowel sounds	Sounds present within minutes after birth in healthy term infants	Sepsis Scaphoid, with bowel sounds in chest and respiratory distress	Infection Diaphragmatic hernia
Stools	Meconium stool passing within 24-48hr after birth	No stool	Imperforate anus
Color	Linea nigra possibly apparent		Hormone influence during pregnancy
Movement with respiration	Respirations primarily diaphragmatic, abdominal and chest movement synchronous	Decreased abdominal breathing "Seesaw"	Intrathoracic disease, phrenic nerve palsy, diaphragmatic hernia Respiratory distress
GENITALIA **Female** General appearance	Female genitalia	Ambiguous genitalia—enlarged clitoris with urinary meatus on tip, fused labia	Chromosomal disorder, maternal drug ingestion
Clitoris	Usually edematous	Virilized female; extremely large clitoris	Congenital adrenal hyperplasia pregnancy hormones
Labia majora	Usually edematous, covering labia minora in term newborns		

	Increased pigmentation		
Labia minora	Edema and ecchymosis after breech birth	Labia majora widely separated and labia minora prominent	Prematurity
	Possible protrusion over labia majora	Absence of vaginal orifice	
	Smegma	Bladder exstrophy	
Discharge	Open orifice	Fecal discharge	Fistula
Vagina	Some vernix caseosa between labia possible		Pregnancy hormones
	Blood-tinged discharge from pseudomenstruation		
	Mucoid discharge		
	Hymenal or vaginal tag		
	Beneath clitoris, difficult to see (to watch for voiding)		
Urinary meatus		Stenosed meatus	
Male			
General appearance	Male genitalia	Increased size and pigmentation	Ambiguous genitalia
Penis			Pregnancy hormones
—Urinary meatus as slit	Meatus at tip of penis	Urinary meatus not on tip of glans penis	Hypospadias, epispadias
			Round meatal opening

Continued

TABLE 15-2

Physical Assessment of Newborn—cont'd

AREA ASSESSED	NORMAL FINDINGS	DEVIATIONS FROM NORMAL RANGE	ETIOLOGY
Male—cont'd			
—Prepuce	Prepuce (foreskin) covering glans penis and not retractable	Prepuce removed if circumcised	
		Wide variation in size of genitalia	
Scrotum			
—Rugae (wrinkles)	Large, edematous, pendulous in term infant; covered with rugae	Scrotal edema and ecchymosis	Breech birth
		Scrotum smooth	Prematurity
—Testes	Palpable on each side	Testes undescended	Prematurity, cryptorchidism
		Hydrocele, small, noncommunicating	Prematurity
		Bulge palpable in inguinal canal	Inguinal hernia
Check urination	Voiding within 24 hr, stream adequate, amount adequate	No voiding	Absence of kidneys, obstruction
	Rust-stained urine		Uric acid crystals

Reflex	Testes retract, especially when newborn is chilled	
—Cremasteric		
EXTREMITIES		
Degree of flexion	Assuming of position maintained in utero	Limited motion
Range of motion	Transient (positional) deformities	Poor muscle tone
Symmetry of motion	Attitude of general flexion	Positive scarf sign
Muscle tone	Full range of motion, spontaneous movements	Malformations
		Prematurity, maternal medications, CNS anomalies
	Slight tremors sometimes apparent	Fracture or crepitus, brachial nerve trauma, malformations
	Contours and movement symmetric	Asymmetry of movement
Arms and hands	Longer than legs in newborn period	Asymmetry of contour
—Intactness		Amelia or phocomelia
—Appropriate placement	Some acrocyanosis, especially when chilled	Palmar creases
—Color		Simian line with short, incurved little fingers
		Malformations, fracture
		Teratogens
		Down syndrome

Continued

TABLE 15-2

Physical Assessment of Newborn—cont'd

AREA ASSESSED	NORMAL FINDINGS	DEVIATIONS FROM NORMAL RANGE	ETIOLOGY
EXTREMITIES—cont'd			
Fingers	Five on each hand	Webbing of fingers: syndactyly	Familial
	Fist often clenched with thumb under fingers	Absence or excess of fingers	
		Strong, rigid flexion; persistent fists; positioning of fists in front of mouth constantly	CNS disorder
Joints	Full range of motion, symmetric contour	Increased tonicity, clonus, prolonged tremors	CNS disorder
Grasp (palmar and plantar)	Intact		
Humerus	Appearance of bowing because lateral muscles more developed than medial muscles	Fractured humerus	Trauma
Legs and feet	Feet appearing to turn in but can be easily rotated	Amelia (absence of limbs), phocomelia (shortened limbs)	Chromosomal deficiency, teratogenic effect
		Temperature of one leg different from that of the other	Circulatory deficiency CNS disorder

	externally, positional defects tending to correct while infant is crying		
	Acrocyanosis		
Number of toes	Five on each foot	Webbing, syndactyly	Chromosomal defect
		Absence or excess of digits	Chromosomal defect, familial trait
Femur	Intact femur	Femoral fracture	Difficult breech birth
	Ortolani maneuver: no click heard, femoral head not overriding acetabulum (Box 15-1)	Developmental dysplasia or dislocation	
Soles of feet	Major gluteal folds even	Soles of feet	Prematurity
	Soles well lined (or wrinkled) over two thirds of foot in term infants	Few lines	Postmaturity
		Covered with lines	
	Plantar fat pad giving flat-footed effect	Congenital clubfoot	
Joints	Full range of motion, symmetric contour	Hypermobility of joints	Down syndrome
		Asymmetric movement	Trauma, CNS disorder

Continued

TABLE 15-2

Physical Assessment of Newborn—cont'd

AREA ASSESSED	NORMAL FINDINGS	DEVIATIONS FROM NORMAL RANGE	ETIOLOGY
BACK Spine Shoulders Scapulae Iliac crests	Spine straight and easily flexed Infant able to raise and support head momentarily when prone Temporary minor positional deformities, correction with passive manipulation Shoulders, scapulae, and iliac crests lining up in same plane	Limitation of movement	Fusion or deformity of vertebra
Base of spine—pilonidal area		Spina bifida cystica Pigmented nevus with tuft of hair	Meningocele, myelomeningocele Often associated with spina bifida occulta

	Normal	Abnormal
ANUS		
Patency	One anus with good sphincter tone Passage of meconium within 24-48 hr after birth	Low obstruction: anal membrane High obstruction: anal or rectal atresia Absence of anal opening
Sphincter response (active "wink" reflex)	Good "wink" reflex of anal sphincter	Drainage of fecal material from vagina in female or urinary meatus in male Rectal fistula
STOOLS		
Patency	Meconium followed by transitional and soft yellow stools	No stool
Frequency, color, consistency		Frequent watery stools Obstruction Infection, phototherapy

BOX 15-1

Ortolani's Maneuver

The examiner places the index and middle fingers of each hand over the greater trochanters of the hips at the same time.

—Downward pressure is exerted on the hips while the neonate's knees are flexed. The hips are flexed at least 70 degrees and then abducted. The motion should be smooth without any unusual clicks.

—The presence of a click, unequal movement, or uneven gluteal skin folds is considered a positive response, indicating that the hip is dislocated, and the physician should be notified.

Relieving airway obstruction

Repositioning the infant and suctioning the mouth and nose with the bulb syringe may eliminate the problem.

• Position the infant with the head slightly lower than the body to facilitate gravity drainage.

• Auscultate the infant's respiration and lung sounds with a stethoscope to determine whether there are crackles, ronchi, or inspiratory stridor. Fine crackles may be auscultated for several hours after birth.

• If air movement is adequate, the bulb syringe may be sufficient to clear the mouth and nose. If the bulb syringe does not clear mucus interfering with respiratory effort, use mechanical suction.

• If the newborn has an obstruction that is not cleared with suctioning, investigate further to determine if there is a mechanical defect (e.g., tracheoesophageal fistula or choanal atresia) causing the obstruction (see Emergency box, Relieving Airway Obstruction).

All personnel working with infants must have current infant cardiopulmonary resuscitation (CPR) certification. Many institutions offer infant CPR courses to new parents before discharge (see Emergency box, CPR).

EMERGENCY

Relieving Airway Obstruction

Back blow and chest thrusts are used to clear an airway obstructed by a foreign body.

BACK BLOWS

Position the infant prone over forearm with the head down and the infant's jaw firmly supported.

Rest the supporting arm on the thigh.

Deliver four back blows forcefully between the infant's shoulder blades with the heel of the free hand.

TURN INFANT

Place the free hand on the infant's back to sandwich the baby between both hands; one hand supports the neck, jaw, and chest, while the other supports the back.

Turn the infant over, and place the head lower than the chest, supporting the head and neck.

Alternative position: Place the infant face down on your lap with the head lower than the trunk; firmly support the head. Apply back blows, and then turn the infant as a unit.

See Maternity Nursing text, p. 612

CHEST THRUSTS

Provide four downward chest thrusts on the lower third of the sternum.

Remove foreign body if it is visible.

See Maternity Nursing text, p. 612

OPEN AIRWAY

Open airway with the head tilt–chin lift maneuver, and attempt to ventilate.

Repeat the sequence of back blows, turning, and chest thrusts.

Continue these emergency procedures until signs of recovery occur:

Palpable peripheral pulses return.

The pupils become normal in size and are responsive to light.

Mottling and cyanosis disappear.

Record the time and duration of the procedure and the effects of this intervention.

EMERGENCY

Cardiopulmonary Resuscitation (CPR)

Wash hands before and after touching infant and equipment. Wear gloves if possible.

ASSESS RESPONSIVENESS

Observe color; tap or gently shake shoulders.

Yell for help; if alone, perform CPR for 1 minute before calling for help again.

POSITION INFANT

Turn the infant onto back, supporting the head and neck.

Place the infant on firm, flat surface.

AIRWAY

Open the airway with the head tilt–chin lift method.

Place one hand on the infant's forehead, and tilt the head back.

Place the fingers of other hand under the bone of the lower jaw at the chin.

See Maternity Nursing text, p. 613

BREATHING

Assess for evidence of breathing:

Observe for chest movement.

Listen for exhaled air.

Feel for exhaled air flow.

To breathe for infant:

Take a breath.

Place mouth over the infant's nose and mouth to create a seal.

NOTE: When available, a mask with a one-way valve should be used.

Give two breaths (1 to 1½ sec/breath), pausing to inhale between breaths.

NOTE: Gently puff the volume of air in your cheeks into infant. Do not force air. The infant's chest should rise slightly with each puff; keep fingers on the chest wall to sense air entry.

CIRCULATION

Assess circulation:

Check pulse of the brachial artery (or pulse at the base of the umbilical cord, if newly born) while maintaining the head tilt.

See Maternity Nursing text, p. 613

If the pulse is present, initiate rescue breathing. Continue doing once every 2 sec or 30 times/min until spontaneous breathing resumes.

If the pulse is absent or <60 bpm, initiate chest compressions and coordinate them with breathing.

CHEST COMPRESSION

There are two systems of chest compression; the 2 thumbs method is preferred.

Maintain the head tilt and

1. Place thumbs side-by-side in the lower third of the sternum (avoiding the xiphoid process) with fingers around the chest and supporting the back.
   —Compress the sternum $1/3$ the anterior-posterior diameter of the chest.
2. Place index finger of hand just under an imaginary line drawn between the nipples. Place the middle and ring fingers on the sternum adjacent to the index finger with the other hand supporting the back.
   —Using the middle and ring fingers, compress the sternum approximately $1/3$ the anterior-posterior diameter of the chest.

Release the pressure without moving the thumbs/fingers from the chest.

There should be a 3 : 1 ratio of compressions to ventilations; each event should take approximately ½ second.

This will result in 90 compressions and 30 ventilations per minute.

Reassess the heart rate approximately every 30 seconds.

Discontinue compressions when the infant's spontaneous heart rate reaches or exceeds 60 beats/min.

Record the time and duration of the procedure and the effects of intervention.

Source: 2005 American Heart Association Guidelines for Cardiopulmonary Resuscitation and Emergency Cardiovascular Care, Part 13. Neonatal resuscitation guidelines, *Circulation*, 112, IV 188-IV 195 (online document available at http://circ.ahajournals.org/content/ vol 12/24– suppl, accessed April 13, 2006).

signs of
POTENTIAL COMPLICATIONS: ABNORMAL NEWBORN BREATHING

Bradypnea: respirations (25 breaths/min or fewer)
Tachypnea: respirations (60 breaths/min or more)
Abnormal breath sounds: crackles, rhonchi, wheezes, or expiratory grunt
Respiratory distress: nasal flaring, retractions, chin tug, or labored breathing

Maintaining Body Temperature

- Cold stress increases the need for oxygen and may deplete glucose stores. The infant may react to exposure to cold by increasing the respiratory rate and becoming cyanotic.
- Ways to stabilize the newborn's body temperature include the following:
  - Place the infant directly on the mother's chest or abdomen, and cover with a warm blanket (skin to skin contact).
  - Dry and wrap the newborn in warmed blankets immediately after birth.
  - Keep the head covered.
  - Maintain the ambient temperature of the nursery at 23.8° C to 26.1° C.
  - If the infant does not remain with the mother during the first 1 to 2 hours after birth, place the thoroughly dried unclothed infant under a radiant warmer until the body temperature stabilizes.
- Use the infant's skin temperature as the point of control in a warmer with a servocontrolled mechanism.
  - The control panel usually is maintained between 36° C and 37° C.
  - Maintain this setting at the healthy newborn's skin temperature of around 36.5° C to 37° C.
  - Tape a thermistor probe (automatic sensor) to the right upper quadrant of the abdomen immediately below the right intercostal margin (never over a bone).
  - A reflector adhesive patch may be used over the probe to provide adequate warming. This will ensure detection of minor changes resulting from external environmental factors

or neonatal factors (peripheral vasoconstriction, vasodilation, or increased metabolism) before a dramatic change in core body temperature develops.

–The servocontroller adjusts the warmer temperature to maintain the infant's skin temperature within the desired range.

–Check the sensor periodically to make sure it is securely attached to the infant's skin.

–Check the axillary temperature of the newborn every hour (or more often as needed) until the newborn's temperature stabilizes.

Because the time needed to stabilize and maintain body temperature varies, each newborn should be allowed to achieve thermal regulation as necessary, and care should be individualized.

Examinations and activities are performed with the newborn under a heat panel to avoid heat loss. The initial bath is postponed until the newborn's skin temperature is stable and can adjust to heat loss from a bath. The exact and optimal timing of the bath for each newborn remains unknown.

Causes of hypothermia
- Birth in a car on the way to the hospital
- A cold birthing room
- Inadequate drying and wrapping immediately after birth

Warming the hypothermic infant is accomplished with care. Rapid warming may cause apneic spells and acidosis in an infant. The warming process is monitored to progress slowly over a period of 2 to 4 hours.

Therapeutic Interventions
Eye prophylaxis
The agent used for prophylaxis varies according to hospital protocols, but the usual agents are erythromycin, tetracycline, or silver nitrate. To instill medication, the thumb and forefinger are used to open the eye; medication is placed in the lower conjunctiva from the inner to the outer canthus (Fig. 15-2). Eye prophylaxis may be delayed until 1 hour or so after birth so that eye contact and parent-infant attachment and bonding are facilitated (see Medication Guide in Appendix B). Eye Prophylaxis: Erythromycin ophthalmic ointment 0.5% and tetracycline opthalmic ointment 1%.

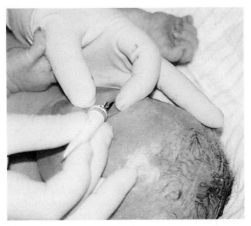

Fig. 15-2 Instillation of medication into eye of newborn. (Courtesy Marjorie Pyle, RNC, Lifecircle, Costa Mesa, CA.)

Vitamin K administration

Administering vitamin K is routine in the newborn period. A single intramuscular dose of 0.5 to 1 mg of vitamin K is given soon after birth to prevent hemorrhagic disorders (Fig. 15-3). By day 8, normal newborns are able to produce their own vitamin K (see Medication Guide in Appendix B–Vitamin K: Phytonadione (AquaMEPHYTON, Konakion)).

Umbilical cord care

The cord is clamped immediately after delivery.

The umbilical cord stump is an excellent medium for bacterial growth and can easily become infected. Hospital protocol directs the time and technique for routine cord care.

- Many hospitals have subscribed to the practice of "dry care," which consists of cleaning the periumbilical area with soap and water and wiping it dry.
- Others apply an antiseptic solution, such as Triple Dye, or alcohol to the cord.
- Current recommendations for cord care by the Association of Women's Health, Obstetric and Neonatal Nurses (AWHONN) include cleaning the cord with sterile water or a neutral pH cleanser. Subsequent care entails cleaning with water.
- The stump and base of the cord should be assessed for edema, redness, and purulent drainage with each diaper change.

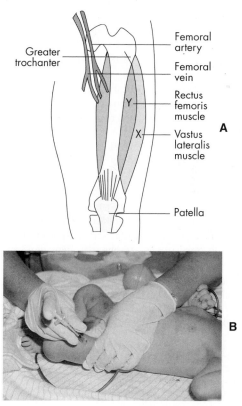

Fig. 15-3 Intramuscular injection. **A,** Acceptable intramuscular injection site for newborn infant. *X,* Injection site. **B,** Infant's leg stabilized for intramuscular injection. Nurse is wearing gloves to give injection. (**B** courtesy Marjorie Pyle, RNC, Lifecircle, Costa Mesa, CA.)

- The cord clamp is removed after 24 hours when the cord is dry.
- The average cord separation time is 10 to 14 days.

CARE MANAGEMENT: FROM 2 HOURS AFTER BIRTH UNTIL DISCHARGE

Gestational Age Assessment

- The simplified Assessment of Gestational Age is commonly used to assess gestational age of infants between 35 and 42 weeks. The total score correlates with a maturity rating of 26 to 44 weeks of gestation. The score is accurate to plus or minus 2 weeks and is accurate for infants of all races.

- The *New Ballard Score,* a revision of the original scale, can be used with newborns as young as 20 weeks of gestation (see Fig. 15-1, *A*). The scale overestimates gestational age by 2 to 4 days in infants younger than 37 weeks of gestation, especially at gestational ages of 32 to 37 weeks.

Classification of newborns by gestational age and birth weight

Classification of infants at birth by both birth weight and gestational age provides a more satisfactory method for predicting mortality risks and providing guidelines for management of the neonate than estimating gestational age or birth weight alone. The infant's birth weight, length, and head circumference are plotted on standardized graphs that identify normal values for gestational age (see Fig. 15-1, *B*).

Birth weights are classified in the following ways:

Large for gestational age (LGA). Weight is above the 90th percentile (or two or more standard deviations above the norm) at any week.

Appropriate for gestational age (AGA). Weight falls between the 10th and 90th percentiles for infant's age.

Small for gestational age (SGA). Weight is below the 10th percentile (or two or more standard deviations below the norm) at any week.

Low birth weight (LBW). Weight is 2500 g or less at birth. These newborns have had either less than the expected rate of intrauterine growth or a shortened gestation period. Preterm birth and LBW commonly occur together (e.g., less than 32 weeks of gestation and birth weight of less than 1200 g).

Very low birth weight (VLBW). Weight is 1500 g or less at birth.

Intrauterine growth restriction (IUGR). This term is applied to the fetus whose rate of growth does not meet expected norms.

Newborns are classified according to their gestational ages in the following ways:

Preterm or premature. The infant is born before completion of 37 weeks of gestation, regardless of birth weight.

Term. The infant is born between the beginning of week 38 and the end of week 42 of gestation.

Postterm (postdate). The infant is born after completion of week 42 of gestation.

Postmature. The infant is born after completion of week 42 of gestation and shows the effects of progressive placental insufficiency.

Maternal effects on gestational age assessment and birth weight

* Some maternal conditions can affect the results of the gestational assessment:
  * Infants deprived of oxygen during labor will show poor muscle tone.
  * Infants in respiratory distress tend to be flaccid and assume a "frog-leg" posture.
  * Even though an infant may look large, such as the infant of a diabetic mother, the infant may respond more like a premature infant.
  * The infant of a mother who has been receiving magnesium sulfate will tend to be somewhat lethargic.

Physical Assessment

A complete physical examination is performed within 24 hours after birth (see Table 15-2).

A neurologic assessment of the newborn's reflexes (see Table 15-3) provides useful information about the infant's nervous system and state of neurologic maturation. The assessment must be carried out as early as possible because abnormal signs present in the early neonatal period may disappear. They may reappear months or years later as abnormal functions.

Common Problems in the Newborn

Physical injuries

Birth trauma includes any physical injury sustained by a newborn during labor and birth. Injury may occur because of obstetric birth techniques such as forceps-assisted birth, vacuum extraction, version and extraction, and cesarean birth. Most injuries are minor and resolve in the neonatal period without treatment; some types of trauma require intervention. A few are serious enough to be fatal.

Text continued on p. 475.

TABLE 15-3

Assessment of Newborn's Reflexes

REFLEX	ELICITING THE REFLEX	CHARACTERISTIC RESPONSE	COMMENTS
Sucking and rooting	Touch infant's lip, cheek, or corner of mouth with nipple	Infant turns head toward stimulus; opens mouth, takes hold, and sucks	Response is difficult if not impossible to elicit after infant has been fed; if response weak or absent, consider prematurity or neurologic defect Parental guidance: avoid trying to turn head toward breast or nipple, allow infant to root; response disappears after 3-4*mo but may persist up to 1yr
Swallowing	Feed infant; swallowing usually follows sucking and obtaining fluids	Swallowing is usually coordinated with sucking and usually occurs without gagging, coughing, or vomiting	If response is weak or absent, this may indicate prematurity or neurologic defect Sucking and swallowing are often uncoordinated in preterm infant

Grasp			
—Palmar	Place finger in palm of hand	Infant's fingers curl around examiner's fingers; toes curl downward	Palmar response lessens by 3-4 mo; parents enjoy this contact with infant; plantar response lessens by 8 mo
—Plantar	Place finger at base of toes		
Extrusion	Touch or depress tip of tongue	Newborn forces tongue outward	Response disappears about fourth month of life
Glabellar (Myerson)	Tap over forehead, bridge of nose, or maxilla of newborn whose eyes are open	Newborn blinks for first four or five taps	Continued blinking with repeated taps is consistent with extrapyramidal disorder

*All durations for persistence of reflexes are based on time elapsed after 40 wk of gestation, that is, if this newborn was born at 36 wk of gestation, add 1 mo to all time limits given.

Continued

TABLE 15-3

Assessment of Newborn's Reflexes—cont'd

REFLEX	ELICITING THE REFLEX	CHARACTERISTIC RESPONSE	COMMENTS
Tonic neck or "fencing"	With infant falling asleep or sleeping, turn head quickly to one side	With infant facing left side, arm and leg on that side extend; opposite arm and leg flex (turn head to right, and extremities assume opposite postures)	Responses in leg are more consistent Complete response disappears by 3-4 mo, incomplete response may be seen until third or fourth yr After 6 wk, persistent response is sign of possible cerebral palsy

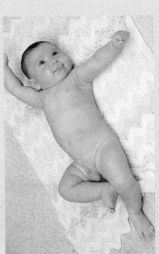

Classic pose in spontaneous tonic neck reflex. (Courtesy Marjorie Pyle, RNC, Costa Mesa, CA.)

Moro

Hold infant in semisitting position, allow head and trunk to fall backward to an angle of at least 30 degrees

Place infant on flat surface, strike surface to startle infant

Symmetric abduction and extension of arms are seen; fingers fan out and form a C with thumb and forefinger; slight tremor may be noted; arms are adducted in embracing motion and return to relaxed flexion and movement

Legs may follow similar pattern of response

Preterm infant does not complete "embrace"; instead, arms fall backward because of weakness

Response is present at birth; complete response may be seen until 8 wk; body jerk is seen only between 8 and 18 wk; response is absent by 6 mo if neurologic maturation is not delayed; response may be incomplete if infant is deeply asleep; give parental guidance about normal response

Asymmetric response may connote injury to brachial plexus, clavicle, or humerus

Persistent response after 6 mo indicates possible brain damage

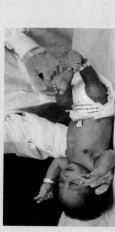

Moro reflex. (From Dickason, E., Silverman, B., & Kaplan, J. (1998). *Maternal-infant nursing care* (3rd ed.). St. Louis: Mosby.)

Continued

TABLE 15-3

Assessment of Newborn's Reflexes—cont'd

REFLEX	ELICITING THE REFLEX	CHARACTERISTIC RESPONSE	COMMENTS
Stepping or "walking"	Hold infant vertically, allowing one foot to touch table surface	Infant will simulate walking, alternating flexion and extension of feet; term infants walk on soles of their feet, and preterm infants walk on their toes	Response is normally present for 3-4 wk

Stepping reflex. (From Dickason, E., Silverman, B., & Kaplan, J. (1998). *Maternal-infant nursing care* (3rd ed.). St. Louis: Mosby.)

Crawling	Place newborn on abdomen	Newborn makes crawling movements with arms and legs	Response should disappear about 6wk of age
Deep tendon	Use finger instead of percussion hammer to elicit patellar, or knee jerk, reflex; newborn must be relaxed	Reflex jerk is present; even with newborn relaxed, nonselective overall reaction may occur	
Crossed extension	Infant should be supine; extend one leg, press knee downward, stimulate bottom of foot; observe opposite leg	Opposite leg flexes, adducts, and then extends	

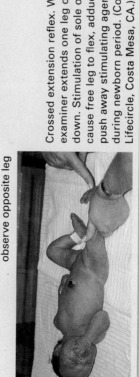

Crossed extension reflex. With the infant in supine position, examiner extends one leg of the infant and presses the knee down. Stimulation of sole of foot of fixated limb should cause free leg to flex, adduct, and extend as if attempting to push away stimulating agent. This reflex should be present during newborn period. (Courtesy Marjorie Pyle, RNC, Lifecircle, Costa Mesa, CA.)

Continued

TABLE 15-3

Assessment of Newborn's Reflexes—cont'd

REFLEX	ELICITING THE REFLEX	CHARACTERISTIC RESPONSE	COMMENTS
Startle	Perform sharp hand clap; best elicited if newborn is 24-36 hr old or older	Arms abduct with flexion of elbows, hands stay clenched	Response should disappear by 4 mo of age Response is elicited more readily in preterm newborn (inform parents of this characteristic)
Babinski sign (plantar)	On sole of foot, beginning at heel, stroke upward along lateral aspect of sole, then move finger across ball of foot	All toes hyperextend, with dorsiflexion of big toe—recorded as a positive sign	Absence requires neurologic evaluation, should disappear after 1 yr of age

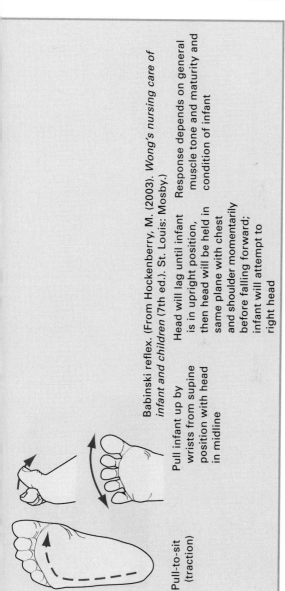

Babinski reflex. (From Hockenberry, M. (2003). *Wong's nursing care of infant and children* (7th ed.). St. Louis: Mosby.)

Pull-to-sit
(traction)

Pull infant up by wrists from supine position with head in midline

Head will lag until infant is in upright position, then head will be held in same plane with chest and shoulder momentarily before falling forward; infant will attempt to right head

Response depends on general muscle tone and maturity and condition of infant

Continued

TABLE 15-3

Assessment of Newborn's Reflexes—cont'd

REFLEX	ELICITING THE REFLEX	CHARACTERISTIC RESPONSE	COMMENTS
Trunk incurvation (Galant)	Place infant prone on flat surface, run finger down back about 4-5 cm lateral to spine, first on one side and then down other	Trunk is flexed, and pelvis is swung toward stimulated side With transverse lesions of cord, no response below the level of the lesion is present	Response disappears by fourth week Absence suggests general depression of nervous system Response may vary but should be obtainable in all infants, including preterm ones

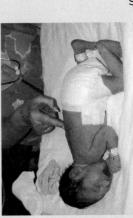

(Courtesy Marjorie Pyle, RNC, Lifecircle, Costa Mesa, CA.)

Magnet

Place infant in supine position, partially flex both lower extremities and apply pressure to soles of feet

Both lower limbs should extend against examiner's pressure

Absence suggests damage to spinal cord or malformation

Reflex may be weak or exaggerated after breech birth

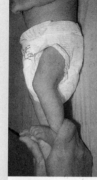
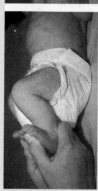

(Courtesy Michael S. Clement, M.D., Mesa, AZ)

Continued

TABLE 15-3

Assessment of Newborn's Reflexes—cont'd

REFLEX	ELICITING THE REFLEX	CHARACTERISTIC RESPONSE	COMMENTS
Additional newborn responses: yawn, stretch, burp, hiccup, sneeze	These are spontaneous behaviors	May be slightly depressed temporarily because of maternal analgesia or anesthesia, fetal hypoxia, or infection	Parental guidance: most of these behaviors are pleasurable to parents Parents need to be assured that behaviors are normal Sneeze is usually response to lint, etc., in nose and not an indicator of a cold No treatment is needed for hiccups; sucking may help

Physiologic jaundice

- The majority of term newborns have some degree of physiologic jaundice (become yellowish) during the first 3 days of life. Jaundice is clinically visible when serum bilirubin levels reach 5 to 7 mg/dl.

- Every newborn is assessed for jaundice. The blanch test helps differentiate cutaneous jaundice from skin color. To do the test, apply pressure with a finger over a bony area (e.g., the nose, forehead, or sternum) for several seconds to empty all the capillaries in that spot. If jaundice is present, the blanched area will look yellow before the capillaries refill. The conjunctival sacs and buccal mucosa also are assessed, especially in darker-skinned infants. It is better to assess for jaundice in daylight, because artificial lighting and reflection from nursery walls can distort the actual skin color.

- Jaundice is noticeable first in the head and then progresses gradually toward the abdomen and extremities because of the newborn infant's circulatory pattern (cephalocaudal developmental progression). If jaundice is suspected, evaluation of serum bilirubin level is needed.

- The intensity of jaundice is not always related to the degree of hyperbilirubinemia.

- Noninvasive monitoring of bilirubin by cutaneous reflectance measurements (transcutaneous bilirubinometry [TcB]) allows for repetitive estimations of bilirubin levels.
  - These devices work well on dark- and light-skinned infants and correlate fairly well with serum measurements of bilirubin levels in term infants.
  - With shorter maternity stays, the TcB measurement can be valuable as an assessment tool for home care follow-up.
  - TcB meters may reduce or obviate the need for blood sampling in certain healthy neonates.
  - TcB monitors provide accurate measurements within 2 to 3 mg/dl in most neonatal populations at serum levels less than 15 mg/dl. After phototherapy has been initiated, TcB is no longer useful as a screening tool.
  - The use of hour-specific serum bilirubin levels to predict newborns at risk for rapidly rising levels has now become

an official recommendation from the American Academy of Pediatrics, Subcommittee on Hyperbilirubinemia, for the monitoring of healthy neonates at 35 weeks of gestation or greater before discharge from the hospital.

- Using a nomogram with three levels (high, intermediate, or low risk) of rising total serum bilirubin may be done at the same time as the routine newborn profile (phenylketonuria [PKU], galactosemia, and others).
- In many institutions the hour-specific bilirubin risk nomogram is used to determine the infant's risk for development of hyperbilirubinemia requiring medical treatment or closer screening.
  - Risk factors recognized to place infants in the high risk category include gestational age less than 38 weeks, breastfeeding, previous sibling with significant jaundice, and jaundice appearing before discharge.
  - Healthy infants (35 weeks or greater) should receive follow-up care and assessment of bilirubin within 3 days of discharge if discharged at less than 24 hours and a risk assessment with tools such as the hour-specific nomogram.
  - Newborns discharged at 24 to 47.9 hours should receive follow-up evaluation within 4 days (96 hours), and those discharged between 48 and 72 hours should receive follow-up within 5 days.

Hypoglycemia

- *Hypoglycemia* in a term infant is defined as a plasma concentration of less than 36 mg/dl during the first 2 to 3 hours after birth (some suggest values of 40 to 45 mg/dl are more appropriate). The glucose level normally declines during the first hours after birth. Hypoglycemia can result if early feedings result in limited intake or if the neonate is stressed. Newborns who are symptomatic and those considered to be at risk for hypoglycemia are tested.
- Signs of hypoglycemia may be transient and recurrent and include the following:
  - Jitteriness
  - Irregular respiratory effort
  - Cyanosis

  −Apnea
  −Weak, high-pitched cry
  −Feeding difficulty
  −Hunger
  −Lethargy
  −Twitching
  −Eye rolling
  −Seizures
- Hypoglycemia in the low risk term infant is usually eliminated by feeding the infant. Occasionally the intravenous administration of glucose is required for newborns with persistently high insulin levels or those with depleted glycogen stores.

Hypocalcemia
- *Hypocalcemia* (serum calcium levels of less than 7.8 to 8 mg/dl in term infants or less than 7 mg/dl in preterm infants) may occur in newborns of diabetic mothers, in newborns who had perinatal asphyxia or trauma, and in LBW and preterm infants. Early-onset hypocalcemia occurs within the first 72 hours after birth.
- Signs of hypocalcemia include the following:
  −Jitteriness
  −High-pitched cry
  −Irritability
  −Apnea
  −Intermittent cyanosis
  −Abdominal distention
  −Laryngospasm
  −Some hypocalcemic infants are asymptomatic
- In most instances, early-onset hypocalcemia is self-limiting and resolves within 1 to 3 days. Treatment includes early feeding and occasionally the administration of calcium supplements. Preterm or asphyxiated infants may require intravenous elemental calcium.
- Jitteriness is a symptom of both hypoglycemia and hypocalcemia; therefore hypocalcemia must be considered if the therapy for hypoglycemia proves ineffective. In many newborns, jitteriness remains despite therapy and cannot be explained by hypoglycemia or hypocalcemia.

BOX 15-2

Standard Laboratory Values in a Term Newborn*

Hemoglobin	14-24 gm/dl
Hematocrit	44%-64%
Glucose	46-65 mg/dl
Leukocytes (white blood cells)	9,000-30,000/mm^3
Bilirubin, total serum	≤2.0 mg/dl
Blood gases	
Arterial	pH 7.32-7.49
	P_{CO_2} 26-41 mm Hg
	P_{O_2} 60-70 mm Hg
Base excess	−10 to −2 mEq/L
	(whole blood)
Bicarbonate, serum	21-28 (arterial)
Anion gap	7-16 mEq/L
Venous	pH 7.31-7.41
	P_{CO_2} 40-50 mm Hg
	P_{O_2} 40-50 mm Hg

Some data from Pagana, K. D., & Pagana, T. J. (2003). *Mosby's diagnostic and laboratory test reference* (6th ed.). St. Louis: Mosby.
*These values may change significantly in the first week of life.

LABORATORY AND DIAGNOSTIC TESTS

Laboratory tests commonly performed in the newborn period include the following:

- Blood glucose levels
- Bilirubin levels
- Complete blood count (CBC)
- Newborn screening tests
- Drug screen

Box 15-2 gives standard laboratory values for a term newborn.

Newborn Genetic Screening

- Before hospital discharge, a heel stick blood sample is obtained to detect a variety of congenital conditions. All states screen for phenylketonuria (PKU) and hypothyroidism, but each state determines whether other tests, such as for galactosemia, cystic fibrosis, maple syrup urine disease, and sickle cell disease, are performed.

- The screening test should be repeated at age 1 to 2 weeks if the initial specimen was obtained when the infant was younger than 24 hours.
- The advent of tandem mass spectrometry holds promise to increase the number of conditions (30 total) that can be tested with the same minimal amount of blood. Information about which tests are required in a state can be obtained from state health departments.

Newborn Hearing Screening

Universal newborn hearing screening is required by law in more than 30 states and is performed routinely in other states. Newborn hearing screening is completed before hospital discharge, and infants who do not pass are referred for repeated testing within the next 2 to 8 weeks. The practice of universal hearing screening reduces the age at which infants with hearing loss are identified and treated.

Collection of Specimens
Heel stick

- Warm the heel before the sample is taken because heat applied for 5 to 10 minutes helps dilate the vessels in the area. A cloth soaked with warm water and wrapped loosely around the foot can effectively warm the foot. Disposable heel warmers are available from a variety of companies but should be used with care to prevent burns.
- Wear gloves when collecting any specimen.
- Cleanse the area with alcohol.
- Restrain the infant's foot with your free hand.
- Identify an appropriate puncture site (Fig. 15-4).
- Make the puncture at the outer aspect of the heel, and do not penetrate deeper than 2.4 mm. A spring-loaded automatic puncture device causes less pain and requires fewer punctures than a manual lance blade.
- After the specimen has been collected, apply pressure with a dry gauze square, but do not apply more alcohol because this will cause the site to continue to bleed.
- Cover the site with an adhesive bandage.

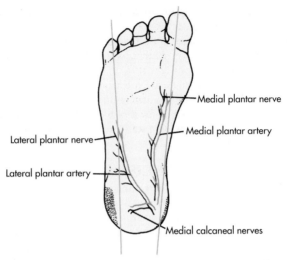

Fig. 15-4 Heel stick sites *(shaded areas)* on infant's foot for obtaining samples of capillary blood.

- Dispose of equipment used properly.
- Review the laboratory slip for correct identification.
- Check the specimen for accurate labeling and routing.

A heel stick is traumatic for the infant and causes pain. After several heel sticks, infants often withdraw their feet when they are touched. To reassure the infant and promote feelings of safety, the neonate should be cuddled and comforted when the procedure is complete and appropriate pain management measures taken to minimize the pain.

Venipuncture

Venous blood samples can be drawn from antecubital, saphenous, superficial wrist, and rarely, scalp veins. If an intravenous site is used to obtain a blood specimen, it is important to consider the type of infusion fluid, because mixing of the blood sample with the fluid can alter the results.

Although regular venipuncture needles may be used, some prefer butterfly needles. A 25-gauge needle is adequate for blood sampling in neonates with minimal hemolysis occurring when the proper procedure is followed. The mummy restraint commonly is used to help secure the infant.

Crying, fear, and agitation will affect blood gas values; therefore every effort must be made to keep the infant quiet during the procedure. For blood gas studies, the blood sample tubes are packed in ice (to reduce blood cell metabolism) and are taken immediately to the laboratory for analysis.

The infant's tolerance of the procedure should be recorded. The infant should be cuddled and comforted when the procedure is completed.

Obtaining a urine specimen

The urine sample should be fresh and analyzed within 1 hour of collection. A variety of urine collection bags are available, including clear plastic, single-use bags with an adhesive material around the opening at the point of attachment.

- Remove the diaper, and place the infant in a supine position.
- Wash the genitalia, perineum, and surrounding skin, and dry thoroughly (the adhesive on the bag will not stick to moist, powdered, or oily skin surfaces).
- Remove the protective paper to expose the adhesive .
- In female infants, stretch the perineum to flatten skin folds, and then press the adhesive area on the bag firmly onto the skin all around the urinary meatus and vagina. Start the application at the bridge of skin separating the rectum from the vagina and work upward.
- In male infants, tuck the penis and scrotum through the opening into the collection bag before removing the protective paper from the adhesive and pressing it firmly onto the perineum, making sure the entire adhesive is firmly attached to skin and the edges of the opening do not pucker. This helps ensure a leakproof seal and decreases the chance of contamination from stool.
- Cutting a slit in the diaper and pulling the bag through the slit also may help prevent leaking.
- Replace the diaper, and check the bag frequently.
- When a sufficient amount of urine (this amount varies according to the test done) appears, remove the bag.
- Observe the infant's skin for signs of irritation while the bag is in place.

• Aspirate the specimen with a syringe, or drain the specimen directly from the bag.

For some types of urine tests, urine can be aspirated directly from the diaper by means of a syringe without a needle. If the diaper has absorbent gel material that traps urine, a small gauze dressing or some cotton balls can be placed inside the diaper and the urine aspirated from them.

CARE MANAGEMENT

Therapeutic and Surgical Procedures

Intramuscular injection

Hepatitis B (Hep B) vaccination is recommended for all infants (see Medication Guide in Appendix B–Hepatitis B Vaccine (Recombivax HB, Engerix-B)). If the infant is born to an infected mother or to a mother who is a chronic carrier, hepatitis vaccine and hepatitis B Immune globulin (HBIG) should be administered within 12 hours of birth (see Medication Guide in Appendix B–Hepatitis B Immune Globulin). The hepatitis vaccine is given in one site and the HBIG in another. For infants born to healthy women, the first dose of the vaccine may be given at birth or at age 1 or 2 months.

Obtain parental consent before administering these vaccines.

Therapy for hyperbilirubinemia

The best therapy for hyperbilirubinemia is prevention. Because bilirubin is excreted primarily through stooling, prevention can be facilitated by early feeding, which stimulates the passage of meconium. The goal of treatment of hyperbilirubinemia is to help reduce the newborn's serum levels of unconjugated bilirubin. The two principal ways of doing this are phototherapy and, rarely, exchange blood transfusion. Exchange transfusion treats those infants whose increased levels of bilirubin cannot be controlled by phototherapy.

Phototherapy

• During phototherapy the unclothed infant is placed beneath a bank of lights. The distance may vary based on unit protocol

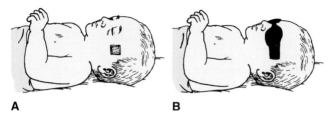

A   **B**

Fig. 15-5 Eye patches for newborns receiving phototherapy. **A,** Small Velcro patch stuck to both sides of head. **B,** Eye cover sticks to Velcro patch, which reduces movement of eye cover and facilitates removal for feedings.

and the type of light used. There should always be a Plexiglas panel or shield between the lights and the infant when conventional lighting is used. The most effective therapy is achieved with lights at 400 to 500 manometers, and blue light spectrum is the most efficient. The lamp energy should be monitored routinely during treatment with a photometer to ensure efficacy of therapy.

- Phototherapy is carried out until the infant's serum bilirubin level decreases to within an acceptable range. The decision to discontinue therapy is based on the observation of a definite downward trend in the bilirubin values. After therapy has been terminated, the infant may have a rebound in bilirubin levels, which is usually harmless.
- Several precautions must be taken while the infant is undergoing phototherapy:
  - Protect the infant's eyes with an opaque mask to prevent overexposure to the light (Fig. 15-5).
  - Cover the eyes completely with the eye shield, but do not occlude the nares.
  - Before applying the mask, gently close the infant's eyes to prevent excoriation of the corneas.
  - Remove the mask during infant feedings so that the eyes can be checked and the parents can have visual contact with the infant.
  - To promote optimal skin exposure during phototherapy, leave the diaper off, or make a "string bikini" from a disposable face mask to cover the infant's genital area.

- Monitor the infant's temperature.
- Phototherapy lights may increase insensible water loss, placing the infant at risk for fluid loss and dehydration; therefore it is important that the infant be adequately hydrated.
- Hydration maintenance in the healthy newborn is accomplished with human milk or infant formula; glucose water and plain water do not promote excretion of bilirubin in the stools and may actually perpetuate enterohepatic circulation, thus delaying bilirubin excretion.
- Urine output may be decreased or unaltered; the urine may have a brown or gold appearance.
- Record all aspects of the phototherapy treatment in the infant's chart.
- Monitor the number and consistency of stools. Bilirubin breakdown increases gastric motility, which results in the formation of loose stools that can cause skin excoriation and breakdown.
- Clean the infant's buttocks after each stool to help maintain skin integrity.
- A fine maculopapular rash may appear during phototherapy, but this is transient.
- Because visualization of the infant's skin color is difficult with blue light, implement appropriate cardiorespiratory monitoring based on the infant's overall condition.
- An alternative device for phototherapy that is safe and effective is a fiberoptic panel attached to an illuminator.
  - The fiberoptic blanket may be wrapped around the newborn's torso or flat in the bed, thus delivering continuous phototherapy.
  - Place a covering pad between the infant's skin and the fiberoptic device.
  - During treatment the newborn can remain in the mother's room in an open crib or in her arms.
  - Follow unit protocol for the use of eye patches.
  - The blanket also may be used for home care.
- Use a combination of conventional lights and fiberoptic blankets when intensive therapy is warranted.

Parent Education. Serum levels of bilirubin in the newborn continue to increase until the fifth day of life. Parents should have written instructions for assessing the infant's condition and the name of the contact person to whom to report their findings and concerns. Some health care agencies have a nurse make a home visit to evaluate the infant's condition. If it proves necessary to measure the infant's bilirubin levels after discharge from the hospital, either the home care nurse may draw the blood specimen or the parents may take the baby to a laboratory for the determination.

Circumcision

Circumcision of newborn males is commonly performed in the United States, although there is controversy over its value. If circumcision is performed, analgesia should be used. Circumcision is a matter of personal parental choice. Parents usually decide to have their newborn circumcised for reasons of hygiene, religious conviction, tradition, culture, or social norms. Parents should be given unbiased information and the opportunity to discuss the benefits and risks of the procedure.

* Suggested medical benefits of circumcision for the infant include the following:
  - Decreased incidence of urinary tract infection
  - Decreased risk for sexually transmitted disease, penile cancer, and human papillomavirus (HPV) infection
  - Possibility of a lower risk of cervical cancer among female partners of circumcised males
* Risks and potential complications associated with circumcision include hemorrhage, infection, and penile injury (removal of excessive skin or damage to the meatus or glans).

Procedure:
  - Circumcision involves removing the prepuce (foreskin) of the glans. The procedure is performed in the hospital before the infant's discharge. The circumcision of a Jewish male is commonly performed on the eighth day after birth and is done at home in a ceremony called a *bris.*
  - Formula feedings are usually withheld up to 4 hours before the circumcision to prevent vomiting and aspiration.
  - Breastfed infants may be allowed to nurse up until the procedure is done; this varies with unit protocol.
  - To prepare the infant for the circumcision, position him on a plastic restraint form (Fig. 15-6), and cleanse the penis

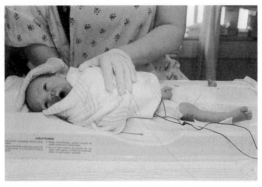

Fig. 15-6 Proper positioning of infant in Circumstraint. (Courtesy Paul Vincent Kuntz, Texas Children's Hospital, Houston, TX.)

with soap and water or a preparatory solution, such as povidone-iodine.

—Drape the infant to provide warmth and a sterile field, and ready the sterile equipment for use.

The procedure itself takes only a few minutes. After it is completed, a small petrolatum gauze dressing or a generous amount of petrolatum may be applied for 1 or 2 days to prevent the diaper from adhering to the site. If a PlastiBell is used for the circumcision, petrolatum need not be applied.

Discomfort

—Circumcision is painful, and the pain is manifested by both physiologic and behavioral changes in the infant. Analgesia or anesthesia should be used during the procedure.

—Three types of anesthesia or analgesia are used in newborns who undergo circumcisions. These include (from most effective to less effective) ring block, dorsal penile nerve block (DPNB), and topical anesthetic. A ring block is the injection of buffered lidocaine administered subcutaneously on each side of the penile shaft. A DPNB includes subcutaneous injections of buffered lidocaine at the 2 o'clock and 10 o'clock positions at the base of the penis. The circumcision should not be done for at least 5 minutes after these injections.

—Nonpharmacologic methods, such as nonnutritive sucking, containment, and swaddling, may be used in addition to pharmacologic use of oral acetaminophen and a concentrated oral glucose solution. A combination of ring block or DPNB, topical anesthetic, nonnutritive sucking, oral acetaminophen, concentrated oral sucrose solution (2 ml of a 24% concentration given during the procedure on a pacifier, with a syringe or nipple), and swaddling has been shown to be the most effective at decreasing the pain associated with circumcision.

–A topical cream containing prilocaine-lidocaine, such as EMLA, can be applied to the base of the penis at least 1 hour before the circumcision.

–Coat the area where the prepuce attaches to the glans well with 1 g of the cream, and then cover with a transparent occlusive dressing or finger cot.

–Just before the procedure, remove the cream. Blanching or redness of the skin may occur.

–After the circumcision, the infant is comforted until he is quieted. If the parents were not present during the procedure, the infant is returned to them. The infant may be fussy for several hours, or he may be sleepy and difficult to awaken for feedings. Oral acetaminophen may be administered after the procedure every 4 hours (as ordered by the practitioner) for a maximum of five doses in 24 hours or a maximum of 75 mg/kg/day.

Care of the newly circumcised infant

• Bleeding is the most common complication of circumcision.

–Check the infant hourly for the next 12 hours to make sure no bleeding is occurring and that voiding is normal.

–If bleeding is noted from the circumcision, apply gentle pressure to the site of bleeding with a folded sterile gauze square.

–Absorbable gelatin sponge (Gelfoam) powder or sponge may be applied to stop bleeding.

–If bleeding is not easily controlled, a blood vessel may require ligation. In this event, one nurse notifies the physician and prepares the necessary equipment (circumcision tray and suture material), while another nurse maintains intermittent pressure until the physician arrives.

–If the parents take the baby home before the end of the 12-hour observation period, instruct them in postcircumcision care and when to notify the physician.

—Before the infant is discharged, check to see that the parents have the physician's telephone number.

- If the PlastiBell technique was used, the parents are instructed to observe the position of the plastic ring on the glans; it should remain on the glans (not on the shaft of the penis) and should fall off within 5 to 7 days. No petrolatum is used in caring for the penis circumcised with the PlastiBell technique. Otherwise, care is the same as for the other types of circumcision.

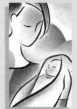

Newborn Nutrition and Feeding

RECOMMENDED INFANT NUTRITION

The American Academy of Pediatrics recommends exclusive breastfeeding or human milk feeding for the first 6 months of life and that breastfeeding or human milk feeding continue as the sole source of milk for the next 6 months.

- During the second 6 months of life, appropriate complementary foods (solids) are added to the infant's diet.
- If infants are weaned from breast milk before 12 months of age, they should receive iron-fortified infant formula, not cow's milk.

Benefits of Breastfeeding

Table 16-1 lists benefits of breastfeeding.

CHOOSING AN INFANT FEEDING METHOD

Breastfeeding is a natural extension of pregnancy and childbirth; it is much more than simply a means of supplying nutrition for infants.

In some situations, breastfeeding is contraindicated.

- Newborns who have galactosemia should not be breastfed.
- Mothers with active tuberculosis or human immunodeficiency virus (HIV) infection and those who are positive for human T-cell lymphotropic virus type I or type II should not breastfeed.
- Breastfeeding is not recommended when mothers are receiving chemotherapy or radioactive isotopes (e.g., with diagnostic procedures).
- Maternal use of drugs of abuse ("street drugs") is incompatible with breastfeeding.

TABLE 16-1

Benefits of Breastfeeding

BENEFITS FOR THE INFANT	BENEFITS FOR THE MOTHER	BENEFITS TO FAMILIES AND SOCIETY
Decreased incidence and severity of infectious diseases: bacterial meningitis, bacteremia, diarrhea, respiratory infection, necrotizing enterocolitis, otitis media, urinary tract infection, late-onset sepsis in preterm infants	Decreased postpartum bleeding and more rapid uterine involution	Convenient; ready to feed
	Reduced risk of breast cancer, uterine cancer, and ovarian cancer	No bottles or other necessary equipment
	Earlier return to prepregnancy weight	Less expensive than infant formula
Reduced postneonatal infant mortality	Decreased risk of postmenopausal osteoporosis	Reduced annual health care costs
Decreased rates of SIDS	Unique bonding experience	Less parental absence from work because of ill infant
Decreased incidence of type 1 and type 2 diabetes	Increases maternal role attainment	Reduced environmental burden related to disposal of formula cans
Decreased incidence of lymphoma,		

leukemia, and Hodgkin disease

Reduced risk of obesity and hypercholesterolemia

Decreased incidence and severity of asthma and other allergies

Slightly enhanced cognitive development

Enhances jaw development, decreasing problems with malocclusions and malalignment of teeth

Analgesic effect for infants undergoing painful procedures, such as venipuncture

Modified from Gartner, L., et al. (2005). Breastfeeding and the use of human milk. *Pediatrics* 115(2), 496-506; Lawrence, R., & Lawrence, R. (2005). *Breastfeeding: A guide for the medical profession* (6th ed.). St. Louis, Mosby.
SIDS, Sudden infant death syndrome.

CARE MANAGEMENT: THE BREASTFEEDING MOTHER AND INFANT

Infant

Before the initiation of breastfeeding, the nurse must consider the following in preparing to assist the breastfeeding infant effectively:

- Maturity level: gestational age, term or preterm, and birth weight (small for gestational age [SGA] or large for gestational age [LGA])
- Labor and birth: length of labor, maternal medications (narcotics, magnesium sulfate), type of birth: vaginal (with or without use of vacuum extraction or forceps) or cesarean, and type of anesthesia
- Birth trauma: fractured clavicle or bruising of face or head
- Maternal risk factors: diabetes, preeclampsia, infection, HIV, herpes, or hepatitis B
- Congenital defects: cleft lip or palate, cardiac anomalies, or Down syndrome or other genetic anomalies
- Physical stability: vital signs within normal limits, unlabored respirations, and bowel sounds present
- State of alertness: awake, sleepy, or crying

Feeding Readiness. Term neonates are born with reflexes that facilitate feeding: rooting, sucking, and swallowing. However, coordination of sucking, swallowing, and breathing in order to feed requires adaptation by the infant. Although the majority of newborns experience minimal hunger or thirst in the first hours after birth, they will suckle when given the opportunity.

Physical assessment of the newborn reveals signs that the baby is physiologically ready to begin feeding:

- Vital signs within normal limits
- Unlabored respirations; nares patent; no cyanosis
- Active bowel sounds
- No abdominal distention

When newborns feel hunger, they usually cry vigorously until their needs are met. Some infants, however, will withdraw into sleep because of discomfort associated with hunger. Babies exhibit feeding-readiness cues that can be recognized;

feeding should begin when the infant exhibits some of these cues:

- Hand-to-mouth or hand-to-hand movements
- Sucking motions
- Rooting—infant moves toward whatever touches the area around the mouth and attempts to suck
- Mouthing

Babies normally consume small amounts of milk during the first 3 days of life. As the baby adjusts to extrauterine life and the digestive tract is cleared of meconium, milk intake increases from 15 to 30 ml per feeding in the first 24 hours to 60 to 90 ml by the end of the first week.

At birth and for several months thereafter, all secretions of the infant's digestive tract contain enzymes especially suited to the digestion of human milk.

- The ability to digest foods other than milk depends on the physiologic development of the infant.
- The capacities for salivary, gastric, pancreatic, and intestinal digestion increase with age, indicating that the natural time for introduction of solid foods may be around 6 months of age.
  - Babies are born with a tongue extrusion reflex that causes them to push out of the mouth anything placed on the tongue.
  - This reflex disappears by 6 months another indication of physiologic readiness for solids.
  - Early introduction of solids may make the infant more prone to food allergies.
  - Regular feeding of solids can lead to decreased intake of breast milk or formula and may be associated with early cessation of breastfeeding.

Assessment. Assessment of the infant for latch-on (attachment of the infant to the breast for feeding), position, alignment, and sucking and swallowing is made by direct observation while the infant is breastfeeding. See Box 16-1 for signs of adequate intake.

During the time in the hospital, the nurse can help the mother to view each breastfeeding session as a "feeding lesson" or "practice session" that will foster maternal confidence and a satisfying breastfeeding experience for mother and baby.

BOX 16-1

Signs of Adequate Intake in the Breastfeeding Infant

- The mother's milk transitions from colostrum to mature milk. Milk "comes in" by 3 to 5 days after birth.
- The infant feeds at least eight times per day: approximately every 2 to 3 hours in the day and every 4 hours at night.
- After correctly latching on to the breast, the baby feeds for 15 to 20 minutes (per breast) with gliding jaw movements and audible swallowing. At least one breast is softened completely at each feeding.
- The infant appears relaxed and satisfied after feeding and is likely to fall asleep.
- By 24 hours after the milk has "come in," the infant urinates at least six to eight times (pale urine) and has at least two bowel movements per day. The stools transition from meconium to bright yellow, somewhat loose stools with a cottage cheese consistency by the fifth day.
- The infant gains 15 to 30 g/day after the fourth or fifth day and surpasses the birth weight by 10 to 14 days of age.
- The mother reports a "tugging" sensation at the nipple with feeding and feels warm and relaxed during feeding.

Interventions

The ideal time to begin breastfeeding is immediately after birth.

- Newborns without complications should be allowed to remain in direct skin-to-skin contact with the mother until the baby is able to breastfeed for the first time.
- Each mother should receive instruction, assistance, and support in positioning and latching on until she is able to do so independently.

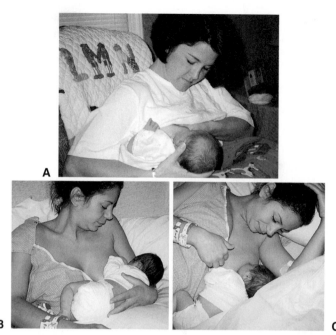

Fig. 16-1 Three breastfeeding positions. **A,** Football hold. **B,** Modified cradle. **C,** Side-lying. (**B** and **C** courtesy Marjorie Pyle, RNC, Lifecircle, Costa Mesa, CA.)

Positioning

The four basic positions for breastfeeding are the football hold, cradle, modified cradle or across-the-lap, and side-lying positions (Fig. 16-1).

- Initially it is advantageous to use the position that most easily facilitates latch-on while allowing maximal comfort for the mother.
- The football hold is often recommended for early feedings because the mother can easily see the baby's mouth as she guides the infant onto the nipple. The football hold is usually preferred by mothers who gave birth by cesarean.
- The modified cradle or across-the-lap hold also works well for early feedings, especially with smaller babies.

- The side-lying position allows the mother to rest while breast-feeding and is often preferred by women with perineal pain and swelling.
- Cradling is the most common breastfeeding position for infants who have learned to latch on easily and feed effectively.

Before discharge from the hospital, assist the mother to try all the positions so that she will feel confident in her ability to vary positions at home.

Whichever position is used, the mother should be comfortable.

- The infant is placed at the level of the breast, supported by pillows or folded blankets, turned completely on his or her side and facing the mother so that the infant is "belly to belly," with the arms "hugging" the breast.
- The baby's mouth is directly in front of the nipple. It is important that the mother support the baby's neck and shoulders with her hand and not push on the occiput.
- The baby's body is held in correct alignment (ears, shoulders, and hips are in a straight line) during latch-on and feeding.

Latch-on

- Manually express a few drops of colostrum or milk, and spread it over the nipple to lubricate the nipple; this may entice the baby to open the mouth as the milk is tasted.
- Support the breast in one hand with the thumb on top and four fingers underneath at the back edge of the areola.
- Compress the breast slightly so that an adequate amount of breast tissue is taken into the mouth with latch-on.
- Tickle the baby's lower lip with the tip of the nipple, stimulating the mouth to open.
- When the mouth is open wide and the tongue is down, quickly pull the baby onto the nipple.

The amount of areola in the baby's mouth with correct latch-on (Fig. 16-2) depends on the size of the baby's mouth and the size of the areola and the nipple. In general, the baby's mouth should cover the nipple and an areolar radius of approximately 2 to 3 cm all around the nipple.

- When the infant is latched on correctly, the following occur:

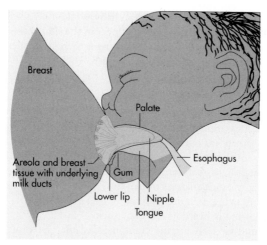

Fig. 16-2 Correct attachment (latch-on) of infant at breast.

—The baby's cheeks and chin are touching the breast.
—The mother reports a firm tugging sensation on her nipples but no pinching or pain.
—The baby sucks with cheeks rounded, not dimpled.
—The baby's jaw glides smoothly with sucking.
—Swallowing is audible.
• Depressing the breast tissue around the baby's nose is not necessary.
—If the mother is worried about the baby's breathing, she can raise the baby's hips slightly to change the angle of the baby's head at the breast.
—If the baby cannot breathe, innate reflexes will prompt the baby to move the head and pull back to breathe.
   Sucking creates a vacuum in the intraoral cavity as the breast is compressed between the tongue and the palate.
• If the mother feels pinching or pain after the initial sucks or does not feel a strong tugging sensation on the nipple, the latch-on and positioning should be evaluated.
• Any time the signs of adequate latch-on and sucking are not present, the baby should be taken off the breast and latch-on attempted again.

- To prevent nipple trauma as the baby is taken off the breast, break the suction by inserting a finger in the side of the baby's mouth between the gums and leaving it there until the nipple is completely out of the baby's mouth.

Milk ejection, or let-down

As the baby begins sucking on the nipple, the let-down, or milk-ejection, reflex is stimulated. The following signs indicate that let-down has occurred:

- The mother may feel a tingling sensation in the nipples, although many women never feel their milk let down.
- The baby's suck changes from quick, shallow sucks to a slower, more drawing, sucking pattern.
- Swallowing is heard as the baby sucks.
- The mother feels uterine cramping and may have increased lochia during and after feedings.
- The mother feels relaxed, even sleepy, during feedings.
- The opposite breast may leak.

Frequency of feedings

Newborns need to breastfeed 8 to 12 times in a 24-hour period. Feeding patterns are variable because every baby is unique. Infants should be fed whenever they exhibit feeding cues.

- Some infants breastfeed every 2 to 3 hours throughout a 24-hour period.
- Others may cluster-feed, breastfeeding every hour or so for three to five feedings and then sleeping for 3 to 4 hours between clusters.
- During the first 24 to 48 hours after birth, most babies do not awaken this often to feed.
- Parents should awaken the baby to feed at least every 3 hours during the day and at least every 4 hours at night. (Feeding frequency is determined by counting from the beginning of one feeding to the beginning of the next.)
- Once the infant is feeding well and gaining weight adequately, it is more appropriate to go to demand feeding, in which the infant determines the frequency of feedings. (With demand feeding, the infant should still receive at least eight feedings in 24 hours.)

- Parents should be cautioned about attempting to place newborn infants on strict feeding schedules.
- Parents can keep a feeding diary, writing down the frequency and length of time of feedings for the first week or so. The wet diapers and bowel movements the baby is having can also be recorded. This record can be taken with the baby for the first pediatrician visit.

Duration of feedings

The duration of breastfeeding sessions is highly variable because the timing of milk transfer differs for each mother-baby pair.

- The average time for feeding is 30 to 40 minutes, or approximately 15 to 20 minutes per breast.
- Some mothers do one-sided nursing, in which the baby nurses only one breast at each feeding. The first breast offered should be alternated at each feeding to ensure that each breast receives equal stimulation and emptying.

If a baby seems to be feeding effectively and the urine output is adequate but the weight gain is not satisfactory, the mother may be switching to the second breast too soon.

- The high-lactose, low-fat foremilk may cause the baby to have explosive stools, gas pains, and inconsolable crying.
- Feeding on the first breast until it softens ensures that the baby will receive the hindmilk, which usually results in increased weight gain.

Supplements, bottles, and pacifiers

The AAP recommends that, unless a medical indication exists, no supplements should be given to breastfeeding infants.

- Situations that may necessitate supplementary feeding include things such as low birth weight, hypoglycemia, dehydration, or inborn errors of metabolism.
- Mothers may be unable to breastfeed because of severe illness or complications of birth, or they may be taking medications incompatible with breastfeeding.

Offering formula to a baby after breastfeeding just to "make sure the baby is getting enough" is normally unnecessary and should be avoided.

- Supplementation interferes with the supply-meets-demand system of milk production.
- Babies who receive supplementary feedings in the early days of breastfeeding may develop nipple confusion (i.e., difficulty knowing how to latch on to the breast).
- If supplementation is needed, devices such as supplemental nursing systems may be used, in which the baby can be supplemented while breastfeeding.
- Syringe feeding, finger feeding, and cup feeding are other methods for offering supplements to breastfed infants.
- If parents choose to use bottles, a slow-flow nipple is recommended. Although some parents combine breastfeeding and bottle feeding, many babies never take a bottle and go directly from the breast to a cup as they grow.
- Pacifiers are not recommended until breastfeeding is well established. Their use has been associated with shorter duration of breastfeeding, sore nipples, and insufficient milk supply.

Special Considerations

Waking the sleepy newborn

- Lay the baby down, and unwrap.
- Change the diaper.
- Hold the baby upright, and turn from side to side.
- Talk to the baby.
- Gently, but firmly, massage the chest and back.
- Rub the baby's hands and feet.
- Do baby "sit-ups." Gently rock the baby from a lying to sitting position and back again until the eyes open.
- Adjust lighting up for stimulation or down to encourage the baby to open the eyes.
- Apply cool cloth to face.

    Babies sometimes awaken from sleep crying frantically. Although they may be hungry, they cannot focus on feeding until they are calmed.

- Infant fussiness during feeding may be the result of birth injury, such as bruising of the head or fractured clavicle. Changing the feeding position may alleviate this problem.
- Infants who were suctioned extensively or intubated at birth may demonstrate an aversion to oral stimulation. The baby may scream and stiffen if anything approaches the mouth.

Parents may need to spend time holding and cuddling the baby before attempting to breastfeed.

- An infant may become fussy and appear discontented when sucking if the nipple does not extend far enough into the mouth. It may be helpful for the mother to support her breast throughout the feeding so that the nipple stays in the same position as the feeding proceeds and the breast softens.
- Fussiness may be related to gastrointestinal (GI) distress (i.e., cramping and gas pains). This can be related to the following:
  - Occasional feeding of infant formula may cause GI distress.
  - Most mothers can consume their normal diet without affecting the baby; however, foods such as broccoli, cabbage, or onions may irritate some babies.
  - Others may react to cow's-milk protein ingested by the mother.
- No standard foods should be avoided by all mothers when breastfeeding; each mother-baby couple responds individually.
- If gas is a problem, the physician may suggest giving the baby liquid simethicone drops before feeding.
- Persistent crying or refusing to breastfeed can indicate illness, and the health care provider should be notified.
- Ear infections, sore throat, or oral thrush may cause the infant to be fussy and not breastfeed well.

Calming the fussy baby
- Swaddle the baby.
- Hold closely.
- Move or rock gently.
- Talk soothingly.
- Reduce environmental stimuli.
- Allow baby to suck on adult finger.
- Place baby skin-to-skin with mother.

Slow weight gain
Newborn infants typically lose 5% to 10% of body weight before they begin to show weight gain.
- Weight loss of 7% in a breastfeeding infant during the first 3 days of life should be investigated.

- Babies should gain 110 to 200 g/wk, or 20 to 28 g/day, for the first 3 months.
- Breastfed infants usually do not gain weight as quickly as formula-fed infants.
- The infant who continues to lose weight after 5 days, who does not regain birth weight by 14 days, or whose weight is below the 10th percentile by 1 month should be evaluated and closely monitored by a health care provider.
- Most often, slow weight gain is related to inadequate breast-feeding. Feedings may be short or infrequent, or the infant may be latching on incorrectly or sucking ineffectively or inefficiently.
- Other possibilities are illness or infection, malabsorption, or circumstances that increase the baby's energy needs, such as congenital heart disease, cystic fibrosis, or simply being SGA.

Maternal factors may be the cause of slow weight gain:

- Inadequate emptying of the breasts, pain with feeding, or inappropriate timing of feedings may occur.
- Inadequate glandular breast tissue or previous breast surgery may affect milk supply.
- Severe intrapartum or postpartum hemorrhage, illness, or medications may decrease milk supply.
- Stress and fatigue also may negatively affect milk production.

Usually the solution to slow weight gain is to improve the feeding technique. Positioning and latch-on are evaluated, and adjustments are made.

- Add one or two feedings in a 24-hour period.
- If the problem is a sleepy baby, parents are taught waking techniques.
- Using alternate breast massage during feedings may help increase the amount of milk going to the infant.
  - The mother massages her breast from the chest wall to the nipple whenever the baby has sucking pauses. This may increase the fat content of the milk, which aids in weight gain.
- When babies are calorie deprived and need supplementation, expressed breast milk or formula can be given with a nursing supplementer, cup, syringe, or bottle.

- If the baby's slow weight gain is related to the mother's milk supply, it must be determined if this is an actual or perceived problem and whether it is related to milk production or milk transfer to the infant.
- Maternal health habits should be assessed because medications, smoking, stress, fatigue, or infection can decrease milk supply.

Jaundice

Physiologic jaundice usually occurs after age 24 hours and peaks by the third day.

- Breastfeeding-associated jaundice (early-onset jaundice) begins at 2 to 4 days of age and occurs in approximately 10% to 25% of breastfed newborns.
- Early-onset jaundice or breastfeeding jaundice is associated with insufficient feeding and infrequent stooling.
- Colostrum has a natural laxative effect and promotes early passage of meconium. Bilirubin is excreted from the body primarily through the intestines. Infrequent stooling allows bilirubin in the stool to be reabsorbed into the infant's system, thus promoting hyperbilirubinemia.
- Infants who receive water or glucose water supplements are more likely to have hyperbilirubinemia because only small amounts of bilirubin are excreted through the kidneys.
- Decreased caloric intake (less milk) is associated with decreased stooling and increased jaundice.
- To *prevent* early-onset breastfeeding jaundice, babies should be breastfed frequently during the first several days of life. More frequent feedings are associated with lower bilirubin levels.
- To *treat* early-onset jaundice, breastfeeding is evaluated in terms of frequency and length of feedings, positioning and latch-on, and the infant's ability to empty the breast.
- Factors such as a sleepy or lethargic baby or breast engorgement may interfere with effective breastfeeding and should be corrected.
- If the infant's intake of milk needs to be increased, a supplemental feeding device may be used to deliver additional breast milk or formula while the infant is nursing.

- Hyperbilirubinemia may reach levels that require treatment with phototherapy.
- Breast milk jaundice (late-onset jaundice) is a progressive indirect hyperbilirubinemia beyond the first week of life typically occurring after 3 to 5 days of age and peaking by about 2 weeks.
  - Affected infants are typically thriving, gaining weight, and stooling normally; all pathologic causes of jaundice have been ruled out.
  - The jaundice may be caused by factors in the breast milk that either inhibit the conjugation or decrease the excretion of bilirubin. Less frequent stooling by breastfed infants may allow for extended time for reabsorption of bilirubin from stools.
  - In most cases, no intervention is necessary, although some experts recommend temporary interruption of breastfeeding for 12 to 24 hours to allow bilirubin levels to decrease. During this time, the mother pumps her breasts, and the baby is offered alternative nutrition, usually formula.

Preterm infants

Human milk is the ideal food for preterm infants, with benefits that are unique and in addition to those received by term, healthy infants. Depending on gestational age and physical condition, many preterm infants are capable of breastfeeding for at least some feedings each day.

- Mothers of preterm infants who are not able to breastfeed their infants should begin pumping their breasts as soon as possible after birth with a hospital-grade electric pump.
- The mother should use a dual collection kit and pump 8 to 10 times daily for 10 to 15 minutes and/or until the milk flow has ceased for a few minutes.
- These women are taught proper handling and storage of breast milk to minimize bacterial contamination and growth.

Breastfeeding multiple infants

Breastfeeding is especially beneficial to twins, triplets, and other higher-order multiples because of the immunologic and nutritional advantages, as well as the opportunity for the mother to interact with each baby frequently.

- Most mothers are capable of producing an adequate milk supply for multiple infants.
- Parenting multiples may be overwhelming, and mothers, as well as fathers, need extra support and assistance learning how to manage feedings.

Expressing Breast Milk

In the following situations, expression of breast milk is necessary or desirable:
- Engorgement occurs.
- The mother and baby are separated (e.g., preterm or sick infant).
- The mother is employed outside the home and needs to maintain her milk supply.
- The nipples are severely sore or damaged.
- The mother is leaving the infant with a caregiver and will not be present for feeding.

Because pumping and hand expression are rarely as efficient as a baby in removing milk from the breast, the milk supply should never be judged based on the volume expressed.

Hand expression
- Wash hands thoroughly.
- Place one hand on the breast at the edge of the areola.
- With the thumb above and fingers below, press in toward the chest wall and gently compress the breast while rolling the thumb and fingers forward toward the nipple.
- Repeat these motions rhythmically until the milk begins to flow.
- Maintain steady, light pressure while the milk is flowing easily.
- The thumb and fingers should not pinch the breast or slip down to the nipple, and the hand should be rotated to reach all sections of the breast.

Pumping
- For most women, it is advisable to initiate pumping only after the milk supply is well established and the infant is latching on and breastfeeding well.

- When breastfeeding is delayed after birth, pumping is started as soon as possible and continued regularly until the infant is able to breastfeed effectively.
- Some women pump on awakening in the morning or when the baby has fed but did not completely empty the breast.
- Others choose to pump after feedings or may pump one breast while the baby is feeding from the other.
- Double pumping (pumping both breasts at the same time) saves time and may stimulate the milk supply more effectively than single pumping.
- The amount of milk obtained when pumping depends on the type of pump being used, the time of day, how long it has been since the baby breastfed, the mother's milk supply, how practiced she is at pumping, and her comfort level (pumping is uncomfortable for some women).
- Breast milk may vary in color and consistency, depending on the time of day, the age of the baby, and foods the mother has eaten.

Types of Pumps. Many types of breast pumps are available, varying in price and effectiveness.

- Manual or hand pumps are the least expensive and may be the most appropriate where portability and quietness of operation are important. These are most often used by mothers who are pumping for an occasional bottle.
- Full-service electric pumps or hospital-grade pumps most closely duplicate the sucking action and pressure of the breastfeeding infant.
  - When breastfeeding is delayed after birth (e.g., preterm or ill newborn), or when mother and baby are separated for lengthy periods, these pumps are most appropriate.
  - Portable versions of these pumps can be rented for home use.
- Electric, self-cycling double pumps are efficient and easy to use. These pumps were designed for working mothers. Some of these pumps come with carrying bags containing coolers to store pumped milk.
- Smaller electric or battery-operated pumps also are available.
  - Some have automatic suck/release cycling, and others require use of a finger to regulate strength and speed of suction.

–These are typically used when pumping is done occasionally.

–Some models are satisfactory for working mothers or others who pump on a regular basis.

Breast milk storage guidelines for home use

• Before expressing breast milk, wash your hands.

• Containers for storing milk should be washed in hot, soapy water and rinsed thoroughly; they can also be washed in a dishwasher. Plastic bags designed specifically for breast milk storage can be used.

• Write the date of expression on the container before storing the milk.

• It is acceptable to store breast milk in the refrigerator or freezer with other food items.

• When storing milk in a refrigerator or freezer, place the containers in the middle or back of the freezer, not on the door.

• Freeze milk in serving sizes of 2 to 4 oz to avoid waste.

• When filling a storage container that will be frozen, allow space at the top of the container for expansion.

• To thaw frozen breast milk, place the container in the refrigerator for gradual thawing or place the container under warm, running water for quicker thawing.

NURSE ALERT *Frozen milk is never thawed or heated in a microwave oven. Putting frozen milk in a microwave oven does not heat the milk evenly and can cause encapsulated boiling bubbles to form in the center of the liquid. This may not be detected when drops of milk are checked for temperature. Babies have sustained severe burns to the mouth, throat, and upper GI tract as a result of milk heated in a microwave oven.*

• Milk thawed in the refrigerator can be stored for 24 hours. Milk thawed in warm water can be refrigerated for use within 4 hours.

• Thawed breast milk should never be refrozen.

• Shake the milk container before feeding baby, and test the temperature of the milk on the inner aspect of your wrist.

- Any unused milk left in the bottle after feeding must be discarded.
- Freshly expressed breast milk can be stored at room temperature (less than 77° F [25° C]) for up to 8 hours.
- Breast milk can be stored in the refrigerator for 5 days.
- Frozen breast milk can be stored for 2 weeks in a freezer compartment within a refrigerator.
- Frozen breast milk can be stored for up to 6 months in a freezer section with a separate door.
- Frozen breast milk can be stored for 6 to 12 months in a deep freeze (32° F [0° C] or lower).

Milk Banking

For those infants who cannot be breastfed but who also cannot survive except on human milk, banked donor milk is critically important. Because of the antiinfective and growth-promoting properties of human milk, as well as its superior nutrition, donor milk is used in many neonatal intensive care units for preterm or sick infants when the mother's own milk is not available. Banked milk is dispensed only by prescription. A per-ounce fee is charged by the bank to pay for the processing costs.

Medications and breastfeeding

Few drugs are absolutely contraindicated during lactation (Table 16-2).

- Breastfeeding mothers should be cautioned about taking any medications except those that are deemed essential; they should be advised to check with their physician before taking any medication.
- A breastfeeding mother who is taking a medication that has a questionable effect on the infant can be advised to take the medication just after nursing the baby or just before the infant is expected to sleep for a long time.
- Alcohol consumed by the breastfeeding mother is transferred to the infant in significant amounts, although it is not deemed harmful if the amount and duration are limited.
  - A mother who chooses to consume alcohol should be advised to minimize its effects by having only an occasional drink and not breastfeeding for 2 hours after the drink.

TABLE 16-2

Selected Drugs Excreted in Milk

DRUG	AAP RATING
Acetaminophen (Datril, Tylenol, Darvocet, Excedrin)	6
Alcohol (ethanol)	6
Aspirin (Bayer, Anacin, Bufferin, Excedrin, Fiorinal, Empirin)	5
Caffeine	6
Cocaine	2
Codeine	6
Heroin	2
Ibuprofen (Advil, Nuprin, Motrin)	6
Indomethacin (Indocin)	6
Ketorolac tromethamine (Toradal)	6
Marijuana	2
Medroxyprogesterone acetate (Depo- Provera)	6
Meperidine (Demerol, Mepergan)	6
Methadone	6
Morphine	6
Naproxen (Naproxyn, Anaprox, Naprosyn, Aleve)	6
Oxycodone	Not rated
Phenobarbitol (Luminal, Donnatal, Tedral)	5
Phenytoin (Dilantin)	6
Propylthiouracil	6
Thyroid and thyroxine	6
Tolbutamide (Orinase)	6

American Academy of Pediatrics (AAP) Committee on Drugs rated drugs that transfer into human milk. The ratings are as follows:
1. Drugs that are contraindicated during breastfeeding
2. Drugs of abuse that are contraindicated during breastfeeding
3. Radioactive compounds that require temporary cessation of breastfeeding
4. Drugs with unknown effects on breastfeeding but may be of concern
5. Drugs that have been associated with significant effects on some breastfeeding infants and should be given to breastfeeding mothers with caution
6. Maternal medication usually compatible with breastfeeding
7. Food and environmental agents that have an effect of breastfeeding

—The mother who is pumping for a sick or preterm infant should avoid alcohol entirely until her infant is healthy.

- Women who smoke are less likely to breastfeed than non-smokers; smokers who choose to breastfeed tend to do so for shorter durations than nonsmokers.
  - Nicotine is transferred to the infant in breast milk, whether the mother smokes or uses a nicotine patch, although the effect on the infant is uncertain.
  - Exposing the infant to secondhand smoke is of concern, and breastfeeding mothers are encouraged to stop smoking.
  - Mothers who smoke should be advised to limit smoking, to smoke after feeding the infant, and to consider switching to the nicotine patch.
- Maternal intake of caffeine may cause infant irritability and poor sleeping patterns.
  - For most women, two servings of caffeine per day do not cause untoward effects; however, some infants are sensitive to even small amounts of caffeine.
  - Mothers of such infants should limit caffeine intake.
  - Caffeine is found in coffee, tea, chocolate, and many soft drinks.
- Herbs and herbal teas are becoming more widely used during lactation.
  - Although some are considered safe, others contain pharmacologically active compounds that may have detrimental effects.
  - Each remedy should be evaluated for its compatibility with breastfeeding. The regional poison control center may provide information on the active properties of herbs.

Common Problems of the Breastfeeding Mother
Engorgement
- Engorgement is characterized by painful overfilling of the breasts and typically occurs 3 to 5 days after birth when the milk "comes in" and lasts about 24 hours.
- The breasts are firm, tender, and hot and may appear shiny and taut.
- The areolae are firm, and the nipples may flatten. The unyielding areolae make it difficult for the infant to latch on.

- Because back pressure on full milk glands inhibits milk production, if milk is not removed from the breasts, the milk supply may diminish.

Prevention

- Breastfeeding the baby frequently, at least every 2 to 3 hours, as the milk is coming in may help prevent engorgement.
- The baby should be encouraged to feed at least 15 to 20 minutes on each breast or until one breast softens per feeding.

Treatment

- Feed every 2 hours, massaging the breasts as the baby is feeding.
- The baby should feed on the first breast until it softens before switching to the other side.
- If the infant does not soften the second breast, the mother may use a breast pump to empty the breast. Pumping during engorgement will not cause a problematic increase in milk supply.
- A warm shower just before feeding or pumping can aid in relaxation and let-down.
- Cold compresses (ice packs) may reduce swelling, vascularity, and pain.
- Raw cabbage leaves placed over the breasts for 15 or 20 minutes between feedings may help reduce the swelling.
  - The cabbage leaves are washed, placed in the refrigerator until they are cool, and then crushed.
  - This can be repeated for two or three sessions; frequent application of cabbage leaves can decrease milk supply.
  - Cabbage leaves should not be used if the mother is allergic to cabbage or sulfa drugs or develops a skin rash.
- Antiinflammatory medications, such as ibuprofen, may help reduce the pain and swelling associated with engorgement.

Sore nipples

- Mild nipple tenderness during the first few days of breastfeeding is common.
- Severe soreness and abraded, cracked, or bleeding nipples are not normal and most often result from poor positioning, incorrect latch-on, improper suck, or a monilial infection.
- Correct breastfeeding technique is key to prevention.
  - Express a few drops of colostrum or milk to moisten the nipple and areola before latch-on.

—Evaluate the latch-on and baby's position at the breast.

—Reposition as necessary to try to resolve the nipple discomfort.

—Often sore nipples are the result of the mother latching the baby onto the breast before the mouth is open wide.

- The treatment for sore nipples is to correct the cause.
- When sore nipples occur, start the feeding on the least sore nipple.
- After feeding, the nipples are wiped with water to remove the baby's saliva.
- A few drops of milk can be expressed, rubbed into the nipple, and allowed to air dry.
- Sore nipples should be open to air as much as possible.
- Rapid healing of sore nipples is critical to relieve the mother's discomfort, maintain breastfeeding, and prevent mastitis.
- Warm water, purified lanolin, and hydrogel are the only treatments that have been studied and shown to have some effect.
- An antibiotic ointment may be recommended if nipples are cracked, abraded, or bleeding; this must be washed off before the feeding.
- If nipples are extremely sore or damaged, and the mother cannot tolerate breastfeeding, she can use an electric breast pump for 24 to 48 hours to allow the nipples to begin healing before resuming breastfeeding.

Monilial infections

Nipple soreness may be caused by a monilial (yeast) infection.

- The mother usually reports sudden onset of severe nipple pain and tenderness, burning, or stinging and may have sharp, shooting, burning pains into the breasts during and after feedings.
- The nipples appear somewhat pink and shiny or may be scaly or flaky; there may be a visible rash, small blisters, or thrush.
- The pain is out of proportion to the appearance of the nipple.
- Yeast infections of the nipples and breast can be excruciatingly painful and can lead to early cessation of breastfeeding if not recognized and treated promptly.

- Babies may or may not exhibit symptoms of monilial infection. Oral thrush and a red, raised diaper rash are common indications of a yeast infection.
- Mothers and babies must be treated simultaneously with antifungal medication, even if the infant has no visible signs of infection.

Plugged milk ducts

- A milk duct may become plugged or clogged, causing a red, tender area or small lump in the breast, which may or may not be tender.
- Plugged milk ducts are most often the result of inadequate emptying of the breast.
- Application of warm compresses to the affected area and to the nipple before feeding helps promote emptying of the breast and release of the plug. (A disposable diaper filled with warm water makes an easy compress.)
- Soaking in a warm bath before feeding may be helpful.
- Frequent feeding is recommended, with the baby beginning the feeding on the affected side to foster more complete emptying.
- Massaging the affected area while the baby nurses or while pumping is helpful.
- Varying feeding positions and feeding without wearing a bra may be useful in resolving a plugged duct.

FORMULA FEEDING

Readiness for Feeding

- The first feeding of formula is ideally given after the initial transition to extrauterine life is made. This may be sips of sterile water to assess patency of the GI tract and absence of tracheoesophageal fistula. If the infant sucks and swallows the water without difficulty, formula is then offered.
- Feeding-readiness cues include things such as stability of vital signs, presence of bowel sounds, an active sucking reflex, and those described earlier for breastfed infants.

- The type of formula is usually determined by the pediatrician. Parents are advised to avoid switching formulas unless instructed to do so by the physician.

Feeding Patterns

- Typically, a newborn will drink 15 to 30 ml of formula per feeding during the first 24 hours, with the intake gradually increasing during the first week of life.
- Most newborn infants should be fed every 3 to 4 hours, even if that requires waking the baby for the feedings.
- The infant showing an adequate weight gain can be allowed to sleep at night and fed only on awakening.
- Most newborns need six to eight feedings in 24 hours, and the number of feedings decreases as the infant matures.
- Usually by 3 to 4 weeks after birth, a fairly predictable feeding pattern has developed.
- Scheduling feedings arbitrarily at predetermined intervals may not meet a baby's needs, but initiating feedings at convenient times often moves the baby's feedings to times that work for the family.
- Mothers will usually note increases in the infant's appetite at 7 to 10 days, 3 weeks, 6 weeks, 3 months, and 6 months. These appetite spurts correspond to growth spurts. The amount of formula per feeding should be increased by about 30 ml to meet the baby's needs at these times. See Box 16-2 for tips on feeding technique.

Common Concerns

Spitting up

Parents need to know what to do if the infant is spitting up.

- They may need to decrease the amount of feeding or feed smaller amounts more frequently.
- Burping the infant several times during a feeding, such as when the infant's sucking slows down or stops, may decrease spitting.
- The parent can hold the baby upright for 30 minutes after feeding and avoid bouncing or placing the infant on the abdomen soon after the feeding is finished. Spitting may be a result of overfeeding or may be symptomatic of gastroesophageal reflux (GER).

BOX 16-2

Bottle-Feeding Techniques and Tips

- Newborns should be fed at least every 3 to 4 hours and should never go longer than 4 hours without feeding until a satisfactory pattern of weight gain is established. This may take 2 weeks. If a baby cries or fusses between feedings, check to see if the diaper should be changed and if the baby needs to be picked up and cuddled. If the baby continues to cry and acts hungry, feed him or her. Babies do not get hungry on a regular schedule.
- Babies should be held and never left alone while feeding. Never prop the bottle. The baby might inhale formula or choke on any that was spit up. Babies who fall asleep with a propped bottle of milk or juice may be prone to cavities when the first teeth come in.
- Babies gradually increase the amount of milk they drink with each feeding. The first day or so, most newborns consume 15 to 30 ml ($^1/_2$ to 1 ounce) with each feeding. This amount increases as the infant grows. If any formula remains in the bottle as the feeding ends, that milk must be thrown away, because saliva from the baby's mouth can cause the formula to spoil.
- For feeding, hold the baby close in a semi-reclining position. Talk to the baby during the feeding. This is a great time for social interaction and cuddling.
- Place the nipple in the baby's mouth on the tongue. It should touch the roof of the mouth to stimulate the baby's sucking reflex. Hold the bottle like a pencil. Keep the bottle tipped so that the nipple stays filled with milk and the baby does not suck in air.
- It is normal for babies to take a few sucks and then pause briefly before continuing to suck again. Some newborns take longer to feed than others. Be patient. It may be necessary to keep the baby awake and to encourage sucking. Moving the nipple gently in the baby's mouth may stimulate sucking.
- Newborns are apt to swallow air when sucking. Give the baby opportunities to burp several times during a feeding. As the baby gets older, you will know better when it is necessary to stop for burping.

Continued

BOX 16-2

Bottle-Feeding Techniques and Tips—cont'd

- When the infant falls asleep, turns aside the head, or ceases to suck, it is usually an indication that enough formula has been taken to satisfy the baby.
- After the first 2 or 3 days, the stools of a formula-fed infant are yellow and soft but formed. The baby may have a stool with each feeding in the first 2 weeks, although this may decrease to one or two stools each day.

- Vomiting one third or more of the feeding at most feeding sessions or projectile vomiting should be reported to the health care provider.

Bottles and nipples
- Most babies will feed well with any bottle and nipple.
- Bottles and nipples should be washed in warm soapy water, using a bottle and nipple brush to facilitate thorough cleansing, followed by careful rinsing.
- Boiling of bottles and nipples is not needed unless there is some question about the safety of the water supply.

Infant Formulas
Commercial formulas
Commercial infant formulas are designed to resemble human milk as closely as possible, although none has ever duplicated it.
- Infants who are not breastfed should be given commercial formulas fortified with iron.
- The WIC program provides iron-fortified commercial infant formula for low-income families.
- Cow's milk is the basis for most infant formulas, although soy-based and other specialized formulas are available for the infant who cannot tolerate cow's milk.

- Commercial formulas are available in three forms: powder, concentrate, and ready-to-feed. All are equivalent in terms of nutritional content, but they vary considerably in cost:
  - Powdered formula is the least expensive type. It is easily mixed by using one scoop for every 60 ml of water.
  - Concentrated formula is more expensive than powder. It is diluted with equal parts of water and can be stored in the refrigerator for 48 hours after opening.
  - Ready-to-feed formula is the most expensive but easiest to use. The desired amount is poured into the bottle. The opened can is safely refrigerated for 48 hours. This type of formula can be purchased in individual disposable bottles for the most convenient feeding.

Special formulas
- Some infants have an allergic reaction to cow's-milk formula.
- Some may better tolerate a soy-milk formula, although some may be allergic to soy protein.
- Some women may be able to begin breastfeeding or, in life-threatening cases, obtain human milk through a milk bank, at least temporarily.
- Other special formulas are available for infants with a variety of disorders, such as protein allergy, malabsorption syndromes, and inborn errors of metabolism.
- Formulas for preterm infants contain higher calorie concentration (22 to 24 cal/oz) and higher concentrations of some nutrients, such as protein, vitamin A, folic acid, and zinc.

Evaporated Milk

Although evaporated milk is concentrated and less expensive than commercial formula, the mixing of evaporated milk and water to feed a baby is no longer recommended because evaporated milk does not provide adequate nutrition for an infant.

Unmodified Cow's Milk

Unmodified cow's milk is not suited to the nutritional needs of the human infant in the first year of life because it contains the following:

- Excessive amounts of calcium, phosphorus, and other minerals
- An imbalance of calcium and phosphorus
- An excessive protein content
- Poorly absorbed fat
- Low iron concentration

It causes microscopic hemorrhages that lead to GI blood loss, increasing the likelihood of iron deficiency anemia.

Formula Preparation

Commercial infant formula includes directions for preparation and use with pictures and symbols for the benefit of persons who cannot read. Some manufacturers are translating the directions into various languages, such as Spanish, French, Vietnamese, Chinese, and Arabic, to prevent misunderstanding and errors in formula preparation.

- Wash your hands and clean the bottle, nipple, and can opener carefully before preparing formula.
- If new nipples seem too firm or stiff, they can be softened by boiling them in water for 5 minutes before use.
- Read the label on the container of formula, and mix it exactly according to the directions.
- Use tap water to mix concentrated or powdered formula unless directed otherwise by the baby's physician or nurse.
- Test the size of the nipple hole by holding a prepared bottle upside down.
  - The formula should drip from the nipple. If it runs in a stream, the hole is too big and should not be used.
  - If it has to be shaken for the formula to come out, the hole is too small.
  - Either buy a new nipple or enlarge the hole by boiling the nipple for 5 minutes with a sewing needle inserted in the hole.
- If a nipple collapses when the baby sucks, loosen the nipple ring a little to let in air.
- Opened cans of ready-to-feed or concentrated formula should be covered and refrigerated. Any unused portions must be discarded after 48 hours.
- Bottles or cans of unopened formula can be stored at room temperature.

- If the formula is refrigerated, warm it by placing the bottle in a pan of hot water.
- Never use a microwave to warm any food to be given to a baby.
- Test the temperature of the formula by letting a few drops fall on the inside of your wrist. If the formula feels comfortably warm to you, it is the correct temperature.

> **NURSE ALERT** *It is important to impress on families that the proportions must not be altered—neither diluted to expand the amount of formula nor concentrated to provide more calories.*

- It is important that formula be mixed properly. The newborn's kidneys are immature, and giving the infant overly concentrated formula may provide protein and minerals in amounts that exceed the kidney's excretory ability.
  - If the formula is diluted too much (sometimes done in an effort to save money), the infant does not consume enough calories and does not grow well.
- Sterilization of formula rarely is recommended for those families with access to a safe public water supply.
  - The formula is prepared with attention to cleanliness.
  - When water from a private well is used, parents should be advised to contact the health department to have a chemical and bacteriologic analysis of the water done before using the water in formula preparation. The presence of nitrates, excess fluoride, or bacteria may be harmful to the infant.
  - If the sanitary conditions in the home appear unsafe, it would be better to recommend the use of ready-to-feed formula or to teach the mother to sterilize the formula.

Vitamin and Mineral Supplementation

Commercial iron-fortifed formula has all the nutrients the infant needs for the first 6 months of life. After 6 months, the only mineral supplementation required is fluoride if the local water supply is not fluoridated.

Chapter 17

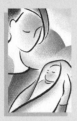

Problems of the Newborn

Classification of high risk infants according to birth weight, gestational age, and predominant pathophysiologic problems is presented in Box 17-1.

THE PRETERM INFANT

Preterm infants, those born before 37 weeks of gestation, are at risk because their organ systems are immature and they lack adequate physiologic reserves to function in an extrauterine environment.

COMPLICATIONS ASSOCIATED WITH PREMATURITY

Respiratory Distress Syndrome (RDS)

RDS is a lung disorder affecting mostly preterm infants, although a small percentage of term or near-term infants may also be affected.

Clinical Manifestations and Etiology

- Maternal and fetal conditions associated with a decreased incidence and severity of RDS include the following:
  - Female infant
  - African-American race
  - Maternal steroid (betamethasone) therapy
  - Stressors such as maternal gestational hypertension, maternal drug abuse, chronic retroplacental abruption, prolonged rupture of membranes, and intrauterine growth restriction (IUGR)
- The incidence and severity of RDS increase with a decrease in gestational age. Perinatal asphyxia, hypovolemia, male infant, Caucasian race, maternal diabetes, second-born twin,

BOX 17-1

Classification of High Risk Infants

CLASSIFICATION ACCORDING TO SIZE

Low-birth-weight (LBW) infant—An infant whose birth weight is less than 2500 g, regardless of gestational age

Very low-birth-weight (VLBW) infant—An infant whose birth weight is less than 1500 g

Extremely low-birth-weight (ELBW) infant—An infant whose birth weight is less than 1000 g

Appropriate for gestational age (AGA) infant—An infant whose birth weight falls between the 10th and 90th percentiles on intrauterine growth curves

Small-for-date (SFD) or small for gestational age (SGA) infant—An infant whose rate of intrauterine growth was restricted and whose birth weight falls below the 10th percentile on intrauterine growth curves

Large for gestational age (LGA) infant—An infant whose birth weight falls above the 90th percentile on intrauterine growth charts

Intrauterine growth restriction (IUGR)—Found in infants whose intrauterine growth is restricted (sometimes used as a more descriptive term for the SGA infant)

Symmetric IUGR—Growth restriction in which the weight, length, and head circumference are all affected

Asymmetric IUGR—Growth restriction in which the head circumference remains within normal parameters while the birth weight falls below the 10th percentile

CLASSIFICATION ACCORDING TO GESTATIONAL AGE

Premature (preterm) infant—An infant born before completion of 37 weeks of gestation, regardless of birth weight

Full-term infant—An infant born between the beginning of 38 weeks and the completion of 42 weeks of gestation, regardless of birth weight

Postmature (postterm) infant—An infant born after 42 weeks of gestation, regardless of birth weight

CLASSIFICATION ACCORDING TO MORTALITY

Live birth—Birth in which the neonate manifests any heartbeat, breathes, or displays voluntary movement, regardless of gestational age

Fetal death—Death of the fetus after 20 weeks of gestation and before birth, with absence of any signs of life after birth

Neonatal death—Death that occurs in the first 27 days of life; early neonatal death occurs in the first week of life; late neonatal death occurs at 7 to 27 days

Perinatal mortality—Total number of fetal and early neonatal deaths per 1000 live births

familial predisposition, maternal hypotension, cesarean birth without labor, hydrops fetalis, and third-trimester bleeding are all factors that place an infant at increased risk for RDS.

- RDS is caused by a lack of pulmonary surfactant, which leads to progressive atelectasis, loss of functional residual capacity, and ventilation/perfusion imbalance with an uneven distribution of ventilation.
- Surfactant deficiency may be caused by insufficient surfactant production, abnormal composition and function, disruption of surfactant production, or a combination of these factors.
- The sequence of events that occurs is further compromised by weak respiratory muscles and an overly compliant chest wall, which are common to premature infants.
- Lung capacity is compromised by the presence of proteinaceous material and epithelial debris in the airways. The resulting decreased oxygenation, cyanosis, and metabolic or respiratory acidosis can increase pulmonary vascular resistance (PVR).
- This increased PVR can lead to right-to-left shunting and a reopening of the ductus arteriosus and foramen ovale.
- Respiratory distress of a nonpulmonary origin in neonates may also be caused by sepsis, cardiac defects (structural or functional), exposure to cold, airway obstruction (atresia), intraventricular hemorrhage, hypoglycemia, metabolic acidosis, acute blood loss, and drugs. Pneumonia in the neonatal period may present as respiratory distress caused by bacterial or viral agents and may occur alone or as a complication of RDS.
- Clinical symptoms of RDS include tachypnea, grunting, nasal flaring, intercostal or subcostal retractions, hypercapnia, respiratory or mixed acidosis, hypotension, and shock.
  - These respiratory symptoms usually present immediately after birth or within 6 hours of birth.
  - Physical examination reveals crackles, poor air exchange, pallor, use of accessory muscles (retractions), and occasionally apnea.
  - Radiographic findings include uniform reticulogranular appearance and air bronchograms.
- The infant's clinical course varies. There is usually an increased oxygen requirement and increased respiratory effort as atelectasis, loss of functional residual capacity, and ventilation/perfusion imbalance worsen.

- Severe RDS is often associated with a shocklike state, as manifested by diminished cardiac inflow and low arterial BP.
  - The ELBW or VLBW infant, as a result of extreme pulmonary immaturity, decreased glycogen stores, and lack of accessory muscles, may have severe RDS at birth.
- RDS is a self-limiting disease with respiratory symptoms abating after 72 hours. The disappearance of respiratory symptoms coincides with the production of surfactant in type II cells of the alveoli.

Interventions

The treatment for RDS is supportive.
- Adequate ventilation and oxygenation must be established and maintained in an attempt to prevent ventilation/perfusion mismatch and atelectasis.
- Exogenous surfactant, which alters the typical course of RDS, may be administered at or shortly after birth.
- Positive-pressure ventilation, CPAP, and oxygen therapy may be needed during the respiratory illness.
- Prevention of complications associated with mechanical ventilation is critical.
  - These complications include pulmonary interstitial emphysema, pneumothorax, pneumomediastinum (accumulation of air in the mediastinum), and pneumopericardium (accumulation of air in the space surrounding the heart).
- Acid-base balance is evaluated by monitoring ABG values (Table 17-1). Frequent blood sampling requires arterial access either by umbilical artery catheter (UAC) or by a peripheral arterial line.
  - Pulse oximetry and transcutaneous carbon dioxide and oxygen monitors document trends in ventilation and oxygenation.
  - Capillary blood gas values may be used to evaluate pH and PCO_2 in infants whose condition is more stable.
- The maintenance of a neutral thermal environment (NTE) continues to be of critical importance in infants with RDS; infants with hypoxemia are unable to increase their metabolic rate when cold stressed.
- Sepsis evaluation, including blood culture, complete blood count (CBC) with differential, and occasionally a lumbar

TABLE 17-1

Normal Arterial Blood Gas Values for Neonates

VALUE	RANGE
pH	7.35-7.45
Arterial oxygen pressure (PaO$_2$)	60-80 mmHg
Carbon dioxide pressure (PacO$_2$)	35-45 mmHg
Bicarbonate (HCO$_3$)	22-26 mEq/L
Base excess	(−4) to (+4)
Oxygen saturation	92%-94%

From Parry, W., & Zimmer, J. (2002). Acid-base homeostasis and oxygenation. In G. Merenstein & S. Gardner (Eds.), *Handbook of neonatal intensive care* (5th ed.). St. Louis: Mosby.

puncture, is done in infants with RDS to rule out systemic infection.

- Laboratory and radiographic tests rarely confirm the diagnosis of neonatal pneumonia; rather, it is the clinical history and presenting clinical signs that provide a basis for the diagnosis and treatment.
- Broad-spectrum antibiotics are begun while the results of cultures are awaited.
- Fluid and nutrition must be maintained for the infant critically ill with RDS.
  - Parenteral nutrition can provide protein and fat to promote a positive nitrogen balance.
  - Daily monitoring of electrolytes, urine output, specific gravity, and weight assists in the evaluation of hydration status.

Patent Ductus Arteriosus (PDA)

The ductus arteriosus is a muscular contractile structure in the fetus connecting the left pulmonary artery and the dorsal aorta. The ductus constricts after birth as oxygenation, the levels of circulating prostaglandins, and the muscle mass increase. Other factors that promote ductal closure include catecholamines, low pH, bradykinin, and acetylcholine. When the fetal ductus arteriosus fails to close after birth, PDA occurs. Ductal closure usually occurs within hours or days in the term infant but may be delayed in preterm infants as a result of oxygenation and circulating hormones (prostaglandins).

- The clinical presentation in an infant with a PDA includes systolic murmur, active precordium, bounding peripheral pulses, tachycardia, tachypnea, crackles, and hepatomegaly.
- The systolic murmur is heard best at the second or third intercostal space at the upper left sternal border.
- An active precordium is caused by an increased left ventricular stroke volume.
- A widened pulse pressure may result in an increase in peripheral pulses.
- Radiographic studies of infants with a large shunting PDA typically show cardiac enlargement and pulmonary edema; with a smaller PDA the radiograph may appear normal for the infant's age.
- ABG findings reveal hypercarbia and metabolic acidosis. A color flow Doppler echocardiogram can demonstrate a PDA, identify the direction of the shunting (left-to-right, right-to-left, or both), and quantitate the amount of blood shunting across the PDA.

   The PDA can be managed medically or surgically.

- Medical management consists of ventilatory support, fluid restriction, and the administration of diuretics and indomethacin.
   - Indomethacin is a prostaglandin synthetase inhibitor that blocks the effect of the arachidonic acid products on the ductus and causes the PDA to constrict.
   - Ventilatory support is adjusted based on ABG levels.
   - Fluid restriction is implemented to decrease cardiovascular volume overload in association with the diuretic therapy.
   - The nonsteroidal antiinflammatory drug (NSAID) ibuprofen has been used with some success in the medical closure of PDA in preterm infants. This drug has fewer side effects than indomethacin and acts by inhibiting prostaglandin formation.

Surgical ligation is performed when PDA is clinically significant and medical management has failed.

- Nursing care of the infant with PDA focuses on supportive care. The infant needs an NTE, adequate oxygenation, meticulous fluid balance, and parental support.

Periventricular-Intraventricular Hemorrhage (PV-IVH)

PV-IVH is one of the most common types of brain injury that occurs in neonates and is among the most severe in both short-term and long-term outcomes.

- The true incidence of PV-IVH is unknown, but the general estimate is 15% in infants at less than 32 weeks of gestation or weighing under 1501 g.
- PV-IVH occurs in approximately 3.5% to 5% of term infants, with 50% of those cases caused by asphyxia or trauma. In term infants the symptoms appear within 48 hours of birth.

The pathogenesis of PV-IVH includes intravascular factors (e.g., fluctuating or increasing cerebral blood flow, increases in cerebral venous pressure, and coagulopathy), vascular factors, extravascular factors (hypoglycemia and acidosis), and routine nursery care (rapid volume expansion and blood transfusion). PV-IVH events typically occur within the first week of life. PV-IVH is classified according to severity, which determines long-term neurodevelopmental outcomes.

Nursing care focuses on recognition of factors that increase the risk of PV-IVH, interventions to decrease the risk of bleeding, and supportive care to infants who have bleeding episodes.

- The infant is positioned with the head in midline and the head of the bed elevated slightly to prevent or minimize fluctuations in intracranial BP.
- An NTE is maintained, as well as oxygenation.
- Rapid infusions of fluids should be avoided.
- BP is monitored closely for fluctuations.
- The infant is monitored for signs of pneumothorax because it often precedes PV-IVH.

Necrotizing Enterocolitis (NEC)

NEC is an acute inflammatory disease of the GI mucosa, commonly complicated by perforation. This often fatal disease occurs in about 2% to 5% of newborns in NICUs.

- Three factors appear to play an important role in the development of NEC:
  - Intestinal ischemia
  - Colonization by pathogenic bacteria
  - Substrate (formula feeding) in the intestinal lumen

- The precise cause of NEC is still uncertain, but it appears to occur in infants whose GI tract has suffered vascular compromise.
- Prematurity remains the most prominent risk factor in the development of NEC.
   The onset of NEC in the full-term infant usually occurs between 4 and 10 days after birth. In the preterm infant the onset may be delayed for up to 30 days.
- Signs of developing NEC are nonspecific, which is characteristic of many neonatal disease processes.
   - Some generalized signs include decreased activity, hypotonia, pallor, recurrent apnea and bradycardia, decreased oxygen saturation, respiratory distress, metabolic acidosis, oliguria, hypotension, decreased perfusion, temperature instability, and cyanosis.
   - GI symptoms include abdominal distention, increasing or bile-stained residual gastric aspirates, vomiting (bile or blood), grossly bloody stools, abdominal tenderness, and erythema of the abdominal wall.
- Diagnosis of NEC is confirmed by radiographic examination that reveals bowel loop distention, pneumatosis intestinalis, pneumoperitoneum, portal air, or a combination of these findings.
   - The abnormal radiographic findings are caused by the bacterial colonization of the GI tract associated with NEC, resulting in an ileus.
   - Pneumatosis intestinalis, pneumoperitoneum, and portal air are caused by gas produced by the bacteria that invade the wall of the intestines and escape into the peritoneum and portal system when perforation occurs.
- Laboratory evaluation includes a CBC with differential, coagulation studies, ABG analysis, serum electrolyte levels, and blood culture.
   - The white blood cell (WBC) count may be either increased or decreased.
   - The platelet count and coagulation studies may be abnormal, with thrombocytopenia and disseminated intravascular coagulation (DIC).
   - Electrolyte levels may be abnormal, with leaking capillary beds and fluid shifts with the infection.

- Treatment of infants with NEC is supportive and preventive for bowel perforation.
  - Oral or tube feedings are discontinued to rest the GI tract.
  - A nasogastric tube is inserted and placed to low suction to provide gastric decompression.
  - Parenteral therapy (often by TPN) is begun.
  - NEC is an infectious disease; control of infection is imperative, with an emphasis on careful handwashing before and after infant contact.
  - Systemic antibiotic therapy is instituted.
  - Surgical resection is performed if perforation or clinical deterioration occurs.
- With early recognition and treatment, medical management is increasingly successful.
- If there is progressive deterioration under medical management or evidence of perforation, surgical resection and anastomosis are performed.
  - Intestinal transplantation has been successful in some former preterm infants with NEC-associated short-gut syndrome who had already developed life-threatening TPN-related complications.
- Therapy may be prolonged and recovery may be delayed by adhesions, complications of bowel resection, short-gut syndrome (especially if the ileocecal valve is removed), fat malabsorption intolerance of oral feedings, and failure to thrive.

NURSE ALERT *Observe for indications of early development of NEC by checking the appearance of the abdomen for distention (measuring abdominal girth, measuring residual gastric contents before feedings, and listening for the presence of bowel sounds) and performing all routine assessments for high risk neonates.*

- Minimal enteral feedings (trophic feeding and GI priming) may be protective against NEC in nonasphyxiated preterm infants.
- There is evidence that human milk may have a protective effect against the development of NEC.

Complications of Oxygen Therapy
Retinopathy of prematurity

- Retinopathy of prematurity (ROP) is a complex, multicausal disorder that affects the developing retinal vessels of premature infants.
- Normal retinal vessels begin to form in utero at approximately 16 weeks of gestation in response to an unknown stimulus.
- The retinal vessels continue to develop until they reach maturity at approximately 42 to 43 weeks after conception.
- Once the retina is completely vascularized, the retinal vessels are not susceptible to ROP.
- The mechanism of injury in ROP is unclear.
  - Oxygen tensions that are too high for the level of retinal maturity initially result in vasoconstriction.
  - After oxygen therapy is discontinued, neovascularization occurs in the retina and vitreous, with capillary hemorrhages, fibrotic resolution, and possible retinal detachment.
  - Scar tissue formation and consequent visual impairment may be mild or severe.
  - The entire disease process in severe cases may take as long as 5 months to evolve.
- The key to management of ROP is prevention and early detection.
  - Although exposure to bright light has not proven to contribute to ROP, such exposure is nevertheless undesirable from a neurobehavioral developmental perspective.
  - All caregivers should use supplemental oxygen judiciously, monitor oxygen blood levels carefully, attend to saturation monitor alarms promptly, and prevent wide fluctuations in oxygen blood levels (hyperoxemia and hypoxemia).
  - Circumferential cryopexy, laser photocoagulation, vitamin E therapy, and decreased intensity of ambient light are used in the treatment of ROP with varying results.
- Early screening for ROP should be provided for infants born at less than 28 weeks of gestation and whose weight is less than 1500 g and for infants weighing between 1500 and 2000 g who are believed to be at high risk for development of ROP.
  - Examination by an ophthalmologist before discharge and a schedule for repeat examinations thereafter are recommended for the parents' guidance.

Chronic lung disease (CLD) (formerly bronchopulmonary dysplasia)

CLD is a chronic pulmonary iatrogenic condition caused by barotrauma from pressure ventilation and oxygen toxicity.

- The etiology of CLD is multifactorial and includes pulmonary immaturity, surfactant deficiency, lung injury and stretch, barotrauma, inflammation caused by oxygen exposure, fluid overload, ligation of a PDA, and genetic predisposition.
- The incidence of CLD in infants weighing less than 1500 g who require mechanical ventilation for RDS ranges from 23% to 80%.

Clinical signs of CLD include tachypnea, retractions, nasal flaring, increased work of breathing, exercise intolerance (to handling and feeding), and tachycardia. Auscultation of lung fields in affected infants reveals crackles, decreased air movement, and occasionally expiratory wheezing.

Treatment for CLD includes oxygen therapy, nutrition, fluid restriction, and medications (e.g., diuretics, corticosteroids, and bronchodilators).

- The use of corticosteroids to prevent or treat CLD is controversial because of the side effects and varied results in clinical trials; however, corticosteroids are used in many centers to treat or prevent CLD.
- The key to the management of CLD is prevention by reducing the incidence of prematurity and RDS and by using surfactant and antenatal steroids and minimizing lung trauma from mechanical ventilation and high oxygen concentrations.
- The prognosis for infants with CLD depends on the degree of pulmonary dysfunction.
- Most deaths occur within the first year of life as a result of cardiorespiratory failure, sepsis, or respiratory infection; in some infants the deaths are sudden and unexplained.

THE POSTMATURE INFANT

Postterm infants are those whose gestation is prolonged beyond 42 weeks, regardless of birth weight; the infant is called *postmature*.

- These infants may be large for gestational age (LGA) or small for gestational age (SGA), but most often their weight is appropriate for gestational age (AGA).

- There may be meconium staining of the fingernails, the hair and nails may be long, and vernix may be absent. The skin may peel off.
- Insufficient gas exchange in the postmature placenta increases the likelihood of intrauterine hypoxia, which may result in the passage of meconium in utero, thereby increasing the risk for MAS.

Meconium Aspiration Syndrome (MAS)

Meconium staining of the amniotic fluid can indicate a nonreassuring fetal status, especially in a vertex presentation. It appears in 8% to 20% of all births.

- Many infants with meconium staining exhibit no signs of depression at birth; however, the presence of meconium in the amniotic fluid necessitates careful supervision of labor and close monitoring of fetal well-being.
- The presence of a team skilled in neonatal resuscitation is required at the birth of any infant with meconium-stained amniotic fluid.
- The mouth and nares of the infant are routinely suctioned on the perineum before the infant's first breath.
- Meconium in the airway at birth can migrate down to the terminal airways, causing mechanical obstruction leading to MAS.
- The fetus may have aspirated meconium in utero, which can cause a chemical pneumonitis.
- These infants may develop PPHN, further complicating their management.
- Infants with moderate-to-severe MAS may receive surfactant replacement to improve alveolar function.

Persistent Pulmonary Hypertension of the Newborn (PPHN)

Persistent pulmonary hypertension of the newborn is a term applied to the combined findings of pulmonary hypertension, right-to-left shunting, and a structurally normal heart.

- PPHN may occur either as a single entity or as the main component of MAS, congenital diaphragmatic hernia, RDS, hyperviscosity syndrome, or neonatal pneumonia or sepsis.

- PPHN is also called persistent fetal circulation (PFC) because the syndrome includes reversion to fetal pathways for blood flow.
- The infant with PPHN is typically born at term or post-term, has tachycardia and cyanosis as presenting signs, and within minutes or hours progresses to severe respiratory compromise with concomitant acidosis, which further compromises pulmonary perfusion and deteriorating oxygenation.
- Management depends on the underlying cause of the PPHN. The use of inhaled nitric oxide (INO) and extra-corporeal membrane oxygenation (ECMO) (oxygenation of blood external to the body using cardiopulmonary bypass and a membrane oxygenator) has improved the chances of survival of these infants.
- Another mode of treatment for PPHN and other respiratory disorders of the newborn is high-frequency ventilation, an assisted-ventilation method that delivers small volumes of gas at high frequencies and limits the development of high airway pressure, thus theoretically reducing barotrauma.

OTHER PROBLEMS RELATED TO GESTATION

Small for Gestational Age Infants and Intrauterine Growth Restriction

Infants who are SGA (i.e., weight is below the 10th percentile expected at term) or infants who have IUGR (i.e., rate of growth does not meet expected growth pattern) are considered high risk, with the perimortality rate 10 to 20 times greater than that for the normal term infant.

Care of the SGA infant is based on the clinical problems present and is the same given to preterm infants with similar problems.

Common problems that affect SGA infants who experienced IUGR are as follows:

  –Perinatal asphyxia
  –Meconium aspiration (discussed previously)
  –Immunodeficiency

−Hypoglycemia
−Polycythemia
−Temperature instability

Perinatal asphyxia

Commonly, IUGR infants have been exposed to chronic hypoxia for varying periods before labor and birth. The chronically hypoxic infant is severely compromised by a normal labor and has difficulty compensating after birth. The alert, wide-eyed appearance of the newborn is attributed to prolonged fetal hypoxia. Appropriate management and resuscitation are essential for the depressed infant.

Sequelae to perinatal asphyxia include MAS and hypoglycemia.

Hypoglycemia

All high risk infants are at risk for the development of hypoglycemia. Infants who are asphyxiated or have other physiologic stress may experience hypoglycemia as a result of a decreased glycogen supply, inadequate gluconeogenesis, or overuse of glycogen stored during fetal life. The concept of hypoglycemia as being a single cutoff value has received criticism because of the wide variability of glucose values from one newborn to another, expressed along a continuum of falling blood glucose values.

Suggested operational thresholds at which interventions to increase serum blood glucose levels should be implemented to prevent serious effects are as follows:

- At-risk infants (neonatal factors: IDM, hypothermia, hyperinsulinism, respiratory distress, congenital abnormalities, SGA, prematurity; maternal factors: gestational hypertension, terbutaline administration for preterm labor) should have glucose values equal to 36 mg/dl within the first few hours of life, with a therapeutic objective of 45 mg/dl. In these infants it is recommended that close observation and blood glucose levels be monitored within 2 to 3 hours of birth. If the newborn has a blood glucose below 36 mg/dl (2 mmol/L), intervention such as breastfeeding or bottle-feeding should be instituted; if levels remain low despite feeding, IV dextrose is warranted.

- Blood glucose levels for infants with severe hyperinsulinism may need to be higher (60 mg/dl [3.3 mmol/L]) to prevent serious effects.
- Hypoglycemia in preterm infants requires further studies, but it has been suggested that values be maintained above 47 mg/dl (2.6 mmol/L).

Because hypoglycemia is often asymptomatic in newborns, dependence on clinical signs or a single blood glucose value alone is inadequate.

Symptoms of hypoglycemia include poor feeding, hypothermia, and diaphoresis. CNS symptoms can include tremors and jitteriness, weak cry, lethargy, floppy posture, seizures, or coma. Diagnosis is confirmed by laboratory blood glucose determinations or glucose reflectance meter. The use of reagent strips alone is reported to be unreliable, especially at values lower than 40 to 50 mg/dl, and may be affected by the hematocrit.

Large for Gestational Age Infants

The LGA infant is defined as an infant weighing 4000 g or more at birth. An infant is considered LGA despite gestation when the weight is above the 90th percentile on growth charts or two standard deviations above the mean weight for gestational age. Certain fetal disorders, including transposition of the great vessels and Beckwith-Wiedemann syndrome, can also result in LGA status.

Birth trauma, especially associated with breech or shoulder presentation, is a serious hazard for the oversized neonate. Asphyxia, CNS injury, or both may occur.

- All large fetuses are monitored during a trial of labor, and preparation is made for a cesarean birth if nonreassuring fetal status or poor progress of labor occurs.
- LGA newborns may be preterm, term, or postdate; they may be infants of diabetic mothers (IDMs); or they may be postmature.
- Each of these problems carries special concerns.
- Regardless of coexisting potential problems, the LGA infant is at risk by virtue of size alone.

The nurse assesses the LGA infant for hypoglycemia and trauma resulting from vaginal or cesarean birth. The blood glucose levels of LGA infants are monitored, and hypoglycemia is corrected. Any specific birth injuries are identified and treated appropriately.

Infants of Diabetic Mothers

All infants born to mothers with diabetes are at some risk for complications. The degree of risk is influenced by the severity and duration of maternal disease. Problems seen in IDMs include congenital anomalies, macrosomia, birth trauma and perinatal asphyxia, RDS, hypoglycemia, hypocalcemia and hypomagnesemia, cardiomyopathy, hyperbilirubinemia, and polycythemia.

Hyperinsulinemia accounts for many of the problems the fetus or infant develops.

Congenital anomalies

Congenital anomalies occur in about 7% to 10% of IDMs. The most commonly occurring anomalies involve the cardiac system, musculoskeletal system, and CNS.

- The incidence of congenital heart lesions in these infants is five times higher than that in the general population. Coarctation of the aorta, transposition of the great vessels, and atrial or ventricular septal defects are the most common lesions encountered in the IDM.
- CNS anomalies include anencephaly, encephalocele, meningomyelocele, and hydrocephalus.
- The musculoskeletal system may be affected by caudal regression syndrome (i.e., sacral agenesis, with weakness or deformities of the lower extremities, malformation and fixation of the hip joints, and shortening or deformity of the femurs).
- Hypertrichosis on the pinnae (excessive hair growth on the external ear) has been added to the list of characteristic clinical features.
- Other defects noted in this population include GI atresia and urinary tract malformations.

Macrosomia

Despite improvements in the control of maternal blood sugar levels, the incidence of macrosomia in the infants of insulin-dependent diabetic mothers is higher than in infants born of mothers who are not diabetic.

- At birth the typical LGA infant has a round, cherubic ("tomato" or cushingoid) face, a chubby body, and a plethoric or flushed complexion.
- The infant has enlarged internal organs (i.e., hepatospleno-megaly, splanchnomegaly, and cardiomegaly) and increased body fat, especially around the shoulders.
- The placenta and umbilical cord are larger than average.
- The brain is the only organ that is not enlarged. IDMs may be LGA but physiologically immature.
- The macrosomic infant is at risk for hypoglycemia, hypocal-cemia, hyperviscosity, and hyperbilirubinemia.
- The excessive shoulder size in these infants often leads to dystocia, particularly because the head may be smaller in proportion to the shoulders than in a nonmacrosomic infant.
- Macrosomic infants born vaginally or by cesarean birth after a trial of labor may incur birth trauma.

Nursing care

Ideally, planning for the IDM begins during the antenatal period. Pediatric staff members are present at the birth. Implementation of care depends on the neonate's particular problems. If the maternal blood glucose level was well controlled throughout the pregnancy, the infant may require only monitoring. Because euglycemia is not always possible, the nurse must promptly recognize and treat any consequences of maternal diabetes that arise.

BIRTH TRAUMA

Birth trauma (injury) is physical injury sustained by a neonate during labor and birth. In theory, most birth injuries may be avoidable. Fetal ultrasonography for antepartum diagnosis and elective cesarean birth can prevent significant birth injury. The prompt reporting of signs that indicate deviations from normal permits early initiation of appropriate therapy. Table 17-2 provides an overview of neurologic birth injuries and the sites in which they occur.

Soft Tissue Injuries

See Table 17-3 for a description of soft tissue injuries, their causes and treatment.

Skeletal Injuries

- Considerable force is required to fracture the newborn's skull. Two types of skull fractures in the newborn are linear fractures and depressed fractures. The location of the fracture and involvement of underlying structures determine its significance.
  - If an artery is torn as a result of the fracture, increased intracranial pressure (ICP) will follow. Unless a blood vessel is involved, linear fractures, which account for 70% of all fractures for this age group, heal without special treatment.
  - Depressed fractures (or ping-pong ball indentations) may be elevated by using a hand breast pump or vacuum extractor.
- The clavicle is the bone most often fractured during birth. Generally the break is in the middle third of the bone.
  - Dystocia, particularly shoulder impaction, may be the predisposing problem. Limitation of motion of the arm, crepitus over the bone, and the absence of the Moro reflex on the affected side are diagnostic.
  - Except for use of gentle rather than vigorous handling, no accepted treatment for fractured clavicle in the newborn exists, and the prognosis is good.
- The humerus and femur are other bones that may be fractured during a difficult birth. Fractures in newborns generally heal rapidly. Immobilization is accomplished with slings, splints, swaddling, and other immobilization devices.

Care management

The parents need support in handling these infants because they often are fearful of hurting them. Parents are encouraged to practice handling, changing diapers, and feeding the affected neonate under the guidance of nursery personnel. A plan for follow-up therapy is developed.

TABLE 17-2
Neurologic Birth Injuries

SITE OF INJURY	TYPE OF INJURY
Scalp	Caput succedaneum
	Subgaleal hemorrhage
	Cephalhematoma
Skull	Linear fracture
	Depressed fracture
	Occipital osteodiastasis
Intracranial	Epidural hematoma
	Subdural hematoma (laceration of falx, tentorium, or superficial veins)
	Subarachnoid hemorrhage
	Cerebral contusion
	Cerebellar contusion
	Intracerebellar hematoma
Spinal cord (cervical)	Vertebral artery injury
	Intraspinal hemorrhage
	Spinal cord transection or injury
Plexus	Erb palsy
	Klumpke paralysis
	Total (mixed) brachial plexus injury
	Horner syndrome
	Diaphragmatic paralysis
	Lumbosacral plexus injury
Cranial and peripheral nerve	Radial nerve palsy
	Medial nerve palsy
	Sciatic nerve palsy
	Laryngeal nerve palsy
	Diaphragmatic paralysis
	Facial nerve palsy

From Paige, P.L., & Carney, P.R. (2002). Neurologic disorders. In G.B. Merenstein & S.L. Gardner (Eds.), *Handbook of neonatal intensive care* (5th ed.). St. Louis: Mosby.

TABLE 17-3

Soft-Tissue Injuries

SOFT-TISSUE INJURY	CAUSE	TREATMENT
Subconjunctival and retinal hemorrhages	Rupture of capillaries caused by increased pressure during birth	Hemorrhages clear within 5 days after birth and present no further problems. Parents need explanation and reassurance.
Erythema, ecchymoses, petechiae, abrasions, lacerations, or edema of buttocks and extremities	Application of forceps or the vacuum extractor Bruises on face from face presentation Bruising and swelling on buttocks or genitalia from breech presentation Ecchymosis and petechiae on head from tight nuchal cord Petechiae may extend over the upper trunk and face	Lesions are benign if they disappear within 2 or 3 days of birth and no new lesions appear. Ecchymoses and petechiae may be signs of a more serious disorder, such as thrombocytopenic purpura.
Bruised caput or a linear mark across both sides of the face in the shape of the forceps blades	Application of vacuum cup or forceps	Keep areas clean to minimize the risk of infection.
Lacerations on the face, scalp, buttocks, and thighs	Accidental cuts with scalpel during a cesarean birth	Keep clean. Liquid skin adhesive or butterfly adhesive strips can hold together the edges of more serious lacerations. Rarely are sutures needed.

Peripheral Nervous System Injuries

Erb palsy (Erb-Duchenne paralysis) is caused by damage to the upper plexus and usually results from a stretching or pulling away of the shoulder from the head, such as might occur with shoulder dystocia or with a difficult vertex or breech delivery. The less common lower plexus palsy, or Klumpke palsy, results from severe stretching of the upper extremity while the trunk is relatively less mobile.

Clinical manifestation

In Erb palsy, the arm hangs limp alongside the body. The shoulder and arm are adducted and internally rotated. The elbow is extended, and the forearm is pronated, with the wrist and fingers flexed; a grasp reflex may be present because finger and wrist movement remains normal. In lower plexus palsy, the muscles of the hand are paralyzed, with consequent wrist drop and relaxed fingers. In a third and more severe form of brachial palsy, the entire arm is paralyzed and hangs limp and motionless at the side. The Moro reflex is absent on the affected side for all forms of brachial palsy.

Care management

Treatment is aimed at preventing contractures of the paralyzed muscles and maintaining correct placement of the humeral head within the glenoid fossa of the scapula.

- Complete recovery from stretched nerves usually takes 3 to 6 months. However, avulsion of the nerves (complete disconnection of the ganglia from the spinal cord that involves both anterior and posterior roots) results in permanent damage. In some cases botulinum toxin A may be injected into the triceps muscle to reduce muscle contractures.
- The primary concern is proper positioning of the affected arm. It should be gently immobilized on the upper abdomen; passive range-of-motion exercises of the shoulder, wrist, elbow, and fingers are initiated in the latter part of the first week. Wrist flexion contractures may be prevented with the use of supportive splints. Dressing the infant begins with the affected arm, and undressing begins

with the unaffected arm to prevent unnecessary manipulation and stress on the paralyzed muscles.

- Parents are taught to use the "football" position when holding the infant and to avoid picking the child up from under the axillae or by pulling on the arms.

Central Nervous System Injuries

All types of intracranial hemorrhage (ICH) occur in newborns. ICH as a result of birth trauma is more likely to occur in the full-term, large infant. The frequency and degree of severity of ICH differ in the newborn from older children or adults. In the newborn, more than one type of hemorrhage can and does commonly occur.

Subdural hematoma

A subdural hematoma is a life-threatening collection of blood in the subdural space and is most often produced by the stretching and tearing of the large veins in the tentorium of the cerebellum, the dural membrane that separates the cerebrum from the cerebellum. The typical history includes a primiparous mother, with labor and birth lasting less than 2 or 3 hours; a difficult birth involving high- or mid-forceps application; or a large for gestational age infant. Subdural hematoma occurs infrequently because of improvements in obstetric care. However, it is especially serious because of its inaccessibility to aspiration by subdural tap.

Subarachnoid hemorrhage

Subarachnoid hemorrhage, the most common type of ICH, occurs in term infants as a result of trauma and in preterm infants as a result of hypoxia. Small hemorrhages are the most common. Bleeding is of venous origin, and underlying contusion also may occur.

Clinical Manifestation. The presentation of hemorrhage in the full-term infant can vary considerably. In many infants, signs are absent, and hemorrhaging is diagnosed only because of abnormal findings, such as red blood cells (RBCs), on lumbar puncture. A hemorrhage may be seen on a computerized tomography (CT) scan. The initial clinical manifestations of neonatal subarachnoid hemorrhage may be the early onset of alternating central nervous system (CNS) depression and irritability, with refractory seizure. Poor feeding, apnea, and unequal pupils may suggest an intracranial insult. Occasionally the infant appears normal initially and then has seizures on the second or third day of life, followed by no apparent sequelae.

Care management. In general, nursing care of an infant with ICH is supportive and includes monitoring neurologic signs and intravenous therapy, observation and management of seizures, and prevention of increased ICP. Replacement of lost blood and clotting factors is required in acute cases of hemorrhage.

NEONATAL INFECTIONS

Sepsis

Sepsis (the presence of microorganisms or their toxins in the blood or other tissues) continues to be one of the most significant causes of neonatal morbidity and mortality. Maternal immunoglobulin M (IgM) does not cross the placenta. Immunoglobulin A (IgA) and IgM require time to reach optimum levels after birth. Phagocytosis is less efficient. Serum complement levels are inadequate; serum complement (C1 through C6) is involved in immunologic reactions, some of which kill or lyse bacteria and enhance phagocytosis. Dysmaturity seen with intrauterine growth restriction (IUGR) and preterm and postdate birth further compromises the neonate's immune system.

Clinical manifestation

Table 17-4 outlines risk factors for neonatal sepsis. Special precautions for preventing infection, as well as prompt recognition when it occurs, are necessary for optimum newborn care. Neonatal infections may be acquired in utero, during birth or resuscitation, or nosocomially. Table 17-5 outlines the clinical signs associated with neonatal sepsis.

Early-Onset or Congenital Sepsis. Early-onset or congenital sepsis usually manifests within 24 to 48 hours of birth, progresses more rapidly than later-onset infection, and carries a mortality rate as high as 50%. Early-onset infection is usually caused by microorganisms from the normal flora of the maternal vaginal tract, including group B streptococci, *Haemophilus*

TABLE 17-4

Risk Factors for Neonatal Sepsis

SOURCE	RISK FACTORS
Maternal	Low socioeconomic status
	Poor prenatal care
	Poor nutrition
	Substance abuse
Intrapartum	Premature rupture of fetal membranes
	Maternal fever
	Chorioamnionitis
	Prolonged labor
	Rupture of membranes >12-18 hr
	Premature labor
	Maternal urinary tract infection
Neonatal	Twin or multiple gestation
	Male
	Birth asphyxia
	Meconium aspiration
	Congenital anomalies of skin or mucous membranes
	Galactosemia
	Absence of spleen
	Low birth weight or prematurity
	Malnourishment
	Prolonged hospitalization

influenzae, Listeria monocytogenes, Escherichia coli, and *Streptococcus pneumoniae. Coagulase-negative staphylococcus* (CONS) is also a common pathogen. Early-onset sepsis is associated with preterm labor, prolonged rupture of membranes (more than 18 hours), maternal fever during labor, and chorioamnionitis.

Late-Onset Infection. Nosocomial infection (late onset) is most commonly seen after 2 weeks of age and is slower in progression. Bacteria responsible for late-onset sepsis are varied, may be acquired from the birth canal or from the external environment, and include *Staphylococcus aureus, Staphylococcus epidermidis, Pseudomonas organisms,* and group B streptococci.

TABLE 17-5

*Signs of Sepsis**

SYSTEM	SIGNS
Respiratory	Apnea, bradycardia
	Tachypnea
	Grunting, nasal flaring
	Retractions
	Decreased oxygen saturation
	Metabolic acidosis
Cardiovascular	Decreased cardiac output
	Tachycardia
	Hypotension
	Decreased perfusion
Central nervous	Temperature instability
	Lethargy
	Hypotonia
	Irritability, seizures
Gastrointestinal	Feeding intolerance (decreased suck strength and intake; increasing residuals)
	Abdominal distention
	Vomiting, diarrhea
Integumentary	Jaundice
	Pallor
	Petechiae
	Mottling

Adapted from Askin, D.F. (1995). Bacterial and fungal sepsis in the neonate. *Journal of Obstetric, Gynecologic, and Neonatal Nursing, 24*(7), 635-643.
*Laboratory findings include neutropenia, increased bands, hypoglycemia or hyperglycemia, metabolic acidosis, and thrombocytopenia.

Viral Infections

Viral infections may cause miscarriage, stillbirth, intrauterine infection, congenital malformations, and acute neonatal disease. These pathogens also may cause chronic infection. It is important to recognize and treat the acute infection, to prevent nosocomial infections in other infants, and to anticipate effects on the infant's subsequent growth and development.

Fungal Infections

Fungal infections are of greatest concern in the immunocompromised or premature infant. Occasionally, fungal infections such as thrush are found in otherwise healthy term infants.

Septicemia

Septicemia refers to a generalized infection in the bloodstream. Pneumonia, the most common form of neonatal infection, is one of the leading causes of perinatal death. Bacterial meningitis affects 1 in 2500 live-born infants. Gastroenteritis is sporadic, depending on epidemic outbreaks. Local infections such as conjunctivitis and omphalitis occur commonly. Infection continues to be a significant factor in fetal and neonatal morbidity and mortality.

Care management

Care of the infant with neonatal sepsis is described in Table 17-6.

TORCH Infections Affecting Newborns

T   Toxoplasmosis
O   Other: gonorrhea, hepatitis B, syphilis, varicella-zoster virus, parvovirus B19, and HIV
R   Rubella
C   Cytomegalovirus
H   Herpes simplex virus (HSV)

Toxoplasmosis

Toxoplasmosis is a multisystem disease caused by the protozoan *Toxoplasma gondii.* Question pregnant women about contact with cats who hunt birds and mice or about eating raw meat. The transplacental transmission rate increases as pregnancy progresses: 20% in the first trimester, 50% in the second trimester, and 65% in the third trimester. More than 70% of affected infants are free of symptoms.

Clinical manifestation. Severe toxoplasmosis is associated with preterm birth, growth restriction, microcephaly or hydrocephaly, microphthalmos, chorioretinitis, CNS calcification,

TABLE 17-6

Protocol for Suspected Neonatal Sepsis

ASSESSMENTS
- Potential maternal risk factors and unstable vital signs, especially temperature instability
- Sepsis screen in first hour (CBC with differential, platelets, and CRP level) if there are significant maternal risk factors (prolonged rupture of membranes, maternal temperature) or if infant demonstrates physiologic signs of sepsis

TREATMENT
- Start IV administration of antibiotics by peripheral IV line
- Provide other treatments as needed for additional physiologic problems (supplemental oxygen or ventilator for respiratory distress, incubator for temperature instability)

POSSIBLE CONSULTATIONS
- Neonatologists and advanced practice nurses for care of unstable infants
- Medical specialists for care of infants with additional problems (congenital deformities)
- Lactation consultant, interpreter, social worker, and chaplain as needed or requested

ADDITIONAL ASSESSMENTS
- Weight and measurements
- Blood culture, chest x-ray, urinalysis, and lumbar puncture, if infant is symptomatic or CRP level is positive
- Repeat determination of CRP level in the morning for 2 days; if negative and infant not symptomatic, stop antibiotic treatment
- Continuous cardiac and oxygen saturation monitor assessment if infant's condition is unstable

DIRECT INFANT CARE
- Vital signs q1-2 hr for the first 4 hr, then every 4 hr
- Advance oral feedings as tolerated (infant NPO only if condition is physiologically unstable)
- Bath and cord care done per unit protocols

TABLE 17-6

Protocol for Suspected Neonatal Sepsis—cont'd

> **TEACHING AND DISCHARGE PLANNING**
> • Initiate on admission; provide parents with written and oral information on suspected sepsis
> • Reinforce information and determine parents' understanding of information before discharge; include information on well-baby care and community follow-up with the family's primary health care provider

From Lucile Salter Packard Children's Hospital at Stanford, CA.
CBC, Complete blood count; *CRP,* C-reactive protein; *IV,* intravenous; *NPO,* nothing by mouth.

thrombocytopenia, jaundice, and fever. Petechiae or a maculopapular rash may also be evident.

NURSE ALERT *To differentiate hemorrhagic areas from skin rashes and discolorations, try to blanch the skin with two fingers. Petechiae and ecchymoses do not blanch because extravasated blood remains within the tissues, whereas skin rashes and discolorations do.*

Care management. Maternal treatment with spiramycin may prevent fetal infection. The affected infant may be treated with pyrimethamine, as well as oral sulfadiazine, but folic acid supplement will be required to prevent anemia.

Gonorrhea

Gonorrhea is caused by *Neisseria gonorrhoeae.* The incidence of gonococcal infection in pregnant women ranges from 2.5% to 7.3%. The infant may be infected in utero or at birth.

Clinical manifestation. After rupture of membranes, ascending infection can result in orogastric contamination of the fetus. The organism also may invade mucosal surfaces, such as the conjunctiva (ophthalmia neonatorum), rectal mucosa, and pharynx, as the infant passes through the birth canal. Neonatal gonococcal arthritis, septicemia, meningitis, vaginitis, and scalp abscesses can also develop.

Care management. Eye prophylaxis (e.g., with 0.5% erythromycin ointment) is administered at or shortly after birth to prevent ophthalmia neonatorum. The infant with a mild infection often recovers completely with appropriate treatment (e.g., single dose of IM or IV ceftriaxone). Occasionally, infants die of overwhelming infection in the early neonatal period.

Syphilis

Syphilis is caused by the spirochete *Treponema pallidum.* If syphilis during pregnancy is untreated, 40% to 50% of neonates born to these women will have symptomatic congenital syphilis. If maternal infection is treated adequately before the eighteenth week, neonates seldom demonstrate signs of the disease.

Clinical manifestation. Organs develop normally. Later the liver, spleen, kidneys, adrenal glands, and bone covering and marrow may be affected. By the end of the first week of life, a copper-colored maculopapular dermal rash appears in untreated newborns. The rash is characteristically first noticeable on the palms of the hands, the soles of the feet, the diaper area, and around the mouth and anus. The maculopapular lesions may become vesicular and confluent and extend over the trunk and extremities. Poor feeding, slight hyperthermia, and snuffles may be nonspecific signs.

Care management. A 10-day course of aqueous penicillin G or procaine penicillin G (consult drug references for dosage and administration route for each) is the usual treatment for congenital syphilis. Erythromycin is the substitute antibiotic of choice for infants sensitive to penicillin. The infant is checked for antibody titer (received from the mother by way of the placenta) every 2 weeks for 3 months, at which time the test result should be negative.

Varicella Zoster

The varicella zoster virus responsible for chickenpox and shingles is a member of the herpes family. About 90% of women in their childbearing years are immune; therefore the risk of infection in pregnancy is low.

Clinical manifestation. When transmission to the fetus occurs in the early part of pregnancy, especially between weeks 13 and 20, the effects on the fetus include limb atrophy, neurologic abnormalities, eye abnormalities, and IUGR. When maternal infection occurs in the last few days of pregnancy, 20% of infants born to these mothers will develop clinical varicella. The severity of the infant's illness increases greatly if maternal infection occurred within 5 days before or 2 days after birth. The mortality in severe illness is 30%.

Care management. Infants born to mothers who develop chickenpox between 5 days before birth and 48 hours after birth should be given varicella-zoster immune globulin (VZIG) at birth because of the risk of severe disease. Acyclovir can be used to treat infants with generalized involvement and pneumonia.

Hepatitis B Virus (HBV)

Transmission of HBV occurs transplacentally; serum to serum; and by contact with contaminated blood, urine, feces, saliva, semen, or vaginal secretions during birth. The transmission rate of HBV to the newborn is high when the mother is seropositive for both hepatitis B surface antigen (HB_sAg) and hepatitis B e antigen (HB_eAg). Diagnosis is made by viral culture of amniotic fluid as well as the presence of HB_sAg and IgM in the cord blood or newborn's serum.

Clinical manifestation. There is no association between infection during pregnancy and an increase in malformations, stillbirths, or IUGR; however, there is a significant risk for preterm birth. Infants may be symptom free at birth or show evidence of acute hepatitis with changes in liver function. The mortality for full-blown hepatitis is 75%. Infants who become carriers are at high risk for chronic hepatitis, cirrhosis of the liver, or liver cancer even years later.

Care management. Infants whose mothers have antibodies for HB_sAg or who have developed hepatitis during pregnancy or the postpartum period should be treated with hepatitis B immunoglobulin (HBIG), 0.5 ml intramuscularly, as soon as possible after birth or within the first 12 hours of life. The hepatitis B vaccine should also be given concurrently but at a different site. After the infant has been cleansed thoroughly and has received the vaccine, breastfeeding may be initiated. Vaccination for infants not exposed to maternal HBV is recommended before discharge from the birth hospital; breastfeeding for these infants may begin before the vaccine is given.

Human Immunodeficiency Virus (HIV)

Transmission of HIV from the mother to the infant may occur transplacentally at various gestational ages. The majority of cases of pediatric acquired immune deficiency syndrome (AIDS) (90% or more) result from maternal-to-fetal transmission. Postpartum transmission may also occur, with an additional risk of 14% attributed to breast milk contact. Diagnosis of HIV infection in the neonate is complicated by the presence of maternal IgG antibodies, which cross the placenta after 32 weeks of gestation. The most accurate test for newborns and infants younger than 18 months is the HIV DNA PCR assay, which is performed on neonatal blood, not cord blood; results may be obtained by 24 hours.

Clinical manifestation

Typically the HIV-infected neonate is asymptomatic at birth. Early-onset illness (i.e., virus detected within 48 hours of birth) is attributed to prenatal infection and occurs in 10% to 15% of infected infants. The presenting signs and symptoms of HIV infection vary from severe immunodeficiency to nonspecific findings, such as failure to thrive, parotitis, and recurrent or persistent upper respiratory infections.

Care management

Universal counseling and screening of pregnant women are recommended in the United States and Canada.

- With antepartum, intrapartum, and neonatal zidovudine treatment the incidence of neonatal HIV infection is decreased to 5% to 8%, and compliance with highly active antiretroviral therapy (HAART) is said to further reduce newborn infection rates to 1% to 2%.
- Standard Precautions are used. The infant is protected from further exposure to maternal blood and body fluids.
- Breastfeeding in the HIV-positive mother is contraindicated.
- Neonates may be treated with a combination of zidovudine (ZDV), didanosine, and nevirapine. In some cases lamivudine or stavudine may be used instead of didanosine for neonatal treatment.
- Counseling regarding the care of the mothers themselves, the family's care of the infant, and future pregnancies should be

provided. The risk for transmission among members of the same household is minimal. Social services are required in these cases. If the parent chooses to keep the infant, home health care may be arranged.

Rubella Infection

Since rubella vaccination was begun in 1969, cases of congenital rubella have been reduced dramatically. Vaccination failures, lack of compliance, and the immigration of nonimmunized persons result in periodic outbreaks of rubella, also known as German or 3-day measles. The risk for congenital anomalies varies with the gestational age of the fetus at the time maternal infection occurs. Abnormalities are most severe if the mother contracts the virus during the first trimester.

Clinical manifestation

More than two thirds of infected infants have no symptoms apparent at birth, but sequelae may develop years later. Hearing loss, the most common result, appears to be progressive after birth. Initially the newborn may present with hepatospleno-megaly, lymphedema, IUGR, jaundice, hepatitis, thrombocyto-penic purpura with petechiae, and the characteristic blueberry muffin lesions. Congenital rubella syndrome often includes chronic problems, such as cataracts or glaucoma, sensorineural hearing impairment, hypogammaglobulinemia, peripheral pulmonary stenosis, and diabetes mellitus type 1.

Care management

The rubella virus has been cultured in infants up to 18 months after their birth. These infants are a serious source of infection to susceptible individuals, particularly women in the childbearing years. Extended pediatric isolation is mandatory until the noncontagious stage of rubella has been reached (i.e., the infant should be isolated until pharyngeal mucus and the urine are free of virus).

Cytomegalovirus (CMV) Infection

CMV infection during pregnancy may result in miscarriage, stillbirth, or congenital illness. It is the most common cause of congenital viral infections in the United States.

Clinical manifestation. The neonate with full-blown CMV displays IUGR, has microcephaly, and may have a rash, jaundice, and hepatosplenomegaly. Anemia, thrombocytopenia, and hyperbilirubinemia are common. Intracranial, periventricular calcification often is noted on radiography. Inclusion bodies ("owl's eye" figures) in cells sedimented from freshly voided urine or in liver biopsy specimens are typical. Most (90% to 95%) of the affected infants are asymptomatic at birth. The virus may be isolated from urine or saliva of the newborn using the PCR assay. CMV can be transmitted through breast milk while the mother is experiencing acute CMV syndrome. In preterm infants, postnatal acquisition of CMV can result in pneumonia, hepatitis, thrombocytopenia, and long-term neurologic sequelae.

Care management. The infected newborn is treated with ganciclovir. Treatment demands careful monitoring of the infant because the drug is toxic to bone marrow.

Herpes Simplex Virus

- The neonate may acquire the virus by any of four modes of transmission:
  - –Transplacental infection
  - –Ascending infection by way of the birth canal
  - –Direct contamination during passage through an infected birth canal
  - –Direct transmission from infected personnel or family
- Nursery personnel with cold sores should practice strict hand-washing and wear a mask, but no evidence indicates they should be removed from the nursery unless they have a herpetic whitlow (primary HSV infection of the terminal segment of a finger).

Clinical manifestation. Congenital infection is rare and is characterized by in utero destruction of normally formed organs. Affected infants are growth restricted. They have severe psychomotor restriction, with intracranial calcifications, microcephaly, hypertonicity, and seizures. They experience eye involvement, including microphthalmos, cataracts, chorioretinitis, blindness, and retinal dysplasia. Some infants have patent ductus arteriosus, limb anomalies, and recurrent skin vesicles, with a short life expectancy. Most infants are infected directly during passage through the birth canal.

Care management. Standard Precautions should be observed when caregivers have contact with these infants.

- The neonate's eyes, oral cavity, and skin are inspected carefully for the presence of any lesions. Cultures are obtained from the mouth, eyes, and any lesions.
- Circumcision, if performed, is delayed until the infant is ready to be discharged. The infant may be discharged with the mother if the infant's cultures are negative for the virus.
- As long as no suspicious lesions are on the mother's breasts, breastfeeding is allowed.
- For the infant at risk, a prophylactic topical eye ointment (vidarabine or trifluridine) is administered for 5 days to prevent keratoconjunctivitis. Acyclovir should also be given to infants with ocular involvement.
- Blood, urine, and CSF specimens should be cultured when indicated clinically.
- Therapy includes general supportive measures, as well as treatment with intravenous acyclovir. Ophthalmic ointment should be administered simultaneously.

Bacterial Infections

Group B streptococcus

Antepartum maternal screening and administration of penicillin have significantly decreased the incidence of group B streptococcus (GBS). Early-onset GBS infection in the neonate occurs in the first 7 days of life but most commonly manifests in the first 24 hours following birth. Risk factors for the development of early-onset GBS include low birth weight, preterm birth, rupture of membranes of more than 18 hours, maternal fever, previous GBS infant, maternal GBS bacteriuria, and multiple gestation. Early-onset disease usually results from vertical transmission from the birth canal and causes a respiratory illness that mimics the symptoms of severe respiratory distress syndrome. The infant may rapidly develop septic shock, which has a significant mortality rate.

Escherichia coli

E. coli is the second most common cause of neonatal sepsis and meningitis in the United States. *E. coli* is found in the GI tract soon after birth and makes up the bulk of human fecal flora. In addition to meningitis, *E. coli* can also cause infections in other body systems, including the urinary tract. There is concern that increasing the use of ampicillin in labor as prophylaxis against GBS infection will result in more virulent *E. coli* infection because of ampicillin-resistant organisms.

Tuberculosis

The incidence of tuberculosis (TB), which is caused by *Mycobacterium tuberculosis,* is increasing in Canada and the United States. Congenitally acquired TB, although rare, can cause otitis media, pneumonia, hepatosplenomegaly, enlarged lymph glands, or disseminated disease. After birth, exposed infants contract TB through droplets expelled by infected individuals, which results in pneumonia and necrosis of lung tissue. Untreated neonatal tuberculosis is almost always fatal.

Chlamydia infection

Chlamydia trachomatis is an intracellular bacterium that causes neonatal conjunctivitis and pneumonia. The conjunctivitis, with minimal watery discharge, develops 5 to 14 days after birth. Inclusion conjunctivitis is usually self-limiting, but if it is untreated, chronic follicular conjunctivitis (trachoma) with conjunctival scarring and corneal microgranulations has been reported. The organism may spread to the lungs from nasal secretions if left untreated, causing chlamydia pneumonia in about 33% of infected infants with symptoms of a repetitive staccato cough, tachypnea, rales, hyperinflation, and bilateral diffuse infiltrates on radiographic examination.

Ophthalmic silver nitrate, 0.5% erythromycin, and 1% tetracycline are not effective against *C. trachomatis;* therefore it is recommended that infants born to mothers who are positive for *Chlamydia* be observed closely for the development of symptoms. The neonate with positive cultures should be treated with oral erythromycin or oral sulfonamide for 2 to 3 weeks. Erythromycin administration in infants younger than 6 weeks has been associated with an increased risk of infantile hypertrophic pyloric stenosis (IHPS); therefore parents should be educated regarding the symptoms of the condition (feeding intolerance, projectile vomiting, and abdominal distention).

SUBSTANCE ABUSE

Maternal habits hazardous to the fetus and neonate include recreational drug abuse, smoking, and alcohol abuse. Newborns who have been exposed to drugs in utero are not addicted in a behavioral sense, yet they may have mild to strong physiologic signs as a result of the exposure and are described as *drug exposed,* which implies intrauterine drug exposure.

- The adverse effects of exposure of the fetus to drugs are varied. They include transient behavioral changes, such as fetal breathing movements, and irreversible effects, such as fetal death, IUGR, structural malformations, cognitive and motor delay, and behavioral problems.
- Critical determinants of the effect of the drug on the fetus include the specific drug, the dosage, the route of administration, the genotype of the mother or fetus, and the timing of the drug exposure.

Table 17-7 summarizes the effects of commonly abused substances on the fetus and neonate.

Care management

- Use a multidisciplinary approach that includes home health or community resource personnel (e.g., regulatory agencies such as child protective services). Involve the parents in the care.
- Review the mother's prenatal record. Note any history of drug abuse and detoxification.
- Note infant's gestational age and maturity.
- Observe infant for signs of drug withdrawal.
- Assess infant for neonatal abstinence syndrome (NAS) (Table 17-8) (Fig. 17-1).
- Newborn urine, hair, or meconium sampling may be required to identify drug exposure and implement appropriate early interventional therapies aimed at minimizing the consequences of intrauterine drug exposure.

Text continued on p. 559.

TABLE 17-7

Neonatal Effects of Commonly Abused Substances

SUBSTANCE	NEONATAL EFFECTS	NURSING CONSIDERATIONS
Alcohol	Alcohol-related birth defects (ARBD) formerly *fetal alcohol syndrome [FAS]*: craniofacial features vary, may include short eyelid opening, flat midface, flat upper lip groove, thin upper lip; microcephaly; hyperactivity; developmental delays; attention deficits. *Alcohol-related neurodevelopmental disorder (ARND)*: varying forms of ARBD; cognitive, behavioral, and psychosocial problems without typical physical features	Alcohol enters breast milk.
Cocaine	Prematurity; small for gestational age; microcephaly; poor feeding; irregular sleep patterns; diarrhea; visual attention problems; hyperactivity; difficult to console; hypersensitivity to noise and external stimuli; irritability; developmental delays; congenital anomalies, such as prune belly syndrome (i.e., distended, flabby, wrinkled abdomen caused by lack of abdominal muscles)	Cocaine enters breast milk. Caution mothers about this hazard to their infants.

Heroin	Low birth weight; small for gestational age; irritability; tachypnea; yawning; sneezing; feeding difficulties; vomiting; high-pitched cry; abnormal sleep cycle; seizures	Sudden infant death (SIDS) risk is increased. Usually the following drugs are given, singly or in combination: phenobarbital, diluted tincture of opium (paregoric), methadone, or morphine. Use of naloxone (Narcan) is contraindicated in infants because it may exacerbate narcotic abstinence syndrome and cause seizures.
Marijuana	Possible neonatal tremors; low birth weight; growth restriction	Secondhand smoke is a hazard if mother continues to use.
Methadone	Treatment for heroin addiction; withdrawal resembles heroin withdrawal but tends to be more severe and prolonged; tremors, irritability, state lability, hypertonicity, hypersensitivity, vomiting, mottling, nasal stuffiness, and disturbed sleep pattern; higher birth weight than infants in heroin withdrawal, usually appropriate for gestational age; no increased incidence of congenital anomalies	Methadone crosses the placenta and is found in breast milk, but mothers are allowed to breastfeed. Incidence of SIDS is higher. Late-onset withdrawal occurs at age 2-4wk and may continue for weeks or months. Therapy for methadone withdrawal is similar to that for heroin withdrawal.

Continued

TABLE 17-7

Neonatal Effects of Commonly Abused Substances—cont'd

SUBSTANCE	NEONATAL EFFECTS	NURSING CONSIDERATIONS
Methamphetamine	Small for gestational age; prematurity; bradycardia or tachycardia that resolves as the drug is cleared; poor weight gain lethargy; behavioral problems later in childhood; cleft lip and palate; cardiac defects	Monitor for heart rate abnormalities, encourage oral intake.
Phencyclidine (PCP); "angel dust"	Abnormal motor behavior, such as irritability, jitteriness, and hypertonicity	PCP crosses the placenta and is found in breast milk.
Tobacco	Prematurity; low birth weight; increased risk for SIDS; increased risk for bronchitis, pneumonia, developmental delays	Secondhand smoke is a hazard. Counsel parents about effects.
Polydrug use: opioids, stimulants, depressants, and sedatives	Increased tone; increased respiratory rate; disturbed sleep; fever; frantic and increased sucking; loose or watery stools	Provide a quiet environment, and offer a pacifier for frantic and excessive sucking. Do not overfeed infants who demand frequent sucking as part of the withdrawal process.

TABLE 17-8

Signs of Neonatal Abstinence Syndrome

SYSTEM	SIGNS
Gastrointestinal	Poor feeding, vomiting, regurgitation, diarrhea, excessive sucking
Central nervous	Irritability, tremors, shrill cry, incessant crying, hyperactivity, little sleep, excoriations on face, convulsions
Metabolic, vasomotor, respiratory	Nasal congestion, tachypnea, sweating, frequent yawning, increased respiratory rate (>60 breaths/min), fever (>37.2° C)

- Correct fluid and electrolyte balance; and provide nutrition, infection control, and respiratory care.
  - Loose stools, poor intake, and regurgitation after feeding predispose infants to malnutrition, dehydration, and electrolyte imbalance.
  - Weigh frequently to detect fluid losses or caloric intake.
  - Monitor intake and output and electrolytes.
  - Additional caloric supplementation may be necessary.
- Swaddling, holding, reducing environmental stimuli (dim lights and decreased noise level), and feeding may help to ease withdrawal.

Wrap infants snugly; rock and hold them tightly to limit their ability to self-stimulate.

- Protect hyperactive infants from skin abrasions on the knees, toes, and cheeks that are caused by rubbing on bed linens while awake and in a prone position.
- Drug therapies to decrease withdrawal side effects include phenobarbital, morphine, diluted tincture of opium, or methadone singly or in combination.
- Breastfeeding is encouraged.

NEONATAL ABSTINENCE SCORING SYSTEM

SYSTEM	SIGNS AND SYMPTOMS	SCORE	AM	PM	COMMENTS
	Excessive High Pitched (Or Other) Cry	2			Daily Weight:
	Continuous High Pitched (Or Other) Cry	3			
	Sleeps <1 Hour After Feeding	3			
	Sleeps <2 Hours After Feeding	2			
	Sleeps <3 Hours After Feeding	1			
	Hyperactive Moro Reflex	2			
	Markedly Hyperactive Moro Reflex	3			
	Mild Tremors Disturbed	1			
	Moderate-Severe Tremors Disturbed	2			
	Mild Tremors Undisturbed	3			
	Moderate-Severe Tremors Undisturbed	4			
	Increased Muscle Tone	2			
	Excoriation (Specific Area)	1			
	Myoclonic Jerks	3			
	Generalized Convulsions	5			

CENTRAL NERVOUS SYSTEM DISTURBANCES

	Score													
METABOLIC/VASOMOTOR/RESPIRATORY DISTURBANCES														
Sweating	1													
Fever <101° (99-100.8° F./37.2-38.2° C.) Fever >101° (38.4° C. and Higher)	1 2													
Frequent Yawning (>3 or 4 Times/Interval)	1													
Mottling	1													
Nasal Stuffiness	1													
Sneezing (>3 or 4 Times/Interval)	1													
Nasal Flaring	2													
Respiratory Rate >60/min Respiratory Rate >60/min with Retractions	1 2													
GASTROINTESTINAL DISTURBANCES														
Excessive Sucking	1													
Poor Feeding	2													
Regurgitation Projectile Vomiting	2 3													
Loose Stools Watery Stools	2 3													
TOTAL SCORE														
INITIALS OF SCORER														

Fig. 17-1 Neonatal Abstinence Scoring (NAS) system, developed by L. Finnegan. (From Nelson, N. [1990]. *Current therapy in neonatal-perinatal medicine* [2nd ed.]. St. Louis: Mosby.)

- Parents should be involved in their child's care and opportunities for parent-child attachment encouraged.
- Refer the infants to early intervention programs, including child health care, parental drug treatment, individualized developmental care, and parenting education.

HEMOLYTIC DISORDERS

Hemolytic Disease of the Newborn

Hemolytic disease occurs when the blood groups of the mother and newborn differ; the most common of these are RhD factor and ABO incompatibilities. Hemolytic disorders occur when maternal antibodies are present naturally or form in response to an antigen from the fetal blood crossing the placenta and entering the maternal circulation. The maternal antibodies of the immunoglobulin G (IgG) class cross the placenta, causing hemolysis of the fetal RBCs and resulting in fetal anemia and often neonatal jaundice and hyperbilirubinemia.

Rh Incompatibility

Rh incompatibility, or isoimmunization, occurs when an RhD-negative mother has an RhD-positive fetus who inherits the dominant Rh-positive gene from the father. The Rh blood group consists of several antigens, with D being the most prevalent.

Maternal sensitization may occur during pregnancy, birth, miscarriage or abortion, or amniocentesis. Severe Rh incompatibility results in marked fetal hemolytic anemia because the fetal erythrocytes are destroyed by maternal Rh-positive antibodies. Intrauterine transfusion involves the infusion of Rh-negative, type O blood into the umbilical vein. The frequency of intrauterine transfusions may vary according to institution and fetal status, but it may be as often as every 2 weeks until the fetus reaches pulmonary maturity at approximately 37 to 38 weeks of gestation.

ABO Incompatibility

ABO incompatibility is more common than Rh incompatibility but causes less severe problems in the affected infant. It occurs if the fetal blood type is A, B, or AB and the maternal type is O. It occurs rarely in infants with type B blood born to mothers with type A blood. The incompatibility arises because naturally occurring anti-A and anti-B antibodies are transferred across the placenta to the fetus. Unlike the situation that pertains to Rh incompatibility, first-born infants may be affected because mothers with type O blood already have anti-A and anti-B antibodies in their blood. Such a newborn may have a weakly positive direct Coombs' test (also referred to as a direct antiglobulin test [DAT]). The cord bilirubin level usually is less than 4 mg/dl, and any resulting hyperbilirubinemia usually can be treated with phototherapy.

Glucose-6-Phosphate Dehydrogenase Deficiency.

Glucose-6-phosphate dehydrogenase (G6PD) deficiency may cause an exaggerated jaundice in a newborn within 24 to 48 hours of birth. G6PD red cells hemolyze at a greater rate than healthy red cells, thus overwhelming the immature neonatal liver's ability to conjugate the indirect bilirubin. Some triggers that potentiate hemolysis include vitamin K, acetaminophen, aspirin, sepsis, and exposure to certain chemicals. Treatment is the same as for any newborn with rapidly rising serum bilirubin levels. Other metabolic and inherited conditions that increase hemolysis and may cause jaundice in the infant include galactosemia, Crigler-Najjar disease, and hypothyroidism.

Care management

Coombs' Test. At the first prenatal visit of an Rh-negative woman with a fetus who may be Rh positive, an indirect Coombs' test should be done to determine whether she has antibodies to the Rh antigen (been sensitized). The dilution at which clumping occurs determines the titer, or level, of maternal antibodies. This titer indicates the degree of maternal sensitization. A level of 1:8 rarely results in fetal jeopardy. If the titer reaches 1:16, amniocentesis is performed to determine the delta optical density (ΔOD) of the amniotic fluid to estimate fetal hemolytic process. Rising bilirubin levels may indicate the need for an intrauterine transfusion.

The indirect Coombs' test is repeated at 28 weeks. If the result is negative, indicating that sensitization has not occurred, the woman is given an intramuscular injection of $Rh_o(D)$ immune globulin. If the test result is positive, showing that sensitization has occurred, the test is repeated at 4- to 6-week intervals to monitor the maternal antibody titer.

At birth, the neonate's cord blood is sent to the laboratory to determine the infant's blood type and Rh status. A direct Coombs' test is performed on this cord blood to determine whether there are maternal antibodies in the fetal blood. If antibodies are present, the titer, which indicates the degree of maternal sensitization, is measured. If the titer is 1:64, an exchange transfusion is indicated. In addition, the prevention of or prompt therapy for perinatal asphyxia, acidosis, cold stress, sepsis, and hypoglycemia will decrease the newborn's risk for severe hemolytic disease and susceptibility to kernicterus. Early feeding is initiated to stimulate stooling and facilitate the removal of bilirubin.

Exchange Transfusion. Exchange transfusions are needed infrequently because of the decreased incidence of severe hemolytic disease in newborns resulting from isoimmunization. Guidelines for the initiation of exchange transfusion in relation to serum bilirubin levels in infants of at least 35 weeks of gestation may be found in the 2004 American Academy of Pediatrics Clinical Practice Guideline.

In an exchange transfusion, 5 to 20 ml of the infant's blood is removed at a time and replaced with an equal amount of warmed donor blood. The total amount of blood exchanged is approximately 170 ml/kg of body weight, or 75% to 85% of the infant's total blood volume. If the infant has Rh incompatibility, type O Rh-negative blood is used for transfusion. Preservatives in donor blood lower the infant's serum calcium level; therefore calcium gluconate is often given during the exchange transfusion. The neonate is monitored closely for signs of a blood transfusion reaction as well as hypotension, temperature instability, and cardiorespiratory compromise. Potential complications of exchange transfusion include transfusion reaction, infection, metabolic instability, and complications related to placement of the umbilical catheter.

CONGENITAL ANOMALIES

Congenital anomalies (structural defects) occur in approximately 2% of all live births. Major congenital defects are the leading cause of death in infants younger than 1 year of age in the United States and account for 20% of neonatal deaths. The death rate associated with most congenital anomalies has essentially remained stable since 1932.

- The most common major congenital anomalies that cause serious problems in the neonate are congenital heart disease, choanal atresia, neural tube defects (NTDs), cleft lip or palate, clubfoot, and developmental dysplasia of the hip. These are thought to result from the interaction of multiple genetic and environmental factors.

Central Nervous System (CNS) Anomalies

Most congenital anomalies of the CNS result from defects in the closure of the neural tube during fetal development (Table 17-9). Maternal folic acid deficit has a direct bearing on failure of the neural tube to close; therefore folic acid supplementation is recommended for women of childbearing age.

Cardiovascular System Anomalies

Congenital heart defects (CHDs) are anatomic abnormalities of the heart that are present at birth, although they may not be diagnosed immediately. Ventricular septal defects are the most common type of acyanotic lesion. Tetralogy of Fallot is the most common type resulting in cyanosis. After prematurity, CHDs are the next major cause of death in the first year of life.

- Maternal factors associated with a higher incidence of CHD include maternal rubella, alcohol intake, diabetes mellitus, systemic lupus erythematosus, phenylketonuria, poor nutrition, or antiepileptic medication (AED) use.
- Genetic factors are implicated in the pathogenesis of CHD; a familial occurrence of virtually all forms of CHD has been noted. Chromosomal abnormalities may also be associated with CHDs. One half of the children with trisomy 21, or Down syndrome, have a cardiac defect. Most children who have trisomy 18 have a cardiac anomaly.

Text continued on p. 569.

TABLE 17-9

Central Nervous System Anomalies

ANOMALY	DEFINITION	TREATMENT AND NURSING CONSIDERATIONS
Encephalocele	Herniation of the brain and meninges through a skull defect	Surgical repair and shunting to relieve hydrocephalus. Infant may have cognitive deficit.
Anencephaly	Absence of both cerebral hemispheres and of the overlying skull	Incompatible with life; infant may be stillborn or die within a few days of birth. Comfort measures are provided until the infant dies of temperature instability and respiratory failure.
Spina bifida occulta	Posterior portion of the laminae fails to close, but the spinal cord or meninges do not herniate or protrude through the defect	Usually asymptomatic and may not be diagnosed unless there are associated problems.
Spina bifida cystica	Includes meningocele and myelomeningocele	
Meningocele	External sac that contains meninges and CSF and that protrudes through a defect in the vertebral column	Visible at birth, most often in the lumbosacral area. Sac usually covered with a very fragile, thin membrane that can tear easily, allowing CSF to leak out and providing an entry for infectious agents into the CNS. Motor and

Continued

Myelomeningocele	External sac that contains meninges and CSF and nerves and that protrudes through a defect in the vertebral column	sensory deficits below the lesion in myelomeningocele. Usually develops hydrocephalus. Scheduled cesarean birth to try to prevent rupture of the meningeal sac. Protect sac from injury, rupture, and resultant risk of CNS infection. Before surgical repair (within the first 24-48 hr), position in side-lying or prone position to prevent pressure on the sac. Skin around defect must be cleansed and dried carefully to prevent breakdown. Sac should be covered with a sterile, moist, nonadherent dressing and cared for using sterile technique. Provide support and information to parents.
Hydrocephalus	Ventricles of the brain enlarged as a result of an imbalance between production and absorption of CSF; often occurs in conjunction with myelomeningocele	Bulging anterior fontanel and head circumference that increases at an abnormal rate. Enlargement of the forehead with depressed eyes that are rotated downward, causing a "setting sun" sign, occurs as the condition worsens. Surgical shunting of excess CSF from the brain should be done soon after birth to prevent irreversible neurologic damage from increased ICP, as evidenced by palpably widening sutures and

TABLE 17-9

Central Nervous System Anomalies—cont'd

ANOMALY	DEFINITION	TREATMENT AND NURSING CONSIDERATIONS
		fontanels, distended scalp veins, lethargy, poor feeding, vomiting, irritability, opisthotonic positioning, and a high-pitched, shrill cry. Head circumference is measured frequently. A sheepskin or a special pressure-sensitive air mattress is placed under the infant; position is changed frequently to prevent skin breakdown in the enlarged head.
Microcephaly	Head circumference that measures more than three standard deviations below the mean for age and sex	Mental retardation is common. Infants require supportive nursing care and medical observation to determine the extent of the psychomotor retardation that almost always accompanies this abnormality. There is no treatment. Parents need support to learn to care for a child with cognitive impairment.

CNS, Central nervous system; *CSF*, cerebrospinal fluid; *ICP*, intracranial pressure.

- Some CHDs are often evident immediately after birth, especially those defects that cause central cyanosis despite 100% oxygen administration. Infants with these anomalies are transferred directly to an intensive care nursery or pediatric intensive care unit.
- Affected newborns may be cyanotic and unrelieved by oxygen treatment, with the cyanosis increasing whenever the child cries. Pulse oximetry readings that remain low (below 89%) despite oxygen administration are not unusual, and respiratory distress may be present. In many cases the infant's color is unrelated to the severity of the defect. Other infants may be acyanotic and pale, with or without mottling on exertion, such as crying, feeding, or stooling.

Clinical manifestations
- Heart rate and rhythm: Persistent bradycardia (i.e., resting heart rate below 80 to 100 beats/min) or tachycardia (i.e., rate exceeding 160 to 180 beats/min) may be noted. The cardiac rhythm may be abnormal, and a murmur may be heard.
- Respiratory rate: Assess when the newborn is in a resting state. Abnormal findings may include tachypnea, which is a rate of 60 breaths/min or more; retractions with nasal flaring; grunting occurring with or without exertion; and dyspnea, which may worsen with crying and activity.
- Central cyanosis and poor perfusion: Newborns exhibiting these symptoms require prompt attention and appropriate therapy in a neonatal or pediatric intensive care unit.
- Signs of congestive heart failure, diminished cardiac output, and poor tissue perfusion should be assessed.
- Activity level may vary from restlessness to lethargy and possible unresponsiveness, except to pain.

Care management
Administer oxygen as ordered. Give cardiotonic medications to increase cardiac output, medications (e.g., prostaglandin) to prevent closure of the ductus arteriosus, and diuretic agents as needed for congestive heart failure (CHF). Decrease the workload of the heart by maintaining a thermoneutral environment and feeding by gavage if necessary. Diagnostic tests, such as echocardiography and cardiac catheterization, are performed to

obtain specific information about the defect and the need for surgical intervention.

Respiratory System Anomalies

Respiratory distress at birth or shortly thereafter may be the result of lung immaturity or anomalous development. Congenital laryngeal web and bilateral choanal atresia are readily apparent at birth. Respiratory distress caused by congenital diaphragmatic hernia and tracheoesophageal fistula may appear immediately or be delayed, depending on the severity of the defect.

Laryngeal Web and Choanal Atresia

A laryngeal web results from the incomplete separation of the two sides of the larynx and is most often between the vocal cords. Choanal atresia is the most common congenital anomaly of the nose; it is a bony or membranous septum located between the nose and the pharynx. Inability to pass a suction catheter through the nose into the pharynx or cyanosis without obvious respiratory distress usually leads to its detection. Nearly one half of the infants with choanal atresia have other anomalies. Infants with either a laryngeal web or choanal atresia require emergency surgery.

Gastrointestinal System Anomalies

Cleft lip and palate

Cleft lip or palate is a congenital midline fissure, or opening, in the lip or palate resulting from failure of the primary palate to fuse. Cleft lip with or without cleft palate is more common in males, and cleft palate alone is more common in females. The defect appears more often in Asians and certain tribes of Native Americans than in Caucasians, and less often in African-Americans.

Care Management. Treatment of the infant with cleft lip is surgical; repair usually occurs between 6 and 12 weeks of age. Cleft palate repair is generally postponed until 12 to 18 months of age to take advantage of palatal changes that take place with normal growth.

Parents of infants with a cleft lip or palate need much support, particularly in the case of a cleft lip because this is both a cosmetic and functional defect. These defects may interfere with normal parent-infant bonding in the neonatal period.

- Feeding is difficult because the cleft lip renders the newborn unable to maintain a seal around a nipple; with a cleft palate, the infant is unable to form a vacuum to maintain suction when feeding.
- The inability to suck and swallow allows milk to pool in the nasopharynx, which increases the likelihood of aspiration. Milk may come out through the cleft and out of the nares.
- Feeding problems are greater in infants with a cleft palate than in those with a cleft lip alone. Breastfeeding can be successful in some infants.
- Special nipples, bottles, and appliances are available to aid in feeding.
- Parents of infants with these defects need a great deal of education and support as they learn to feed their baby.

Musculoskeletal System Anomalies

Developmental dysplasia of the hip

Developmental dysplasia of the hip (DDH) (formerly known as congenital hip dysplasia or congenital dislocation of the hip) describes disorders related to abnormal development of the hip that may occur at any time during fetal life, infancy, or childhood. DDH more properly reflects a variety of hip abnormalities in which there is a shallow acetabulum, subluxation, or dislocation. Approximately 30% to 50% of infants with DDH are born breech.

- *Acetabular dysplasia (preluxation)* is the mildest form of DDH, in which there is neither subluxation nor dislocation. The femoral head remains in the acetabulum.
- *Subluxation* is incomplete dislocation of the hip. The femoral head remains in contact with the acetabulum, but a stretched capsule and ligamentum teres cause the head of the femur to be partially displaced. Pressure on the cartilaginous roof inhibits ossification and produces a flattening of the socket.
- In *dislocation* the femoral head loses contact with the acetabulum and is displaced posteriorly and superiorly over the fibrocartilaginous rim. The ligamentum teres is elongated and taut.

DDH is often not detected at the initial examination after birth. In the newborn period, dysplasia usually appears as hip joint laxity rather than as outright dislocation. Subluxation and the tendency to dislocate can be demonstrated by the Ortolani or Barlow tests. These tests must be performed by an experienced clinician to prevent fracture or other damage to the hip. If these tests are performed too vigorously in the first 2 days of life, when the hip subluxates freely, persistent dislocation may occur. The Ortolani and Barlow tests are most reliable from birth to 2 or 3 months of age. Other signs of DDH are shortening of the limb on the affected side (Galeazzi sign or Allis sign), asymmetric thigh and gluteal folds, and broadening of the perineum (in bilateral dislocation).

Care management. Treatment is begun as soon as the condition is recognized. The treatment varies with the age of the child and the extent of the dysplasia. The goal of treatment is to obtain and maintain a safe, congruent position of the hip joint to promote normal hip joint development and ambulation.

The hip joint is maintained by dynamic splinting in a safe position with the proximal femur centered in the acetabulum in an attitude of flexion. Of the numerous devices available, the Pavlik harness is the most widely used, and with time, motion, and gravity, the hip works into a more abducted, reduced position. The harness is worn continuously until the hip is proved stable on clinical and radiographic examination, usually in about 3 to 5 months.

Clubfoot

Deformities of the foot and ankle are described according to the position of the ankle and foot. The more common positions involve the following variations:

- Talipes varus—an inversion or a bending inward
- Talipes valgus—an eversion or bending outward
- Talipes equinus—plantar flexion in which the toes are lower than the heel
- Talipes calcaneus—dorsiflexion, in which the toes are higher than the heel

Most cases of clubfoot are a combination of these positions, and the most frequently occurring type of clubfoot is the composite deformity talipes equinovarus (TEV), in which the foot is pointed downward and inward in varying degrees of severity. Unilateral clubfoot is somewhat more common than bilateral clubfoot and may occur as an isolated defect or in association with other disorders or syndromes, such as chromosomal aberrations, arthrogryposis (a generalized immobility of the joints), cerebral palsy, or spina bifida.

Care management. The goal of treatment for clubfoot is to achieve a painless, plantigrade (able to walk on the sole of the foot with the heel on the ground), and stable foot.

Serial casting is begun shortly after birth, before discharge from the nursery. Successive casts allow for gradual stretching of skin and tight structures on the medial side of the foot. Manipulation and casting are repeated frequently (every week) to accommodate the rapid growth of early infancy. In some cases daily manipulation and stretching of tissues are accomplished with taping and splinting of the affected extremity; a continuous passive motion (CPM) machine may be used several hours daily to stretch and strengthen muscle groups involved. A Denis Browne splint may be used to manage feet that correct with casting and manipulation.

GENETIC DIAGNOSIS AND NEWBORN SCREENING

Diagnostic procedures for the detection of genetic disorders are performed after birth at any time from the postnatal period through adulthood. Many tests are available for various disorders; only the most commonly used ones are discussed here.

Newborns are routinely screened for inborn errors of metabolism (IEMs), such as phenylketonuria (PKU), galactosemia, hemoglobinopathy (sickle cell disease and thalassemias), and hypothyroidism; these are the minimum mandatory newborn screening tests in most states in the United States.

Tandem mass spectrometry has the potential for identifying more than 30 inborn errors of metabolism in addition to the standard IEMs. With tandem mass spectrometry, earlier identification of IEMs may prevent further developmental delays and morbidities in affected children.

Phenylketonuria

PKU results from a deficiency of the enzyme phenylalanine dehydrogenase. The test for PKU is not reliable until the newborn has ingested an ample amount of the amino acid phenylalanine, a constituent of both human and cow's milk. The nurse must document the initial ingestion of milk and perform the test at least 24 hours after that time. For infants who are discharged early, the AAP made the following recommendations:

- Obtain a subsequent sample before 2 weeks of age if the initial specimen is collected before the newborn is 24 hours old.
- Designate a primary care provider for all newborns before discharge for adequate newborn screening follow-up.
- Collect the initial specimen as close as possible to discharge and no later than 7 days after birth.
- If the infant has PKU, a diet low in phenylalanine is begun soon after birth. Breastfeeding or partial breastfeeding may be possible for some infants if the phenylalanine levels are monitored carefully and remain within acceptable limits.
- Many affected children have some intellectual impairment. Successful management and outcome largely depend on early identification of the condition, modifying the diet, and compliance with the treatment regimen throughout the entire life cycle.

Galactosemia

Galactosemia, caused by a deficiency of the enzyme galactose-1-phosphate uridyltransferase, results in the inability to convert galactose to glucose. Galactosemia can be detected by measuring the blood levels of galactose in the urine of newborns suspected of having the disease who have ingested formula containing galactose. Early symptoms are vomiting, weight loss, and CNS symptoms, including poor feeding, drowsiness, and seizures. If the disorder goes untreated, the galactose levels will continue to increase and the affected infant will show failure to thrive, mental retardation, cataracts, jaundice, hepatomegaly, and cirrhosis of the liver, with death possibly occurring in the first month of life. Therapy consists of eliminating galactose from the diet; this condition precludes breastfeeding since lactose is present in breast milk.

Hypothyroidism

Congenital hypothyroidism results from a deficiency of thyroid hormones. Newborns are routinely screened for hypothyroidism by measuring thyroxine (T_4) in a drop of blood obtained from a heel stick at 2 to 5 days of age. At this time the normally expected increase in T_4 would be lacking in newborns with hypothyroidism. Thyroid-stimulating hormone (TSH) is measured in specimens with low T_4 values. Treatment is thyroid replacement.

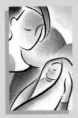
Grieving the Loss of a Newborn

Becoming a parent is an important developmental milestone that is anticipated by most men and women in our society. However, many types of loss can be associated with pregnancy and birth.

- Miscarriage, premature labor and preterm birth, and cesarean birth all involve a loss of the expected pregnancy and birth plans.
- Ectopic pregnancy, fetal death, and stillbirth are other types of loss as well as death of an infant who survives only a few hours or who dies after days, weeks, or months in an intensive care unit.
- Parents may grieve over the sex or appearance of their child or the birth of an infant who has a birth defect or chronic illness.
- Infertility may cause intense feelings of grief. When infertility treatments fail or a pregnancy ends in a miscarriage, feelings of loss are intensified.

CARE MANAGEMENT

Assessment

- The nature of the parental attachment with the pregnancy or infant, the meaning of the pregnancy and infant to the parents, and the related losses they are experiencing need to be addressed.
- The circumstances surrounding the loss, including the level of preparation for the loss and the parents' level of understanding about the cause of the loss or death, and any related unresolved issues are important.
- The immediate response of the mother and father to the loss, whether their responses are complementary or problematic,

and how their responses match with their past experiences, personalities, and behavioral and cultural backgrounds need to be assessed.

- The social support network of the parent (e.g., extended family, friends, co-workers, church) and the extent to which it has been activated are important. Some prefer to handle the tragedy alone for a time. Others want assistance in calling other family members, friends, and clergy to be with them and to help them with decisions.

Interventions

Helping parents actualize the loss

Interventions and support for parents from the nursing and medical staff before and after a perinatal loss or infant death are extremely important in their healing.

- The parents need to be told honestly about the situation by their physician or others on the health care team. It is important for their nurse to be with them during this time.
- Caregivers must use the words "dead" and "died," rather than "lost" or "gone," to assist bereaved persons in accepting this reality.
- Parents need opportunities to tell their story about the events, experiences, and feelings surrounding the loss.
- Knowing the sex and naming the fetus or baby help to actualize the loss. It is important not to create the sense that the parents *have* to name the "baby," especially in the case of a miscarriage when the sex is not known.

> **NURSE ALERT** *Cultural taboos and rules in some religious faiths prohibit the naming of an infant who has died. It is very important to be sensitive to this possibility and not impose naming on such parents.*

- It may be helpful for mothers and fathers to see the fetus or baby. Parents should never be made to feel they "should" see or hold their baby when this is something that they do not really want. A question such as, "Some parents have found it helpful to see their baby. Would you like time to consider this?" is useful.

- In preparation for the visit with the baby, parents appreciate explanations about what to expect. Descriptions of how their baby looks are important. For example, babies may have red, peeling skin that resembles a bad sunburn, dark discoloration similar to bruises, molding of the head that makes the head look soft and swollen, or birth defects.
    - The nurse should make the baby look as normal as possible and remember that parents and health care professionals view the baby differently.
    - Bathing the baby, applying lotion to the baby's skin, combing hair, placing identification bracelets on the arm and leg, dressing the baby in a diaper and special outfit, sprinkling powder in the baby's blanket, and wrapping the baby in a pretty blanket convey to the parents that their baby has been cared for in a special way.
    - It is more complicated if the fetus died several days or weeks before birth or if decapitation or dismemberment occurred. Consultation with a local funeral director can help the nurse prepare the baby to be seen by the parents.
    - A baby that has been in the morgue can be placed underneath a warmer for 20 to 30 minutes and wrapped in a warm blanket before being brought to the parents. Cold cream rubbed over stiffened joints can help in positioning the baby.
    - When bringing the baby to the parents, treat the baby as one would a live baby. Holding the baby close, touching a hand or cheek, using the baby's name, and talking with the parents about the special features of their child convey that it is all right for them to do likewise.
    - If a baby has a congenital anomaly, the nurse can desensitize the family by pointing out aspects of the baby that are normal.
    - Some families may like to have the opportunity to bathe and dress their baby, comb the hair, dress the baby in a special outfit, wrap the baby in a blanket, or place the baby in a crib.
- Parents need to be offered time alone with their baby if they wish. They also need to know when the nurse will return and how to call if they need anything.

- If at all possible the family should be placed in a private room, and when possible the room should have a rocking chair for the parents to sit in when holding their baby.
- Marking the door to the room with a special card can be helpful for reminding the staff that this family has experienced a loss.
- Grandparents should be offered the same opportunities to hold, rock, swaddle, and love their grandchildren so that their grief is started in a healthy way.

Helping the parents with decision making

- One decision might be related to conducting an autopsy. An autopsy can be very important in answering the question "why" if there is a chance that the cause of death can be determined.
- Organ donation can be an aid to grieving and an opportunity for the family to see something positive associated with the experience. The most common donation is of cornea; donation of cornea from a baby can occur if the baby was born alive at 36 weeks of gestation or later.
- Spiritual rituals may be helpful and important to parents. Support from clergy is an option that should be offered to all parents. Members of the clergy may offer the parents the opportunity for baptism when appropriate. Other rituals that may be important include a blessing, naming ceremony, anointing, ritual of the sick, memorial service, or prayer.
- Parents should be given information about the choices for the final disposition of their baby, regardless of gestational age.
  - A baby younger than 20 weeks of gestation is considered a product of conception, whereas embryos, uterine tubes removed with an ectopic pregnancy, and tissue from a pregnancy obtained during a dilation and curettage are all considered tissue.
  - The nurse should know the hospital's policies and procedures and answer the parents' questions honestly.
  - In most states, if a baby is at least 20 weeks and 1 day of gestational age or is born alive, the parents are responsible for making the final arrangements for their baby, although

some hospitals will offer free cremation. In this case, the family would not get the ashes.

LEGAL TIP Defining Live Birth
Laws in all states govern what constitutes a live birth. In most states a live birth is considered to be any products of conception expelled from a woman that show any signs of life. Signs of life are considered to be any muscle irritability, respiratory effort, or heart rate, regardless of gestational age. All nurses should be knowledgeable about their state laws regarding what constitutes a live birth and what forms must be completed and filed in the case of fetal death, stillbirth, or newborn death.

Providing postmortem care

- Preparation of the baby's body and transport to the morgue depend on the procedures and protocols developed by individual hospitals.
- Final disposition of all identifiable babies, regardless of gestational age, includes burial or cremation. Depending on the cemetery's policies, babies in caskets or the ashes from cremated babies can be buried in a special place designated for babies, at the foot of a deceased relative, in a separate plot, or in a mausoleum. Ashes also may be scattered in a designated area; many states have regulations regarding where ashes can be scattered.
- A local funeral director or a state's Vital Statistics Bureau should have information about the state's rules, codes, and regulations regarding live births, burial requirements, transportation of the deceased by parents, and cremation.
- In making final arrangements for their baby, parents may want a special service. They may choose to have a service in the hospital chapel, visitation at a funeral home or their own home, a funeral service, or a graveside service.

Helping the bereaved parents to acknowledge and express their feelings

- One of the most important goals of the nurse is to validate the experience and feelings of the parents by encouraging them to tell their stories and to listen with care.

- At the very least, the nurse should acknowledge the loss with a simple but sincere comment, such as "I'm sorry about the baby."
- Helping the parents to talk about their loss and the meaning it has for their lives and to share their emotional pain is the next step. "Tell me about what happened."
- Because nurses tend to be very focused on the physical and emotional needs of the mother, it is especially important to ask the father directly about his views of what happened and his feelings of loss.
- The nurse should listen patiently during the story of loss or grief, but listening is hard work and can be painful for the listener.
- Bereaved parents have identified many unhelpful responses made to them by well-meaning health care professionals, family, and friends. The nurse should resist the temptation to give advice or to use clichés in offering support to the bereaved individuals (Box 18-1).
- Feelings of anger, guilt, and sadness can occur immediately but often become more problematic in the early days and months after a loss. When a bereaved person expresses feelings of anger, it can be helpful to identify the feeling by simply saying, "You sound angry," or "You look angry."
- The nurse's willingness to sit down and listen to these feelings of anger can help the bereaved family move past those surface feelings into the underlying feelings of powerlessness and helplessness in not being able to control the many aspects of the situation.

Helping parents to normalize the grief process; facilitating use of coping skills

- While helping parents share their feelings of pain, it is critical to help them understand their grief responses and feel they are not alone in these painful responses.
- Reassuring them of the normality of their responses and preparing them for the length of their grief are important.
- Books and pamphlets about grief, if short and sensitive, can be given to parents to take home.

BOX 18-1

What to Say and What Not to Say to Bereaved Parents

WHAT TO SAY
"I'm sad for you."
"How are you doing with all of this?"
"This must be hard for you."
"What can I do for you?"
"I'm sorry."
"I'm here, and I want to listen."

WHAT NOT TO SAY
"God had a purpose for her."
"Be thankful you have another child."
"The living must go on."
"I know how you feel."
"It's God's will."
"You have to keep on going for her sake."
"You're young; you can have others."
"We'll see you back here next year, and you'll be happier."
"Now you have an angel in heaven."
"This happened for the best."
"Better for this to happen now, before you knew the baby."
"There was something wrong with the baby anyway."

Used with permission of Bereavement Services. Copyright Lutheran Hospital–La Crosse, Inc., a Gundersen Lutheran Affiliate, La Crosse, WI.

- Many parents have reported feelings of fear that they were going crazy because of the many emotions and behavioral responses that leave them feeling totally out of control in the months after the loss.
- In the initial days after a loss, other strategies might include follow-up phone calls, referrals to a perinatal grief support group, or provision of a list of publications or websites intended to help parents who have experienced a perinatal loss.
- To reduce relationship problems that can occur in couples who are grieving, it is important to help them understand that they may respond and grieve in very different ways. Nurses should discourage dependence on drugs and alcohol.

Meeting the physical needs of the postpartum bereaved mother

Coping with loss and grief after childbirth can be an overwhelming experience for the woman and her family. One particularly difficult aspect of the loss is the sound of crying babies and the happiness of other families on the unit who have given birth to healthy infants.

- The mother should be given the opportunity to decide if she wants to remain on the maternity unit or be moved to another hospital unit after she hears the advantages and disadvantages of each choice.
- The physical needs of a bereaved mother are the same as those of any woman who has given birth. Postpartum care as well as grief support may not be as good on another hospital unit where staff members are not experienced in postpartum and bereavement care.
- The cruel reality for many bereaved mothers is that their milk may come in with no baby to nurse, their afterpains remind them of their emptiness, and gas pains feel as though a baby is still moving inside. The nurse should ensure that the mother receives appropriate medications to reduce these physical signs and symptoms.
- Adequate rest, diet, and fluids must be offered to replenish the mother's physical strength. Mothers need ideas about how to cope with problems with sleep, such as decreasing food or fluids that contain caffeine, limiting alcohol and nicotine consumption, exercising regularly, using strategies for rest, taking a warm bath or drinking warm milk before bedtime, doing relaxation exercises, listening to restful music, or getting a massage.
- The couple needs to be encouraged and supported in maintaining their relationship and keeping open channels of communication.

Assisting the bereaved couple in communicating with, supporting, and getting support from family

Providing sensitive care to bereaved parents means including their families in the grief process.

- Grandparents and siblings are particularly important when a perinatal loss has occurred.

- Parents need information about how grief affects a family. They may need help in determining ways to let family members know how they feel and what they need.

Creating memories for parents to take home

Parents may want tangible mementos of their baby to allow them to actualize the loss. Some may want to bring in a previously purchased baby book.

- Special memory books, cards, and information about grief and mourning are available for purchase by parents or hospitals or clinics through national perinatal bereavement organizations.
- The nurse can provide information about the baby's weight, length, and head circumference to the family.
- Footprints and handprints can be taken and placed with the other information on a special card or in a memory or baby book.
  - Sometimes it is difficult to obtain good handprints or footprints. Application of alcohol or acetone on the palms or soles can help the ink adhere to make the prints clearer, especially for small babies.
  - When making prints, have a hard surface underneath the paper to be printed. The baby's heel or palm is placed down first, and the foot or hand is rolled forward, keeping the toes or fingers extended.
  - It may be helpful to have assistance in this procedure.
  - If the print does not turn out, tracing around the baby's hands and feet can be done, although this distorts the actual size.
  - A form of plaster of Paris can also be used to make an imprint of the baby's hand or foot.
- Parents often appreciate articles that were in contact with or used in caring for the baby.
  - This might include the tape measure used to measure the baby, baby lotions, combs, clothing, hats, blankets, crib cards, and identification bands.
  - A lock of hair may be another important keepsake. Parents must be asked for permission before cutting a lock of hair, which can be removed from the nape of the neck where it is not noticeable.

- For some, pictures are the most important memento. Photographs should be taken whenever there is an identifiable baby and when it is culturally acceptable to the family.
  - Pictures should include close-ups of the baby's face, hands, and feet.
  - Pictures should be taken of the baby clothed and wrapped in a blanket as well as unclothed.
  - If there are any congenital anomalies, close-ups of the anomalies also should be taken.
  - Flowers, blocks, stuffed animals, or toys can be placed in the background to make the picture more special.
  - Parents may want their pictures taken holding the baby.
  - Keeping a camera nearby and taking pictures when parents are spending special time with their baby can provide special memories.
  - Some parents may have their own camera or video camera and would like the nurse to record them as they bathe, dress, hold, or diaper their baby.

Responding to cultural and spiritual needs of parents

Many of the responses that are described and the interventions suggested in this chapter are based on European-American views of perinatal grief and loss.

- Although it is thought that there are no particular differences in the individual, intrapersonal experiences of grief based on culture, ethnicity, or religion, many differences are found in mourning rituals, traditions, and behavioral expressions of grief that are often ignored or misunderstood.
- The nurse must consider the potential unique responses and needs of parents from different groups. This involves understanding the cultural orientation and beliefs of the individual parent, the partner, the extended family, and the larger community to which they belong.
- Some groups, such as Orthodox Jews, may not support the notion of grieving for perinatal loss because the fetus or stillborn infant is not considered a person.
- In some cultures, such as the Muslim culture, decisions are communal.

- Expressions of grief may range from quiet and stoic to dramatic and hysterical for different Native American groups. Native Americans from many tribes would not respond well to an "interviewing" or "questioning" approach.
- Mexican mothers may be very demonstrative in their grief, while also struggling with the view that hardship is "God's will."
- Some cultural and religious groups do not believe in naming an infant who dies before 30 days of age.
- Picture taking can conflict with beliefs of some cultures, such as some Native American, Eskimo, Amish, Hindu, and Muslim cultures. Families from these cultures should be sensitively offered this opportunity but not pushed into having a picture taken.
- Autopsies are not allowed by some religions except under unusual circumstances.
- Cremation is forbidden by the Jewish religion, Baha'is, and the Greek Orthodox Church. It is discouraged or allowed only under unusual circumstances in the Church of Jesus Christ of Latter-Day Saints.
- Embalming is not allowed for Jews, Baha'is, and Muslims.
- Baptism is extremely important for Roman Catholics and some Protestant groups. Baptism can be performed by a layperson, such as a nurse, in an emergency situation when a priest cannot be there in a timely fashion (Box 18-2).
- Many Protestant groups believe that baptism is conducted at the age of reason, and parents from these religions would not want their baby baptized.
- When bereaved parents need a referral for grief counseling, cultural considerations are paramount. Native Americans, for example, are best referred to native healers and counselors rather than to Western biomedical therapists.

Providing sensitive care at and after discharge

Leaving the hospital without a baby in her arms is a very empty and painful experience for a woman.

- Mothers should not be discharged at a time when other mothers with live babies are leaving whenever possible.

BOX 18-2

Infant Baptism

In an emergency, baptism may be performed by anyone by pouring water over the forehead (or products of conception) and saying "I baptize you in the name of the Father and of the Son and of the Holy Spirit." The person performing the baptism needs only to have the intention of baptizing and does not necessarily have to believe in infant baptism for the baptism to be valid. If the infant has no signs of life, the person performing the baptism can add "If you are alive, I baptize you. . . ."

- Giving the mother a special flower to carry in her arms can be a thoughtful gesture.
- The grief of the mother and her family does not end with discharge; rather it really begins once they return home, attend the funeral, and start to live their lives without their baby.
- Follow-up phone calls after a loss may be helpful to some parents. However, it must be determined when parents do not want a follow-up call, which often is the case after early loss.
- The calls are made at predictably difficult times, such as the first week at home, 4 to 6 weeks later, 4 to 6 months after the loss, and the anniversary of the death.
- A grief conference can be planned when parents return for an appointment with their physician, nurses, and other health care providers.
  - At the conference, the loss or death of the infant is discussed in detail, parents are given information about the baby's autopsy report and genetic studies, and they have opportunities to ask the questions that have arisen since their baby's death.

—Parents appreciate the opportunity to review the events of hospitalization, go over the baby's or mother's chart with their primary health care provider, and talk with those who cared for them and their baby during hospitalization.

—The health care professionals have the opportunity to assess how the family is coping with their loss and provide additional information and education on grief.

- Some parents are very interested in finding a perinatal or parental grief support group. They appreciate the opportunity to talk with others who have been through similar experiences.

- A grief support group also can be helpful for sharing feelings and gaining an understanding of the normality of the grief process.

  —An online perinatal loss *listserv* is a way to connect women who are geographically distant but share similar stories and pain. A group for women experiencing pregnancy after loss is also useful.

  —When referring to a group, it is important to know something about the group and how it operates. For example, if a group has a religious basis for their interventions, a nonreligious parent would not be likely to find the group helpful.

  —If parents experiencing a perinatal loss are referred to a parental grief group, they might feel overwhelmed with the grief of parents whose older children have died of cancer, suicide, or homicide. Their grief might be minimized by participants; therefore the needs of the parents must be matched with the focus of the group.

- Many hospitals have checklists used in providing care, mobilizing members of the multidisciplinary health care team, communicating options the family has chosen, and keeping track of all the details in meeting the needs of bereaved parents (see Maternity Nursing text, p. 950-951).

  —Checklists may be a permanent part of the chart.

  —Documentation in the nursing notes of primary concerns, grief responses, health teaching, health care advice, and any referrals of the mother or other family members is essential to ensure continuity and consistency of care.

SPECIAL LOSSES

Prenatal Diagnoses with Negative Outcome

Early prenatal diagnostic tests, such as ultrasonography, chorionic villus sampling, and amniocentesis, can determine the well-being of the embryo or fetus.

- If the health care provider is certain that the baby has a serious genetic defect that would lead to death in utero or after birth (congenital anomalies incompatible with life or genetic disorders with severe mental retardation), the choice of interruption of a pregnancy may be offered.
- Abortion is controversial, and this may prevent parents from sharing this decision with other family members or friends. This limits their support systems after their loss.
- The decision to terminate a pregnancy paves the way for feelings such as guilt, despair, sadness, depression, and anger.
- The nurse's role is to be a good listener. It is important to assess how these families feel about the experience and to offer options for their memories as appropriate.
- The parent who decides to continue the pregnancy also requires emotional support. The time of labor and birth can be particularly difficult. The nurse should remember that parents may be grieving not only the loss of the perfect child but also the loss of expectations for their child's future.

Loss of One in a Multiple Birth

- The death of a twin or baby in a multifetal gestation during pregnancy, labor, or birth or after birth requires parents to parent and grieve at the same time.
- Such a death results in a confusing and ambivalent induction into parenthood. Parents feel that they cannot do anything right.
  - They cannot parent their surviving child with all the joy and enthusiasm of new parents because their surviving child reminds them of what they have lost.
  - They cannot give over completely and grieve in the manner they need to because their surviving child demands their attention.

- These parents are at risk for altered parenting and complicated bereavement.
  - It is important to help the parents acknowledge the birth of all their babies.
  - Parents should be treated as bereaved families, and all the options previously discussed should be offered.
  - Pictures should be taken of the babies, and parents should be offered the opportunity to hold their babies in their arms and have time to say good-bye to the baby who has died.
- Bereaved parents should be warned that well-meaning family members or friends may say, "Well, at least you have the other baby," implying that there should be no grief because they are lucky to have one at all.
- Parents need to be able to anticipate insensitivity to their loss and be empowered to say to those people, "That is not how I feel."
- By setting a boundary on what their feelings are, they are able to acknowledge the baby who died and then have an opportunity to share more about their feelings if they so choose.
- Bereaved parents of multiples have special problems coping with life without their anticipated "extra special" family, telling their surviving child about his or her twin, dealing with the possibility of that child's feelings of survivor guilt, and deciding how to celebrate birthdays, death days, or special holidays.

Adolescent Grief

Each year, many adolescents experience perinatal loss, including as elective abortion or miscarriage. Adolescents grieve the loss of their babies and need emotional support from the nurses who care for them.

- Nurses and other health care professionals, as well as family members, often believe that the adolescent's loss of her baby was for the best, so that the adolescent can move on with her life. Adolescent girls, then, may not receive the support they need from staff and family.
- Adolescent girls usually do not have the support from the father of the baby as compared with older women who have a perinatal loss; therefore there is a great need to provide sensitive care to all adolescents who experience any type of perinatal loss.

Caring for a bereaved adolescent

- Acknowledge the significance of giving birth, no matter what the mother's age.
- Make additional efforts to develop a trusting relationship with the adolescent.
- Offer options for saying goodbye, anticipatory guidance, support, and information to meet the adolescent at the point of her need.
- It may take longer for adolescents to process their grief because of their level of cognitive and emotional maturation.
- Being patient, saving mementos, and giving the adolescent information on how to contact the nurse are interventions that can help the adolescent accept the reality of the loss and process her grief.

Complicated Bereavement

Some parents have complicated bereavement, that is, extremely intense grief reactions that last for a very long time.

- Evidence of complicated grief includes continued obsession with yearning and loneliness, intense and continued guilt or anger, relentless depression or anxiety that interferes with role functioning, abuse of drugs (including prescription medications) or alcohol, severe relationship difficulties, continued feelings of inadequacy and low self-esteem, and suicidal thoughts or threats.
- Parents showing signs of complicated grief should be referred for counseling to determine whether the parents are experiencing a normal, albeit intense grief response or whether they are also having a serious mental health problem, such as depression.
- It is important to refer to a therapist or counselor who is experienced in grief counseling and knows how to help bereaved people, because some therapists and counselors do not have an understanding of the special needs related to grief.
- Therapy is a big step. The highest number of cancellations and "no shows" in a therapist's practice are intakes, or first visits; therefore anything the nurse can do for a family or individual to help with that major hurdle would be useful.

—It is important to remember that people may have symptoms but may not, for whatever reason, be ready to deal directly with these symptoms or may not have the energy to make the call.

—Enlisting a family member to encourage parents to seek such assistance may be helpful.

English-Spanish Translations

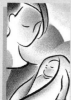

BODY PARTS

Bone	hueso
Blood	sangre
Tongue	lengua
Head	cabeza
Arm	brazo
Finger	dedo
Leg	pierna
Neck	cuello
Elbow	codo
Foot	pie
Ear	oreja, oido
Nose	nariz
Mouth	boca
Bladder	vejiga
Back	espalda
Chest	pecho
Spleen	bazo
Gallbladder	vesícula biliar

SPECIFIC CONDITIONS

Rubella	rubeola
Intensive care	cuidado intensivo
Menstrual period	menstruación
Birth control	anticonceptivo
Allergic reaction	reacción alérgica

EQUIPMENT

Diaper	pañal
Bulb syringe	bombilla
Antibiotic	antibiótico
Pacifier	chupón
Bottle (baby bottle or medicine bottle)	botella
Juice	jugo
Milk	leche

PAIN MANAGEMENT

Please show me where it hurts.	Muéstrame dónde le duele, por favor.
When did it start?	¿Cuándo empegó?
Do you have pain . . . ?	¿Tiene dolor . . . ?
Headache	de cabeza
Stomachache	del estómago
Backache	de la espalda
Chest pain	en el pecho
In the arm	en el brazo
In the legs	en las piernas
In the mouth	en la boca
In the eyes	en los ojos
In the bladder	en la vejiga

PROCEDURES

Injection	inyección
Lumbar puncture	punción lumbar
Start an IV	ponerle suero por vena
To breastfeed, nurse	amamantar
To burp	eructar
X-ray	radiografía

Breastfeeding: Latching-On

Do you want to breastfeed your baby?	¿Desea amamantar a su bebé?
I will help you.	Yo le ayudaré.
Hold your baby's head close to your breast.	Sostenga la cabeza del bebé cerca del pecho.

Lightly touch your nipple to the baby's lower lip until the baby opens his or her mouth.	Con el pezón, toque suavemente el labio inferior del bebé hasta que abra la boca.
Lift your breast to the baby's mouth.	Levante el seno hasta la boca del bebé.
Center your nipple and areola as far in the baby's mouth as possible.	Centre el pezón y la areola lo más que se pueda dentro de la boca del bebé.
Make sure the baby's tongue is under the nipple and the gums close around the areola.	Asegúrese de que la lengua del bebé esté debajo del pezón y que sus encías se cierren sobre la areola.
To change breasts, push one of your fingers into the corner of the baby's mouth.	Para cambiar al otro seno, métase un dedo en la comisura de los labios del bebé.
This will break the suction and prevent the baby from biting the nipple.	Esto interrumpe la aspiración e impide que el bebé muerda el pezón.

Burping

Position #1	**Posición #1**
Hold your baby up, head on your shoulder.	Ponga su bebé con la cabeza muy alta sobre su hombro.
Put one arm under the baby's bottom.	Ponga un brazo debajo de las nalgas del bebé.
With the other hand, pat or rub the baby's back.	Con la otra mano, dé leves palmaditas o sobe la espalda del bebé.
Position #2	**Posición #2**
Sit your baby up in your lap.	Siente al bebé sobre su regazo.
Hold the head and back with one hand.	Con una mano, sostenga la cabeza y la espalda del bebé.
Hold the chin and front with the other.	Con la otra mano, sostenga la barbilla y la parte delantera del bebé.
Rock the baby's upper body back and forth.	Mueva la parte superior del bebé hacia adelante y hacia atrás.

Or pat the baby's back.	O dé suaves palmaditas a la espalda del bebé.
Position #3	**Posición #3**
Lay your baby face down on your lap.	Coloque al bebé boca abajo sobre su regazo.
Hold the baby's head with one hand.	Con una mano, sostenga la cabeza del bebé.
Rub or pat the baby's back.	Sobe o dé suaves palmaditas a la espalda del bebé.
Assess adequacy of intake	
How many times did (he/she) urinate today?	¿Cuántas veces orinó hoy?
How many wet diapers has (he/she) had?	¿Cuántos pañales ha mojado?
How many dirty diapers?	¿Cuántos pañales sucios?

Care During Labor

Lie down, please.	Acuéstese, por favor.
I am going to take your vital signs.	Voy a verificar sus signos vitales.
I am going to listen to the baby's heartbeat.	Voy a escuchar el latido del corazón del bebé.
This is a fetal monitor.	Este es un monitor fetal.
I need to examine you.	Necesito examinarle.
Do you need to use the bathroom?	¿Necesita usar el baño?
Would you like some pain medication?	¿Quisiera medicina para calmar el dolor?
Roll over on your side, please.	Póngase sobre un costado, por favor.
Relax.	Afloje los músculos.
Breathe deeply.	Respire profundamente.
Push.	Puje.
Do not push.	No puje.
Grab your knees, and push.	Agárrese las rodillas, y puje.
You are doing fine.	Bien. Muy bien.
Congratulations!	¡Felicidades!
You have a beautiful boy.	Usted tiene un niño precioso.
You have a beautiful girl.	Usted tiene una niña preciosa.

Cesarean Birth

You need a cesarean.

Necesita una operación cesárea.

Has your doctor discussed with you the reason for needing a cesarean?

¿Ha hablado el doctor con usted sobre la necesidad de tener una operación cesárea?

Do you understand why you need a cesarean?

¿Entiende usted por qué necesita una operación cesárea?

Your signature on this form will allow us to proceed with the surgery.

Su firma en este formulario nos permitirá seguir adelante con la operación.

Please sign this consent form.

Por favor, firme este formulario de autorización.

Contraception

Do you plan to have more children?

¿Piensa tener más hijos?

Are you sexually active?

¿Tiene relaciones sexuales?

Do you have many partners?

¿Tiene muchas parejas sexuales?

Have you had many partners in the past?

¿Ha tenido muchas parejas sexuales en el pasado?

Do you presently use contraception/birth control?

¿Usa anticonceptivos/control de natalidad actualmente?

The pill? Condoms? The diaphragm? The IUD?

¿La píldora anticonceptiva? ¿Los condones (preservativos)? ¿El diafragma? ¿El dispositivo intrauterino (DIU)?

Spermicides? The rhythm method?

¿Los espermaticidas? ¿El método del ritmo?

Injection (Depo-Provera)?

¿La inyección (Depo-Provera)?

How long have you used this method?

¿Por cuánto tiempo ha usado este método?

Do you like this method?

¿Le gusta este método?

Why did you stop using it?

¿Por qué dejó de usarlo?

Do you want to change to a different method?

¿Quiere cambiar a otro método?

Have you had a tubal ligation?

¿Ha tenido una ligadura de trompas?

Has he had a vasectomy?

¿Tuvo él una vasectomía?

Diet and Nutrition

You need to gain weight.	Usted necesita aumentar de peso.
You need to control your weight gain.	Usted necesita controlar su aumento de peso.
Eat nutritious foods.	Coma alimentos nutritivos.
Eat foods high in protein, calcium, vitamins, and iron.	Coma alimentos altos en proteínas, calcio, vitaminas, y hierro.
Eat a lot of fruits and vegetables.	Coma muchas frutas y vegetales.
Drink four glasses of milk each day.	Tome cuatro vasos de leche diariamente.
Drink low-fat instead of whole milk.	Tome la leche baja en grasa en lugar de la leche entera.
Avoid salty foods, such as sausage, hot dogs, and French fries.	Evite alimentos muy salados como calchichas, perros calientes, y papitas fritas.
Avoid fried foods.	Evite las frituras.
Avoid caffeine.	Evite la cafeína.
There is caffeine in Coca-Cola, tea, and chocolate.	Hay cafeína en la Coca-Cola, el té, y el chocolate.
Take prenatal vitamins.	Tome vitaminas prenatales.

Discharge Teaching for Postpartum Woman

When you go to the bathroom, always wipe from front to back.	Cuando vaya al baño, séquese siempre de adelante hacia atrás.
Sit in a warm tub to relieve discomfort.	Siéntese en una bañera con agua tibia para aliviarse.
You will have moderate amounts of vaginal discharge.	Usted tendrá cantidades moderadas de sangrado vaginal.
It may last from 4 to 6 weeks.	Puede durar desde cuatro a seis semanas.
The color may vary from dark brown to red to pink.	El color puede variar entre café oscuro a rojo a rosado.
It may contain blood clots.	Es probable que contenga coágulos.

Use a sanitary pad instead of a tampon.	Use una toalla sanitaria en vez de un tampón.
Your menstrual period will not resume for 4 to 10 weeks.	Su regla no regrasará hasta cuatro a diez semanas más tarde.
If you are breastfeeding, it may take a little longer.	Si está amamantando, puede demorar un poco más.
It is possible to become pregnant while you are breastfeeding.	Es possible quedar embarazada mientras amamanta.
Avoid having sexual relations for 2 to 4 weeks after birth.	Evite las relaciones sexuales por dos a cuatro semanas después del parto.
Gradually increase activity to incorporate everyday routines.	Aumente las actividades gradualmente hasta llegar a su rutina normal.
Do your Kegel exercises.	Haga los ejercicios Kegel.
Do not lift heavy objects (more than 10 pounds).	No levante objetos pesados (de más de diez libras).
Rest as often as possible.	Descanse mucho.
Rest when your baby sleeps.	Descanse cuando duerma su bebé.
Eat daily 4 servings of bread/cereals, fruits/vegetables (green), milk or foods made from milk, and 2 servings of meat. You need to drink 8 glasses of fluids each day to support breastfeeding.	Cómase diariamente cuatro porciones de pan/cereal, frutas/vegetales (verduras), leche o comidas del grupo de leche, y dos porciones de carne. Usted necesita tomar ocho vasos de líquidos diariamente para soportar el dar de pecho.
Call your doctor (obstetrician) if you have:	Llame al médico de obstétricas si tenga cualquier de lo siguiente:
• Fever >38° C (>100.4° F)	• Fiebre >38° C (>100.4° F)
• Increased vaginal bleeding (more than a regular period)	• Aumento de desangre vaginal (más que una regla normal)
• Chills	• Escalofríos
• Painful, burning urination	• Orin que le duele o le quema
• Foul-smelling vaginal discharge	• Desangre vaginal de muy mal olor

- **Increased pain or swelling**

- **Drainage or separation of incision (cesarean)**

- Aumento de dolor o hinchazón

- Desangre o deshecho de la herida

High Risk Factors

HIGH RISK ASSESSMENT		POTENTIAL PROBLEM
Have you had any problems with this pregnancy?	¿Ha tenido problemas con este embarazo?	General assessment
Have you had blurred vision?	¿Ha tenido visión borrosa?	Preeclampsia
Have you had severe headaches?	¿Ha tenido dolores fuertes de cabeza?	Preeclampsia
Have you had difficulty breathing?	¿Ha tenido dificultad para respirar?	Cardiac disease
Have you had heart palpitations?	¿Ha tenido palpitaciones del corazón?	Cardiac disease
Have you been vomiting?	¿Ha tenido vómitos?	Hyperemesis gravidarum
Have you had any infections?	¿Ha tenido alguna infección?	Sexually transmitted infections or vaginal infections
Have you had swelling?	¿Ha tenido hinchazón?	Preeclampsia
Were all your pregnancies term?	¿Llegaron a las cuarenta semanas todos sus embarazos?	Preterm labor
Have you ever had diabetes?	¿Ha tenido diabetes?	Diabetes
Have you ever had high blood pressure?	¿Ha tenido alta presión sanguínea?	Gestational hypertension/ chronic hypertension
Have you ever had anemia?	¿Ha estado anémica?	Anemia

| **Do you take drugs? Prescription medicine?** | ¿Usa drogas? ¿Medicina recetada? | Substance abuse |
| **Do you drink alcohol? Smoke?** | ¿Toma bebidas alcohólicas? ¿Fuma? | Substance abuse |

Induction of Labor

Your labor is not progressing.	Su trabajo de parto no está progresando.
We need to stimulate the contractions.	Necesitamos provocar las contracciones.
I'm going to give you some medication to make your contractions stronger.	Le voy a dar una medicina para hacer más fuertes las contracciones.
I'm going to give you Pitocin through your IV.	Le voy a dar pitufina por medio del suero.

Labor Assessment

What time did the contractions begin?	¿A qué hora le empezaron las contracciones?
How far apart are the contractions?	¿Con qué frecuencia tiene las contracciones?
Have the membranes ruptured? When?	¿Se le rompió la fuente? ¿Cuándo?
What color was the fluid? Red? Pink?	¿Qué color tenía el líquido? ¿Rojo? ¿Rosado?
Have you had bleeding?	¿Ha tenido hemorragia?
How much? A cupful? A tablespoon? A teaspoon?	¿Cuánto? ¿Una taza? ¿Una cucharada? ¿Una cucharadita?
When was the last time you ate or drank anything?	¿Cuándo fue la última vez que comió o tomó algo?
Have you had any problems with this pregnancy?	¿Ha tenido algún problema con este embarazo?
Are you taking any medications?	¿Toma algún medicamento?
Are you allergic to penicillin or other medicines?	¿Es alérgica a la penicilina u otras medicinas?
Please sign this consent form.	Por favor, firme este formulario de autorización.

Menstruation

At what age did you begin to menstruate?	¿A qué edad empezó a menstruar?
When was your last menstrual cycle?	¿Cuándo fue su última menstruación (regla)?
Was it normal?	¿Fue normal?
Do you have pains with your period?	¿Tiene algún dolor con la menstruación (regla)?
How many days does your period last?	¿Por cuántos días dura su menstruación (regla)?
Is the flow light or heavy?	¿Tiene mucha o poquita hemorragia durante su menstruación (regla)?

Pain Management

Pain: **Do you want to get up and walk?**	*Dolor*: ¿Desea levantarse y caminar?
Do you want pain medication?	¿Quiere medicina para el dolor?
I am going to give you the pain medicine in an injection.	Le voy a dar la medicina para el dolor por inyección.
I am going to give you the pain medicine through an IV.	Le voy a dar la medicina para el dolor por el suero.
This is a pain reliever called Demerol/Stadol/Nubain.	Ésta es una medicina para aliviar el dolor que se llama Demerol/Stadol/Nubain.
The effects of this medicine are relatively short.	Los efectos de esta medicina son de corta duración.
The epidural is a stronger method of pain relief.	La anestesia epidural es un método más potente para aliviar el dolor.
You should not be able to feel the contraction pain.	No debe de sentir el dolor de las contracciones.

Pelvic Examination

Take off all your clothes, please.	Quítese toda la ropa, por favor.
Put on the gown, please.	Póngase la bata, por favor.
I am going to examine you.	Le voy a examinar.
You will feel less discomfort if you relax.	Se sentirá más cómoda si se relaja el cuerpo.

Lie down, please.	Acuéstese, por favor.
Put your feet in the stirrups.	Póngase los pies en los estribos.
Open your legs, please.	Sepárese las piernas, por favor.
I am going to take a sample from the lining of the cervix (Pap smear).	Le voy a tomar una muestra del cuello uterino (el examen de Papanicolao).
We will test this sample for cancer.	Haremos un análisis de esta muestra para determinar si hay cáncer.
It won't hurt.	No le va a doler.
Everything looks fine.	Todo está bien.
You may get dressed.	Puede vestirse.

Postpartum Physical Assessment

Are you planning to breastfeed or bottle-feed?	¿Piensa darle pecho o biberón al bebé?
Lie down, please.	Acuéstese, por favor.
I am going to take your vital signs.	Le voy a tomar sus signos vitales.
Open your mouth.	Abra la boca.
Temperature	temperatura
Pulse	pulso
Heartrate	latido del corazón
I need to take your blood pressure.	Necesito tomarle la presión sanguínea.
Do you need to use the bathroom?	¿Necesita usar el baño?
I need to examine you.	Necesito examinarle.
Please spread your knees and legs apart.	Por favor, abra las rodillas and las piernas.
Roll over on your side, please.	Póngase sobre un costado, por favor.
Where does it hurt?	¿Dónde le duele?
Would you like some pain medication?	¿Desea medicina para calmar el dolor?
Would you like to take a sitz bath?	¿Desea tomar un baño de asiento?
Are you sleeping well?	¿Está durmiendo bien?

Prenatal Interview

Have you had a pregnancy test?	¿Ha tenido una prueba del embarazo?
When was your last menstrual cycle?	¿Cuándo fue su última menstruación (regla)?
Have you been pregnant before?	¿Ha quedado embarazada antes?
How many times?	¿Cuántas veces?
How many children do you have?	¿Cuántos hijos tiene usted?
Have you ever had a miscarriage (spontaneous abortion)?	¿Ha perdido un bebé alguna vez? (¿Ha tenido un aborto espontáneo?)
Have you ever had a therapeutic abortion?	¿Ha tenido un aborto provocado?
Have you ever had a stillborn?	¿Ha tenido un niño que nació sin vida?
Have you ever had a cesarean?	¿Ha tenido una operación cesárea?
Have you had any problems with past pregnancies?	¿Ha tenido problemas durante sus embarazos anteriores?
Do you take drugs? Prescription medicine?	¿Usa drogas? ¿Medicina recetada?
If so, which type of medicine do you use and for what?	¿Qué clases de medicina toma? ¿Para qué las toma?
Do you drink alcohol? Do you smoke?	¿Toma bebidas alcohólicas? ¿Fuma?

Prenatal Physical Examination

Get up on the scale, please.	Súbase a la balanza, por favor.
I need a urine sample.	Necesito una muestra de orina.
Go to the bathroom, please.	Vaya al baño, por favor.
I need to take your blood pressure.	Necesito verificar su presión sanguínea.
I am going to listen to the baby's heartbeat.	Voy a escuchar el latido del corazón del bebé.
The doctor is going to examine you.	El doctor le va a examinar.
Don't be afraid.	No tenga miedo.
Lie down, please.	Acuéstese, por favor.
Separate your legs, please.	Sepárese las piernas, por favor.
Relax.	Afloje los músculos.

Go to the laboratory for a blood test, please.	Vaya al laboratorio para un análisis de sangre, por favor.
Go to this office for your ultrasound, please.	Vaya a esta oficina para que se le haga el ultrasonido, por favor.

RECOGNIZING VIOLENCE IN A RELATIONSHIP

ARE YOU IN A RELATIONSHIP IN WHICH YOU ARE...	¿TIENE UNA RELACIÓN CON SU PAREJA EN LA QUE...
afraid of your partner's temper?	tiene miedo de que él pierda los estribos?
afraid to break up because your partner has threatened to hurt someone?	tiene miedo de dejarlo porque él ha amenazado con pegar o lastimar a alguien?
constantly apologizing for or defending your partner's behavior?	constantemente tiene que disculparse por o defender el comportamiento de su pareja?
afraid to disagree with your partner?	tiene miedo de discutir con su pareja?
isolated from your family or friends?	está aislada de su familia o sus amigos?
embarrassed in front of others because of your partner's words or actions?	las palabras o acciones de su pareja delante de otra gente le dan vergüenza?
intimidated by your partner and forced into having sex?	su pareja le intimida a usted y le obliga a tener relaciones sexuales con él?
depressed and jumpy?	está deprimida y/o nerviosa?
A PERSON WHO IS VIOLENT IN A RELATIONSHIP OFTEN...	UNA PERSONA QUE TIENE UN CARÁCTER VIOLENTO EN UNA RELACIÓN A MENUDO...
has an explosive temper.	pierde los estribos.
is possessive or jealous of his partner's time, friends, or family.	es posesivo o tiene celos de que su pareja pase tiempo con la familia o los amigos.
constantly criticizes his partner's thoughts, feelings, or appearance.	critica constantemente los sentimientos, ideas, o apariencia física de su pareja.

pinches, slaps, grabs, shoves, or throws things at his partner.	pellizca, pega, agarra, empuja, o lanza objetos que pueden lastimar a su pareja.
forces his partner into having sex.	obliga a su pareja a tener relaciones sexuales.
causes his partner to be afraid.	causa que su pareja tenga miedo.

What to Do If Symptoms of Preterm Labor Occur

Empty your bladder.	Vacíese la vejiga.
Drink two to three glasses of water or juice.	Tome dos a tres vasos de agua o jugo.
Lie down on your left side for 1 hour.	Acuéstese del lado izquierdo por una hora.
Palpate for contractions like this.	Palpe por contracciones así.
If symptoms continue, call your health care provider or go to the hospital.	Si continúan los síntomas, llame a su proveedor de los servicios de salud/médico o vaya al hospital.
If symptoms abate, resume light activity, but not what you were doing when the symptoms began.	Si se alivian los síntomas, resuma sus actividades livianas, pero no haga lo que estaba haciendo cuando empezaron los síntomas.
If symptoms return, call your health care provider or go to the hospital.	Si se presentan de nuevo los síntomas, llame a su proveedor de los servicios de salud/médico o vaya al hospital.
If any of the following symptoms occur, call your health care provider immediately:	Si le sucede cualquier de los siguientes síntomas, llame inmediatamente a su proveedor de los servicios de salud/médico:
• **Uterine contractions every 10 minutes or less for 1 hour or more**	• Contracciones uterinas cada diez minutos o menos que duran por una hora o más
• **Vaginal bleeding**	• Hemorragia vaginal
• **Odorous vaginal discharge**	• Flujo vaginal con mal olor
• **Fluid leaking from the vagina**	• Flujo que le sale de la vagina

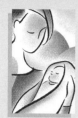

Medication Guides

Women's Health Care

Nonsteroidal Antiinflammatory Agents Used to Treat Dysmenorrhea

DRUG	BRAND NAME AND STATUS	RECOMMENDED DOSAGE*	COMMON SIDE EFFECTS†	COMMENTS	CONTRAINDICATIONS
Diclofenac	Cataflam Rx	50 mg tid or 100 mg initially, then 50 mg tid to 150 mg/day	Nausea, diarrhea, constipation, abdominal distress, dyspepsia, flatulence	Enteric coated: immediate release	For all NSAIDs: do not give if patient has hemophilia or bleeding ulcers; do not give if patient has had an allergic or anaphylactic reaction to aspirin or another NSAID; do not give if patient is taking anticoagulant medication
Ibuprofen	Motrin Rx	400 mg q4-6hr	Nausea, dyspepsia, rash, pruritus	If GI upset occurs, take with food, milk, or antacids; avoid alcoholic beverages; do not take with aspirin	

	Advil OTC, Nuprin OTC, Motrin IB OTC	200 mg q4-6hr to 1200 mg/day		See ibuprofen
Ketoprofen	Orudis Rx Orudis KT OTC Actron OTC	25-50 mg q6-8 hr to 300 mg/day 12.5 mg q6-8 hr to 75 mg/day	Nausea, diarrhea, constipation, abdominal distress, dyspepsia, flatulence	See ibuprofen
Meclofenamate	Meclomen Rx	100 mg tid to 300 mg	See ketoprofen	See ketoprofen
Mefenamic acid	Ponstel Rx	50 mg initially; then 250 mg q6-8 hr to 1000 mg/day	See ketoprofen	Very potent and effective prostaglandin-synthesis inhibitor

References: Clinical Pharmacology. (2004). *Drugs used to treat dysmenorrhea*. Gold Standard Multimedia. Internet document available at http://cp.gsm.com (accessed October 1, 2004); Facts and Comparisons. (2002); *Loose-leaf drug information service*. St. Louis: Facts and Comparisons; Parent-Stevens, L., & Burns, E. (2000). Menstrual disorders. In M. Smith & L. Shimp (Eds.), *20 Common problems in women's health care*. New York: McGraw-Hill.

GI, Gastrointestinal; *NSAID*, nonsteroidal antiinflammatory drugs; *OTC*, over the counter; *Rx*, prescription; *tid*, three times per day.

*Dosages are current recommendations and should be verified before use. Recommended dosages for over-the-counter preparations are generally less than recommendations for therapeutic dosages. As-needed dosing is recommended by manufacturer; scheduled dosing may be more effective.

†Risks with all NSAIDs are gastrointestinal ulceration, possible bleeding, and prolonged bleeding time. Incidence of side effects is dose related. Reported incidence, 3% to 9%.

Continued

Nonsteroidal Antiinflammatory Agents Used to Treat Dysmenorrhea—cont'd

DRUG	BRAND NAME AND STATUS	RECOMMENDED DOSAGE	COMMON SIDE EFFECTS*	COMMENTS	CONTRAINDICATIONS
				Antagonizes already formed prostaglandins Increased incidence of adverse GI side effects	
Naproxen	Naprosyn Rx	500 mg initially, then 250 mg q6-8 hr to 1250 mg/day	See ibuprofen	See ibuprofen	
Naproxen sodium	Anaprox Rx	550 mg initially, then 275 mg q6-8 hr to 1375 mg/day	See ibuprofen	See ibuprofen	
	Aleve OTC	440 mg initially, then 220 mg q6-8 hr to 660 mg/day			

Pregnancy

ANTENATAL GLUCOCORTICOID THERAPY WITH BETAMETHASONE, DEXAMETHASONE

Action

- Stimulates fetal lung maturation by promoting release of enzymes that induce production or release of lung surfactant. NOTE: The FDA has not approved these medications for this use (i.e., this is an off-label use for obstetrics).

Indication

- To prevent or reduce the severity of respiratory distress syndrome in preterm infants between 24 and 34 weeks of gestation.

Dosage and Route

- Betamethasone: 12 mg IM × two doses 12 hours apart.
- Dexamethasone: 6 mg IM × two doses 12 hours apart.
- May be repeated in 7 days if birth has not occurred.

Adverse Reactions

- Possible maternal infection.
- Pulmonary edema (if given with beta-adrenergic medications).
- May worsen maternal condition (diabetes, hypertension).

Nursing Considerations

- Give deep intramuscular injection in gluteal muscle.
- Teach signs of pulmonary edema.
- Assess blood glucose levels and lung sounds.
- Do not give if woman has infection.
- Use in women with preterm premature rupture of membranes (PPROM) not universally recommended.

FDA, U.S. Food and Drug Administration; *IM,* intramuscularly.

Tocolytic Therapy for Preterm Labor

MEDICATION AND ACTION	DOSAGE AND ROUTE	ADVERSE REACTIONS	NURSING CONSIDERATIONS
Magnesium sulfate* CNS depressant; relaxes smooth muscles including uterus	Mix 40 g in 1000 ml IV solution, piggyback to primary infusion, and administer loading dose or bolus of 4-6 g using controller pump over 15-20 min Continue maintenance infusion at 1 g/hr, increasing to a maximum 3 g/hr until contractions stop or intolerable adverse reactions develop	During loading dose: • Hot flushes, sweating, nausea and vomiting, drowsiness, and blurred vision; usually subside when loading dose is completed Intolerable adverse reactions: • Respiratory rate <12 breaths/min • Absent DTRs • Severe hypotension • Extreme muscle weakness • Urine output <25-30 ml/hr • Serum magnesium level ≥10 mEq/L	Assess woman and fetus before and after each rate increase and following frequency of agency protocol Monitor serum magnesium levels; therapeutic level should range between 4 and 7.5 mEq/L Discontinue infusion and notify physician if intolerable adverse reactions occur Ensure that calcium gluconate is available for emergency administration to reverse magnesium sulfate toxicity Limit IV fluid intake to 125 ml/hr

Terbutaline* (Brethine)	Subcutaneous	Similar to Ritodrine	Teach woman and

Terbutaline* (Brethine)

Beta-adrenergic agonist relaxes smooth muscles, inhibiting uterine activity and causing bronchodilation

Subcutaneous injection:
- 0.25 mg q30 min for 2 hr
- Maximum dose: 0.5 mg q4-6 hr

Subcutaneous pump:
- Maintenance dose 0.05-0.1 mg/hr
- Bolus: 0.25 mg q4-6 hr according to contraction pattern
- 3 mg/24 hr maximum dose

Similar to Ritodrine

Teach woman and family:
- Assessment measures: pulse, BP, respiratory effort, insertion site for infection, signs of PTL, and adverse reactions to terbutaline
- Whom to call if problems or concerns arise
- Site care and pump maintenance
- Activity restrictions

Arrange for follow-up and home care

Nifedipine* (Procardia; Adalat)

Calcium channel blocker; relaxes smooth muscles including the uterus

Initial dose: 10-20 mg PO

Maintenance dose: 10-20 mg q4-6 hr PO

Transient tachycardia, palpitations

Hypotension

Dizziness, headache, nervousness

Peripheral edema

Fatigue

Do not use with magnesium sulfate

Assess woman and fetus according to agency protocol, being alert for adverse reactions

*CAUTION: Not FDA approved for PTL (off-label use).

Continued

Tocolytic Therapy for Preterm Labor—cont'd

MEDICATION AND ACTION	DOSAGE AND ROUTE	ADVERSE REACTIONS	NURSING CONSIDERATIONS
by blocking calcium entry	Mix 150 mg in 500 ml isotonic IV solution	Nausea	Do not use sublingual route
Ritodrine (Yutopar)	Attach to controller pump, and piggyback to primary infusion	Facial flushing	Women should be screened with ECG before therapy begins; maternal heart disease and hypertension are contraindications
Beta-adrenergic agonist; relaxes smooth muscles, inhibiting uterine activity and causing bronchodilation	Begin infusion at 0.05-0.1 mg/min	IV adverse reactions:	
	Increase rate by 0.05 mg q10 min until contractions stop, intolerable adverse reactions develop, or a maximum dose of 0.35 mg/min is reached	• Shortness of breath, coughing, tachypnea, pulmonary edema	Use cautiously if woman has type 1 diabetes or hyperthyroidism
		• Tachycardia, palpitations, skipped beats	Validate that woman is in PTL and that pregnancy is >20 wk of gestation
	Maintain effective dose for 12-24 hr	• Chest pains	Assess woman and fetus before and after each rate increase and following
		• Hypotension	
		• Tremors, dizziness, nervousness	
		• Muscle cramps and weakness	
		• Headache	
		• Hyperglycemia; hypokalemia	
		• Nausea and vomiting	
		• Fetal tachycardia	

Oral administration
adverse reactions:
- GI distress
- Significant adverse effects are rare

frequency of agency protocol
Discontinue infusion and notify physician if:
- Maternal heart rate >120-140 beats/min; arrhythmias, chest pain
- BP <90/60 mmHg
- Fetal heart rate >180 beats/min
Ensure that propranolol (Inderal) is available to reverse adverse effects related to cardiovascular function

Continued

Tocolytic Therapy for Preterm Labor—cont'd

MEDICATION AND ACTION	DOSAGE AND ROUTE	ADVERSE REACTIONS	NURSING CONSIDERATIONS
Indomethacin* Prostaglandin inhibitor; relaxes uterine smooth muscle	Initial dose: 50 mg PO or rectally Maintenance dose: 25-50 mg q4-6 hr for 24-48 hr (PO)	Maternal: nausea and vomiting, dyspepsia, dizziness, oligohydramnios Fetal: premature closure of ductus arteriosus Neonate: bronchopulmonary dysplasia, respiratory distress syndrome, intracranial hemorrhage, necrotizing enterocolitis, hyperbilirubinemia	Used when other methods fail; not recommended after 32 wk of gestation Do not use in women with bleeding potential Fetal assessment: amniotic fluid level; function of ductus arteriosus

BP, Blood pressure; *CNS*, central nervous system; *DTRs*, deep tendon reflexes; *ECG*, electrocardiogram; *FDA*, U.S. Food and Drug Administration; *GI*, gastrointestinal; *IV*, intravenously; *PO*, by mouth; *PTL*, preterm labor.
*CAUTION: Not FDA approved for PTL (off-label use).

Labor

CERVICAL RIPENING USING PROSTAGLANDIN E$_1$ (PGE$_1$): MISOPROSTOL (Cytotec)

Action

- PGE$_1$ ripens the cervix, making it softer and causing it to begin to dilate and efface; stimulates uterine contractions.

Indications

- For preinduction cervical ripening (ripening of cervix before oxytocin induction of labor when the Bishop score is 4 or less).
- To induce labor or abortion (abortifacient agent).

Dosage and Route

- Insert 25 to 50 mcg ($\frac{1}{4}$ to $\frac{1}{2}$ of a 100-mcg tablet) intravaginally into the posterior fornix using the tips of index and middle fingers without the use of a lubricant. Repeat every 3 to 6 hours as needed to a maximum of 300 to 400 mcg in a 24-hour period or until an effective contraction pattern is established (three or more uterine contractions in 10 minutes), the cervix ripens (Bishop score of 8 or greater), or significant adverse reactions occur.
- Administer 50 to 100 mcg PO every 4 to 6 hours (GI effects increased; may be less effective; data insufficient to recommend giving orally).

Adverse Reactions

- Higher dosages are more likely to result in adverse reactions, such as nausea and vomiting, diarrhea, fever, tachysystole (12 or more uterine contractions in 20 minutes without alteration of FHR pattern), hyperstimulation of the uterus (tachysystole with nonreassuring FHR patterns), or fetal passage of meconium.

Nursing Considerations

- Explain procedure to woman and her family. Ensure that an informed consent has been obtained as per agency policy.
- Assess maternal-fetal unit before each insertion and during treatment, following agency protocol for frequency. Assess maternal vital signs and health status, FHR and pattern, and status of pregnancy, including indications for cervical ripening or induction of labor, signs of labor or impending labor, and the Bishop score. Recognize that a nonreassuring FHR and/or pattern; maternal fever, infection, vaginal bleeding, or hypersensitivity; and regular, progressive uterine contractions contraindicate the use of misoprostol.

- Use caution if the woman has a history of asthma; glaucoma; or renal, hepatic, or cardiovascular disorders.
- Have woman void before procedure.
- Assist woman to maintain a supine position with lateral tilt or a side-lying position for 30 to 40 minutes after insertion.
- Prepare to swab vagina to remove unabsorbed medication using a saline-soaked gauze wrapped around fingers and to administer terbutaline, 0.25 mg SC or IV, if significant adverse reactions occur.
- Initiate oxytocin for induction of labor no sooner than 4 hours after last dose of misoprostol was administered, following agency protocol, if ripening has occurred and labor has not begun.
- Document all assessment findings and administration procedures.
- Not recommended for use if woman has had previous cesarean birth or if she has a uterine scar.
- Misoprostol (Cytotec) has not yet been approved by the FDA for cervical ripening or labor induction.

FHR, Fetal heart rate; *GI,* gastrointestinal; *IV,* intravenously; *PO,* by mouth; *SC,* subcutaneously.

CERVICAL RIPENING USING PROSTAGLANDIN E$_2$ (PGE$_2$): DINOPROSTONE (Cervidil Insert, Prepidil Gel)

Action

- PGE$_2$ ripens the cervix, making it softer and causing it to begin to dilate and efface; stimulates uterine contractions.

Indications

- PGE$_2$ is used for preinduction cervical ripening (ripening of cervix before oxytocin induction of labor when the Bishop score is 4 or less) and for inducement of labor or abortion (abortifacient agent).

Dosage and Route

Cervidil insert

- Dosage is 10 mg of dinoprostone designed to be released gradually (approximately 0.3 mg/hr) over 12 hours. Insert is placed transversely into the posterior fornix of vagina. The insert is removed at the onset of active labor or after 12 hours.

Prepidil gel

- Dosage is 0.5 mg dinoprostone in 2.5-ml syringe. Gel is administered through a catheter attached to the syringe into the cervical canal just below internal cervical os. Dose may be repeated every 6 hours as needed for cervical ripening up to a maximum of 1.5 mg in a 24-hour period.

Adverse Reactions

- Potential adverse reactions include headache, nausea and vomiting, diarrhea, fever, hypotension, tachysystole (12 or more uterine contractions in 20 minutes without alteration of fetal heart rate [FHR] pattern), hyperstimulation of the uterus (tachysystole with nonreassuring FHR patterns), or fetal passage of meconium.

Nursing Considerations

- Explain procedure to woman and her family. Ensure that an informed consent has been obtained per agency policy.
- Assess maternal-fetal unit before each insertion and during treatment following agency protocol for frequency. Assess maternal vital signs and health status, FHR and pattern, and status of pregnancy, including indications for cervical ripening or induction of labor, signs of labor or impending labor, and the Bishop score. Recognize that a nonreassuring FHR and/or pattern; maternal fever, infection, vaginal bleeding, or hypersensitivity; and regular, progressive uterine contractions contraindicate the use of dinoprostone.
- Use caution if the woman has a history of asthma; glaucoma; or renal, hepatic, or cardiovascular disorders.
- Bring gel to room temperature before administration. Do not force warming process by using a warm water bath or other source of external heat (e.g., microwave).
- Keep insert frozen until immediately before use; no need to warm.
- Have woman void before insertion.
- Assist woman to maintain a supine position with lateral tilt or a side-lying position for 15 to 30 minutes after insertion of gel or for 2 hours after placement of insert.
- Prepare to swab vagina to remove remaining gel using a saline-soaked gauze, or pull string to remove insert and to administer terbutaline 0.25 mg SC or IV, if significant adverse reactions occur.
- Initiate oxytocin for induction of labor within 6 to 12 hours after last instillation of gel or within 30 minutes after removal of the insert or follow agency protocol for induction if ripening has occurred and labor has not begun.
- Document all assessment findings and administration procedures.
- Not recommended for use if woman has had previous cesarean birth or if she has a uterine scar.
- Dinoprostone is the only FDA-approved medication for cervical ripening or labor induction.

FDA, U.S. Food and Drug Administration; *IV,* intravenously; *SC,* subcutaneously.

Opioid Analgesics for Labor

MEPERIDINE (Demerol)

Action

- Opioid agonist analgesic; stimulates mu and kappa opioid receptors to decrease transmission of pain impulses.

Indications

- Labor pain.
- Postoperative pain after cesarean birth.

Dosage and Route

- 25 mg IV; 50 to 75 mg IM or SC.
- May repeat in 1 to 3 hours.
- Use of ataractic or antiemetic drugs may potentiate analgesic effect and decrease nausea and vomiting.

Adverse Reactions

- Nausea and vomiting.
- Sedation.
- Confusion.
- Drowsiness.
- Tachycardia or bradycardia.
- Hypotension.
- Dry mouth.
- Pruritus.
- Urinary retention.
- Respiratory depression (woman and newborn).
- Decreased fetal heart rate (FHR) variability.
- Decreased uterine activity if given in early labor.

Nursing Considerations

- Assess FHR and uterine activity.
- Observe for respiratory depression.
- If birth occurs within 1 to 4 hours of dose, observe newborn for respiratory depression.
- Have naloxone available as antidote.
- Keep side rails up.
- Continue use of nonpharmacologic pain relief measures.

IM, Intramuscularly; *IV,* intravascularly; *SC,* subcutaneously.

BUTORPHANOL TARTRATE (Stadol)

Action

- Mixed agonist-antagonist analgesic; stimulates kappa opioid receptor and blocks mu opioid receptor.

Indications

- Labor pain.
- Postoperative pain after cesarean birth.

Dosage and Route

- 1 mg IV every 3 to 4 hours; 2 mg IM every 3 to 4 hours.

Adverse Reactions

- Confusion, sedation, sweating.
- Transient sinusoidal-like FHR rhythm.
- Less respiratory depression than with meperidine.
- Nausea and vomiting.

Nursing Considerations

- See Meperidine.
- May precipitate withdrawal symptoms in opioid-dependent women and their newborns.

NALBUPHINE (Nubain)

Action

- Mixed agonist-antagonist analgesic; stimulates kappa opioid receptor and blocks mu opioid receptor.

Indications

- Labor pain.
- Postoperative pain after cesarean birth.

Dosage and Route

- 10 mg IV; 10 to 20 mg IM every 3 to 6 hours.

Adverse Reactions

- See Butorphanol.

Nursing Considerations

- See Butorphanol.

IM, Intramuscularly; *IV,* intravenously.

Postpartum

Drugs Used to Manage Postpartum Hemorrhage

DRUG	ACTION	SIDE EFFECTS	CONTRAINDICATIONS	DOSAGE AND ROUTE	NURSING CONSIDERATIONS
Oxytocin (Pitocin)	Contraction of uterus; decreases bleeding	Infrequent; water intoxication; nausea and vomiting	None for postpartum hemorrhage	10-40 units/L diluted in lactated Ringer's solution or normal saline at 125-200 milliunits/min IV or 10-20 units IM	Continue to monitor vaginal bleeding and uterine tone
Methylergonovine (Methergine)*	Contraction of uterus	Hypertension, nausea, vomiting, headache	Hypertension, cardiac disease	0.2 mg IM q2-4hr up to five doses; 0.2 mg IV only for emergency	Check blood pressure before giving and do not give if >140/90 mm Hg; continue monitoring vaginal bleeding and uterine tone
Prostaglandin F$_{2\alpha}$ (Prostin/15M; Hemabate)	Contraction of uterus	Headache, nausea, vomiting, fever	Asthma, hypersensitivity	0.25 mg IM or intramyometrially q15-90 min up to eight doses	Continue monitoring vaginal bleeding and uterine tone

IM, Intramuscularly; IV, intravenously.

*Information about methylergonovine may also be used to describe ergonovine (Ergotrate).

622

RH IMMUNE GLOBULIN, RHOGAM, GAMULIN RH, HYPRHO-D, RHOPHYLAC

Action

- Suppression of immune response in nonsensitized women with Rh-negative blood who receive Rh-positive blood cells because of feto-maternal hemorrhage, transfusion, or accident.

Indications

- Routine antepartum prevention at 20 to 30 weeks of gestation in women with Rh-negative blood.
- Suppress antibody formation after birth, miscarriage or pregnancy termination, abdominal trauma, ectopic pregnancy, amniocentesis, version, or chorionic villi sampling.

Dosage and Route

- Standard dose is 1 vial (300 mcg) IM in deltoid or gluteal muscle; microdose is 1 vial (50 mcg) IM in deltoid muscle; Rhophylac can be given IM or IV (available in prefilled syringes).

Adverse Reactions

- Myalgia, lethargy, localized tenderness and stiffness at injection site, mild and transient fever, malaise, headache.
- Rarely nausea, vomiting, hypotension, tachycardia, possible allergic response.

Nursing Considerations

- Give standard dose to mother at 28 weeks of gestation as prophylaxis or after an incident or exposure risk that occurs after 28 weeks of gestation (e.g., amniocentesis, second-trimester miscarriage or abortion, after external version attempt) and within 72 hours after birth if baby is Rh positive.
- Give microdose for first-trimester miscarriage or abortion, ectopic pregnancy, chorionic villus sampling.
- Verify that the woman is Rh negative and has not been sensitized, that Coombs' test is negative, and that baby is Rh positive. Provide explanation to the woman about procedure, including the purpose, possible side effects, and effect on future pregnancies. Have the woman sign a consent form if required by agency. Verify correct dosage and confirm lot number and woman's identity before giving injection (verify with another nurse or use other procedure per agency policy); document administration per agency policy. Observe patient for at least 20 minutes after administration for allergic response.
- The medication is made from human plasma (a consideration if woman is a Jehovah's Witness). The risk of transmitting infectious agents, including viruses, cannot be completely eliminated.

IM, Intramuscularly; *IV,* intravascularly.

Newborn

EYE PROPHYLAXIS: ERYTHROMYCIN OPHTHALMIC OINTMENT, 0.5%, AND TETRACYCLINE OPHTHALMIC OINTMENT, 1%

Action

- These antibiotic ointments are both bacteriostatic and bactericidal. They provide prophylaxis against *Neisseria gonorrhoeae* and *Chlamydia trachomatis.*

Indication

- These medications are applied to prevent ophthalmia neonatorum in newborns of mothers who are infected with gonorrhea, conjunctivitis, and chlamydia.

Neonatal Dosage and Route

- Apply a 1- to 2-cm ribbon of ointment to the lower conjunctival sac of each eye; also may be used in drop form.

Adverse Reactions

- May cause chemical conjunctivitis that lasts 24 to 48 hours.
- Vision may be blurred temporarily.

Nursing Considerations

- Administer within 1 to 2 hours of birth. Wear gloves. Cleanse eyes if necessary before administration. Open eyes by putting a thumb and finger at the corner of each lid and gently pressing on the periorbital ridges. Squeeze the tube, and spread the ointment from the inner canthus of the eye to the outer canthus. Do not touch the tube to the eye. After 1 minute, excess ointment may be wiped off. Observe eyes for irritation. Explain treatment to parents.
- Eye prophylaxis for ophthalmia neonatorum is required by law in all states of the United States.

VITAMIN K: PHYTONADIONE (AquaMEPHYTON, Konakion)

Action

- This intervention provides vitamin K because the newborn does not have the intestinal flora to produce this vitamin in the first week after birth. It also promotes formation of clotting factors (II, VII, IX, and X) in the liver.

Indication

- Vitamin K is used for prevention and treatment of hemorrhagic disease in the newborn.

Neonatal Dosage and Route

- Administer a 0.5- to 1-mg (0.25- to 0.5-ml) dose IM within 2 hours of birth; may be repeated if newborn shows bleeding tendencies.

Adverse Reactions

- Edema, erythema, and pain at injection site may occur rarely.
- Hemolysis, jaundice, and hyperbilirubinemia have been reported, particularly in preterm infants.

Nursing Considerations

- Wear gloves. Administer in the middle third of the vastus lateralis muscle by using a 25-gauge, 5/8-inch needle. Inject into skin that has been cleaned, or allow alcohol to dry on puncture site for 1 minute to remove organisms and prevent infection. Stabilize leg firmly, and grasp muscle between the thumb and fingers. Insert the needle at a 90-degree angle, release muscle, aspirate, and inject medication slowly if there is no blood return. Massage the site with a dry gauze square after removing needle to increase absorption. Observe for signs of bleeding from the site.

IM, Intramuscularly.

HEPATITIS B VACCINE (Recombivax HB, Engerix-B)

Action

- Hepatitis B vaccine induces protective anti–hepatitis B antibodies in 95% to 99% of healthy infants who receive the recommended three doses. The duration of protection of the vaccine is unknown.

Indication

- Hepatitis B vaccine is for immunization against infection caused by all known subtypes of hepatitis B virus (HBV).

Neonatal Dosage and Route

- The usual dosage is Recombivax HB, 5 mg/0.5 ml, or Engerix-B, 10 mg/0.5 ml IM, at 0, 1, and 6 months.: An alternate dosing schedule is 0, 1, 2, and 12 months and is usually for newborns whose mothers were hepatitis B surface antigen (HBsAg) positive.

Adverse Reactions

- Common adverse reactions are rash, fever, erythema, swelling, and pain at injection site.

Nursing Considerations

- Parental consent must be obtained before administration.
- Wear gloves. Administer in the middle third of the vastus lateralis muscle by using a 25-gauge, 5/8-inch needle. Inject into skin that has been cleaned, or allow alcohol to dry on puncture site for 1 minute to remove organisms and prevent infection. Stabilize leg firmly, and grasp muscle between the thumb and fingers. Insert the needle at a 90-degree angle, aspirate, and inject medication slowly if there is no blood return. Massage the site with a dry gauze square after removing needle to increase absorption.
- If the infant was born to an HBsAg-positive mother, hepatitis B immune globulin (HBIG) should be given within 12 hours of birth in addition to the HB vaccine. Separate sites must be used.

HEPATITIS B IMMUNE GLOBULIN

Action

- Hepatitis B immune globulin (HBIG) provides a high titer of antibody to hepatitis B surface antigen (HBsAg).

Indication

- The HBIG vaccine provides prophylaxis against infection in infants born of HBsAg-positive mothers.

Neonatal Dosage and Route

- Administer one 0.5-ml dose intramuscularly within 12 hours of birth.

Adverse Reactions

- Hypersensitivity may occur.

Nursing Considerations

- Must be given within 12 hours of birth.
- Wear gloves. Administer in the middle third of the vastus lateralis muscle by using a 25-gauge, ⅝-inch needle. Inject into skin that has been cleaned, or allow alcohol to dry on puncture site for 1 minute to remove organisms and prevent infection. Stabilize leg firmly, and grasp muscle between the thumb and fingers. Insert the needle at a 90-degree angle, release muscle, aspirate, and inject medication slowly if there is no blood return. Massage the site with a dry gauze square after removing needle to increase absorption.
- May be given at same time as hepatitis B vaccine but at a different site.

NALOXONE (Narcan)

Action
- Opioid antagonist.

Indications
- Reverses opioid-induced respiratory depression in woman or newborn.
- May be used to reverse pruritus from epidural opioids.

Dosage and Route

Adult
- Narcotic overdose: 0.4 to 2 mg IV, may repeat IV dose at 2- to 3-minute intervals up to 10 mg; if IV route unavailable, IM or SC administration may be used.
- Postoperative narcotic depression: initial dose 0.1 to 0.2 mg IV at 2- to 3-minute intervals to desired degree of reversal; may repeat dose in 1 to 2 hours if needed.

Newborn
- Narcotic-induced depression: initial dose is 0.01 mg/kg IV, IM, or SC; may be repeated at 2- to 3-minute intervals until desired degree of reversal obtained.

Adverse Reactions
- Maternal hypotension and hypertension.
- Maternal tachycardia.
- Maternal nausea and vomiting.
- Maternal sweating.
- Maternal tremulousness.

Nursing Considerations
- Woman should delay breastfeeding until medication is out of system.
- Do not give if woman is opioid dependent—may cause abrupt withdrawal; if given to woman for reversal of respiratory depression caused by opioid analgesic, pain will return suddenly.

IM, Intramuscularly; *IV,* intravenously; *SC,* subcutaneously.

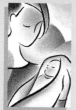

Standard Precautions

Medical history and examination cannot reliably identify all persons infected with human immunodeficiency virus (HIV) or other blood-borne pathogens. Standard Precautions should therefore be used consistently in the care of all persons. These precautions apply to blood, body fluids, and all secretions and excretions, except sweat, nonintact skin, and mucous membranes. Standard Precautions are recommended to reduce the risk of transmission of microorganisms from known and unknown sources of infection.

1. Prompt and thorough handwashing is recommended between patient contacts. Hands and other skin surfaces should be washed immediately and thoroughly if contaminated with blood or other body fluids. Hands should be washed immediately after gloves are removed.

2. In addition to handwashing, all health care workers should routinely use appropriate barrier precautions to prevent skin and mucous membrane exposure when contact with blood or other body fluids of any person is anticipated. Latex gloves should be worn for touching blood and body fluids, mucous membranes, or nonintact skin of all persons; for handling items or surfaces soiled with blood or body fluids; and for performing venipuncture and other vascular access procedures. Gloves should be changed after contact with each patient. Masks and protective eyewear or face shields should be worn during procedures that are likely to generate droplets of blood or other body fluids to prevent exposure of mucous membranes of the mouth, nose, and eyes. Gowns or aprons should be worn during procedures that are likely to generate splashes of blood or other body fluids. Leg coverings, boots, or shoe covers also can be worn to provide protection against splashes and may be recommended for certain procedures, such as surgery.

3. All health care workers should take precautions to prevent injuries caused by needles, scalpels, and other sharp instruments or devices during procedures; when cleaning used instruments; during disposal

629

of used needles; and when handling sharp instruments after procedures. To prevent needlestick injuries, needles should not be recapped, purposely bent or broken by hand, removed from disposable syringes, or otherwise manipulated by hand. After they are used, disposable syringes and needles, scalpel blades, and other sharp items should be immediately placed in a puncture-resistant container for disposal; puncture-resistant containers should be located as close as practical to the use area.

4. Although saliva has not been implicated in HIV transmission, mouthpieces, resuscitation bags, or other ventilation devices should be available for use in areas in which the need for resuscitation is predictable, thus minimizing the chance for emergency mouth-to-mouth resuscitation.

5. Health care workers who have exudative lesions or weeping dermatitis should refrain from all direct patient care and from handling patient care equipment until the condition resolves.

PRECAUTIONS FOR INVASIVE PROCEDURES

An invasive procedure is surgical entry into tissues, cavities, or organs for (1) repair of major traumatic injuries in an operating or birthing room, emergency department, or out-of-hospital setting, including both physicians' and dentists' offices; or (2) a vaginal or cesarean birth or other invasive obstetric procedure during which bleeding may occur. Standard Precautions, combined with the following precautions, should serve as minimum precautions for all such invasive procedures:

1. All health care workers who participate in invasive procedures must routinely use appropriate barrier precautions to prevent skin and mucous membrane contact with blood and other body fluids of all patients. Gloves and surgical masks must be worn for all invasive procedures. Protective eyewear or face shields should be worn for procedures that commonly result in the generation of droplets, splashing of blood or other body fluids, or generation of bone chips. Gowns or aprons made of materials that provide an effective barrier should be worn during invasive procedures that are likely to result in the splashing of blood or other body fluids. All health care workers who perform or assist in vaginal or cesarean births should wear gloves and gowns when handling the placenta or the infant until blood and amniotic fluid have been removed from the infant's skin. Gloves should be worn during infant eye prophylaxis, care of the umbilical cord, circumcision site procedures, parenteral proce-

dures, diaper changes, contact with colostrum, and postpartum assessments.

2. If a glove is torn or a needlestick or other injury occurs, the glove should be removed and a new glove used as promptly as patient safety permits; the needle or instrument involved in the incident also should be removed from the sterile field.

3. Any needlestick or other injury should be reported and appropriate treatment obtained as specified by the health care facility.

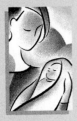

Temperature Equivalents and Conversion of Pounds and Ounces to Grams for Newborn Weights

TEMPERATURE EQUIVALENTS

CELSIUS	FAHRENHEIT	CELSIUS	FAHRENHEIT
34.0	93.2	38.6	101.4
34.2	93.6	38.8	101.8
34.4	93.9	39.0	102.2
34.6	94.3	39.2	102.5
34.8	94.6	39.4	102.9
35.0	95.0	39.6	103.2
35.2	95.4	39.8	103.6
35.4	95.7	40.0	104.0
35.6	96.1	40.2	104.3
35.8	96.4	40.4	104.7
36.0	96.8	40.6	105.1
36.2	97.1	40.8	105.4
36.4	97.5	41.0	105.8
36.6	97.8	41.2	106.1
36.8	98.2	41.4	106.5
<u>37.0</u>	<u>98.6</u>	41.6	106.8
37.2	98.9	41.8	107.2
37.4	99.3	42.0	107.6
37.6	99.6	42.2	108.0
37.8	100.0	42.4	108.3
38.0	100.4	42.6	108.7
38.2	100.7	42.8	109.0
38.4	101.1	43.0	109.4

To convert Fahrenheit to Celsius:

$$(\text{Temperature} - 32) \times 5/9$$

EXAMPLE: To convert 98.6° Fahrenheit to Celsius:

$$98.6 - 32 = 66.6 \times 5/9 = 37° \text{ Celsius}$$

To convert Celsius to Fahrenheit:

$$(9/5 \times \text{Temperature}) + 32$$

EXAMPLE: To convert 40° Celsius to Fahrenheit:

$$9/5 \times 40 = 72 + 32 = 104° \text{ Fahrenheit}$$

Conversion of Pounds and Ounces to Grams for Newborn Weights*

OUNCES

POUNDS	0	1	2	3	4	5	6	7	8	9	10	11	12	13	14	15
0	—	28	57	85	113	142	170	198	227	255	283	312	340	369	397	425
1	454	482	510	539	567	595	624	652	680	709	737	765	794	822	850	879
2	907	936	964	992	1021	1049	1077	1106	1134	1162	1191	1219	1247	1276	1304	1332
3	1361	1389	1417	1446	1474	1503	1531	1559	1588	1616	1644	1673	1701	1729	1758	1786
4	1814	1843	1871	1899	1928	1956	1984	2013	2041	2070	2093	2126	2155	2183	2211	2240
5	2268	2296	2325	2353	2381	2410	2438	2466	2495	2523	2551	2580	2608	2637	2665	2693
6	2722	2750	2778	2807	2835	2863	2892	2920	2948	2977	3005	3033	3062	3090	3118	3147
7	3175	3203	3232	3260	3289	3317	3345	3374	3402	3430	3459	3487	3515	3544	3572	3600
8	3629	3657	3685	3714	3742	3770	3799	3827	3856	3884	3912	3941	3969	3997	4026	4054
9	4082	4111	4139	4167	4196	4224	4252	4281	4309	4337	4366	4394	4423	4451	4479	4508
10	4536	4564	4593	4621	4649	4678	4706	4734	4763	4791	4819	4848	4876	4904	4933	4961
11	4990	5018	5046	5075	5103	5131	5160	5188	5216	5245	5273	5301	5330	5358	5386	5415
12	5443	5471	5500	5528	5557	5585	5613	5642	5670	5698	5727	5755	5783	5812	5840	5868
13	5897	5925	5953	5982	6010	6038	6067	6095	6123	6152	6180	6209	6237	6265	6294	6322
14	6350	6379	6407	6435	6464	6492	6520	6549	6577	6605	6634	6662	6690	6719	6747	6776
15	6804	6832	6860	6889	6917	6945	6973	7002	7030	7059	7087	7115	7144	7172	7201	7228

OUNCES

*To convert pounds and ounces to grams, multiply the pounds by 453.6 and the ounces by 28.35; add the totals. To convert grams into pounds and decimals of a pound, multiply the grams by 0.0022. To convert grams into ounces, divide the grams by 28.35 (16 oz = 1 lb).

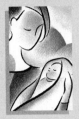

NANDA Nursing Diagnoses 2005-2006

Activity intolerance
Activity intolerance, risk for
Adjustment, impaired
Airway clearance, ineffective
Allergy response, latex
Allergy response, latex, risk for
Anxiety
Anxiety, death
Aspiration, risk for
Attachment, impaired parent/infant/child, risk for
Autonomic dysreflexia
Autonomic dysreflexia, risk for
Body image, disturbed
Body temperature, imbalanced, risk for
Bowel incontinence
Breastfeeding, effective
Breastfeeding, ineffective
Breastfeeding, interrupted
Breathing pattern, ineffective
Cardiac output, decreased
Caregiver role strain
Caregiver role strain, risk for
Comfort, impaired
Communication, verbal, impaired
Communication, readiness for enhanced
Conflict, decisional (specify)
Conflict, parental role
Confusion, acute
Confusion, chronic
Constipation
Constipation, perceived
Constipation, risk for

Coping, ineffective
Coping, readiness for enhanced
Coping, community, ineffective
Coping, community, readiness for enhanced
Coping, defensive
Coping, family, compromised
Coping, family, disabled
Coping, family, readiness for enhanced
Death syndrome, sudden infant, risk for
Denial, ineffective
Dentition, impaired
Development, delayed, risk for
Diarrhea
Disuse syndrome, risk for
Diversional activity, deficient
Energy field, disturbed
Environmental interpretation syndrome, impaired
Failure to thrive, adult
Falls, risk for
Family processes: alcoholism, dysfunctional
Family processes, interrupted
Family processes, readiness for enhanced
Fatigue
Fear
Fluid balance, readiness for enhanced
Fluid volume, deficient
Fluid volume, excess
Fluid volume, deficient, risk for
Fluid volume, imbalanced, risk for
Gas exchange, impaired
Grieving
Grieving, anticipatory
Grieving, dysfunctional
Grieving, risk for dysfunctional
Growth and development, delayed
Growth disproportionate, risk for
Health maintenance, ineffective
Health-seeking behaviors
Home maintenance, impaired
Hopelessness
Hyperthermia
Hypothermia
Identity, personal, disturbed
Incontinence, urinary, functional

Incontinence, urinary, reflex
Incontinence, urinary, stress
Incontinence, urinary, total
Incontinence, urinary, urge
Incontinence, urinary, urge, risk for
Infant behavior, disorganized
Infant behavior, disorganized, risk for
Infant behavior, organized, readiness for enhanced
Feeding pattern, infant, ineffective
Infection, risk for
Injury, risk for
Injury, perioperative positioning, risk for
Intracranial adaptive capacity, decreased
Knowledge, deficient
Knowledge of (specify), readiness for enhanced
Lifestyle, sedentary
Loneliness, risk for
Memory, impaired
Mobility, bed, impaired
Mobility, physical, impaired
Mobility, wheelchair, impaired
Nausea
Neglect, unilateral
Noncompliance
Nutrition, readiness for enhanced
Nutrition: less than body requirements, imbalanced
Nutrition: more than body requirements, imbalanced
Nutrition: more than body requirements, risk for imbalanced
Oral mucous membrane, impaired
Pain, acute
Pain, chronic
Parenting, readiness for enhanced
Parenting, impaired
Parenting, impaired, risk for
Peripheral neurovascular dysfunction, risk for
Poisoning, risk for
Post-trauma syndrome
Post-trauma syndrome, risk for
Powerlessness
Powerlessness, risk for
Protection, ineffective
Rape-trauma syndrome
Rape-trauma syndrome: compound reaction
Rape-trauma syndrome: silent reaction

Religiosity, impaired
Religiosity, readiness for enhanced
Religiosity, risk for impaired
Relocation stress syndrome
Relocation stress syndrome, risk for
Role performance, ineffective
Self-care deficit, bathing/hygiene
Self-care deficit, dressing/grooming
Self-care deficit, feeding
Self-care deficit, toileting
Self-concept, readiness for enhanced
Self-esteem, chronic low
Self-esteem, situational low
Self-esteem, situational low, risk for
Self-mutilation
Self-mutilation, risk for
Sensory perception, disturbed
Sexual dysfunction
Sexuality patterns, ineffective
Skin integrity, impaired
Skin integrity, impaired, risk for
Sleep deprivation
Sleep patterns, disturbed
Sleep, readiness for enhanced
Social interaction, impaired
Social isolation
Sorrow, chronic
Spiritual distress
Spiritual distress, risk for
Spiritual well-being, readiness for enhanced
Suffocation, risk for
Suicide, risk for
Surgical recovery, delayed
Swallowing, impaired
Therapeutic regimen management, effective
Therapeutic regimen management, ineffective
Therapeutic regimen management, readiness for enhanced
Therapeutic regimen management, community, ineffective
Therapeutic regimen management, family, ineffective
Thermoregulation, ineffective
Thought processes, disturbed
Tissue integrity, impaired
Tissue perfusion, ineffective
Transfer ability, impaired

Trauma, risk for
Urinary elimination, readiness for enhanced
Urinary elimination, impaired
Urinary retention
Ventilation, spontaneous, impaired
Ventilatory weaning response, dysfunctional
Violence, other-directed, risk for
Violence, self-directed, risk for
Walking, impaired
Wandering

North American Nursing Diagnosis Association (2005). *Nursing diagnoses: Definitions and classification 2005-2006.* Philadelphia: NANDA.

JCAHO "Do Not Use" List

ABBREVIATION	POTENTIAL PROBLEM	PREFERRED TERM
U (for unit)	Mistaken as zero, four, or cc.	Write "unit."
IU (for international unit)	Mistaken as IV (intravenous) or 10 (ten).	Write "international unit."
Q.D., Q.O.D. (Latin abbreviations for once daily and every other day)	Mistaken for each other. The period after the Q can be mistaken for an "I." The "O" can be mistaken for "I."	Write "daily" and "every other day."
Trailing zero (X.0 mg); lack of leading zero (.X mg)	Decimal point is missed.	Never write a zero by itself after a decimal point (X mg), and always use a zero before a decimal point (0.X mg).
MS MSO₄ MgSO₄	Confused for one another. Can mean morphine sulfate or magnesium sulfate.	Write "morphine sulfate" or "magnesium sulfate."

Source: "Do not use" list required in 2004. (2003). *LTC Update,* Issue 3.

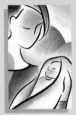

Traditional Cultural Beliefs and Practices: Childbearing and Parenting

Traditional* Cultural Beliefs and Practices: Childbearing and Parenting

PREGNANCY	CHILDBIRTH	PARENTING
HISPANIC (Based primarily on knowledge of Mexican-Americans; members of the Hispanic community have their origins in Spain, Cuba, Central and South America, Mexico, Puerto Rico, and other Spanish-speaking countries.)		
Pregnancy Pregnancy desired soon after marriage Late prenatal care	**Labor** Use of "partera" or lay midwife preferred in some places; may prefer presence of mother rather than husband	**Newborn** Breastfeeding begun after third day; colostrum may be considered "filthy" or "spoiled"

Data from Amaro, H. (1994). Women in the Mexican-American community: Religion, culture, and reproductive attitudes and experiences. *Journal of Comparative Psychology, 16*(1), 6-19; Bar-Yam, N. (1994). Learning about culture: A guide for birth practitioners. *International Journal of Childbirth Education, 9*(2), 8-10; Galanti, G. (1997). *Caring for patients from different cultures: Case studies from American hospitals* (2nd ed.). Philadelphia: University of Pennsylvania Press; D'Avanzo, C., & Geissler, E. (2003). *Pocket guide to cultural assessment* (3rd ed.). St. Louis: Mosby; Mattson, S. (1995). Culturally sensitive prenatal care for Southeastern Asians. *Journal of Obstetric, Gynecologic, and Neonatal Nursing, 24*(4), 335-341; Spector, R. (2004). *Cultural diversity in health and illness* (6th ed.). Upper Saddle River, NJ: Prentice Hall Health; and Williams, R. (1989). Issues in women's health care. In B. Johnson (Ed.), *Psychiatric mental health nursing: Adaptation and growth.* Philadelphia: JB Lippincott.

NOTE: Most of these cultural beliefs and customs reflect the traditional culture and are not universally practiced. These lists are not intended to stereotype patients but rather to serve as guidelines while discussing meaningful cultural beliefs with a patient and her family. Examples of other cultural beliefs and practices are found throughout this text.

*Variations in some beliefs and practices exist within subcultures of each group.

Continued

Traditional Cultural Beliefs and Practices: Childbearing and Parenting—cont'd

PREGNANCY	CHILDBIRTH	PARENTING
Expectant mother influenced strongly by mother or mother-in-law	After birth of baby, mother's legs brought together to prevent air from entering uterus	Olive oil or castor oil given to stimulate passage of meconium
Cool air in motion considered dangerous during pregnancy	Loud behavior in labor	Male infant not circumcised
Unsatisfied food cravings thought to cause a birthmark	**Postpartum**	Female infant's ears pierced
Some pica observed in the eating of ashes or dirt (not common)	Diet may be restricted after birth; for first 2 days only boiled milk and toasted tortillas permitted (special foods to restore warmth to body)	Belly band used to prevent umbilical hernia
Milk avoided because it causes large babies and difficult births	Bed rest for 3 days after birth	Religious medal worn by mother during pregnancy; placed around infant's neck
Many predictions about gender of baby	Keep warm	Infant protected from "evil eye"
May be unacceptable and frightening to have pelvic examination by male health care provider	Delay bathing	Various remedies used to treat "mal ojo" (evil eye) and fallen fontanel (depressed fontanel)
	Mother's head and feet protected from cold air;	

Continued

Use of herbs to treat common complaints of pregnancy

Drinking chamomile tea thought to ensure effective labor

bathing permitted after 14 days

Mother often cared for by her own mother

40-day restriction on sexual intercourse

Newborn

Feeding very important: "Good" baby thought to eat well

Early introduction of solid foods

May breastfeed or bottle-feed; breastfeeding may be considered embarrassing

Parents fearful of spoiling baby

Commonly call baby by nicknames

AFRICAN-AMERICAN

(Members of the African-American community, many of whom are descendants of slaves, have different origins. Today a number of black Americans have emigrated from Africa, the West Indian Islands, the Dominican Republic, Haiti, and Jamaica.)

Pregnancy

Acceptance of pregnancy depends on economic status

Pregnancy thought to be state of "wellness," which is often the reason for delay in seeking prenatal care, especially by lower-income African-Americans

"Old wives' tales" include having a picture taken during pregnancy will cause stillbirth and reaching up will cause cord to strangle baby

Labor

Use of "granny midwife" in certain parts of United States

Varied emotional responses: some cry out, some display stoic behavior to avoid calling attention to selves

Patient may arrive at hospital in far-advanced labor

Emotional support often provided by other women, especially own mother

Traditional Cultural Beliefs and Practices: Childbearing and Parenting—cont'd

PREGNANCY	CHILDBIRTH	PARENTING
Craving for certain foods, including chicken, greens, clay, starch, and dirt Pregnancy may be viewed by African-American men as a sign of their virility Self-treatment for various discomforts of pregnancy, including constipation, nausea, vomiting, headache, and heartburn	**Postpartum** Vaginal bleeding seen as sign of sickness; tub baths and shampooing of hair prohibited Sassafras tea thought to have healing power Eating liver thought to cause heavier vaginal bleeding because of its high "blood" content	May use excessive clothing to keep baby warm Belly band used to prevent umbilical hernia Abundant use of oil on baby's scalp and skin Strong feeling of family, community, and religion

ASIAN-AMERICAN
(Typically refers to groups from China, Korea, the Philippines, Japan, Southeast Asia [particularly Thailand], Indochina, and Vietnam.)

Pregnancy

Pregnancy considered time when mother "has happiness in her body"

Pregnancy seen as natural process

Strong preference for female health care provider

Belief in theory of hot and cold

May omit soy sauce in diet to prevent dark-skinned baby

Prefer soup made with ginseng root as general strength tonic

Milk usually excluded from diet because it causes stomach distress

Inactivity or sleeping late may cause difficult delivery

Labor

Mother attended by other women, especially her own mother

Father does not actively participate

Labor in silence

Cesarean birth not desired

Postpartum

Must protect self from yin (cold forces) for 30 days

Ambulation limited

Shower and bathing prohibited

Warm room

Diet:

Warm fluids

Some patients are vegetarians

Korean mother served seaweed soup with rice

Chinese diet high in hot foods

Chinese mother avoids fruits and vegetables

Newborn

Concept of family important and valued

Father is head of household; wife plays a subordinate role

Birth of boy preferred

May delay naming child

Some groups (e.g., Vietnamese) believe colostrum is dirty; therefore they may delay breastfeeding until milk comes in

Continued

Traditional Cultural Beliefs and Practices: Childbearing and Parenting—cont'd

PREGNANCY	CHILDBIRTH	PARENTING
EUROPEAN-AMERICAN (Members of the European-American [Caucasian] community have their origins in countries such as Ireland, Great Britain, Germany, Italy, and France.)		
Pregnancy Pregnancy viewed as a condition that requires medical attention to ensure health Emphasis on early prenatal care Variety of childbirth education programs available and participation encouraged Technology driven Emphasis on nutritional science	**Labor** Birth is a public concern Technology dominated Birthing process in institutional setting valued Involvement of father expected Physician seen as head of team **Postpartum** Emphasis or focus on early bonding	**Newborn** Increased popularity of breastfeeding Breastfeeding begins as soon as possible after childbirth **Parenting** Motherhood and transition to parenting seen as stressful time Nuclear family valued, although single parenting and other forms of parenting more acceptable than in the past

Involvement of the father valued

Written source of information valued

Medical interventions for dealing with discomfort

Early ambulation and activity emphasized

Self-care valued

Women often deal with multiple roles

Early return to prenatal activities

NATIVE AMERICAN

(Many different tribes exist within the Native-American culture; viewpoints vary according to tribal customs and beliefs.)

Pregnancy
Pregnancy considered as a normal, natural process
Late prenatal care
Avoid heavy lifting
Herb teas encouraged

Labor
Prefers female attendant, although husband, mother, or father may assist with birth
Birth may be attended by whole family
Herbs may be used to promote uterine activity
Birth may occur in squatting position

Postpartum
Herb teas to stop bleeding

Newborn
Infant not fed colostrum
Use of herbs to increase flow of milk
Use of cradle boards for infant
Babies not handled often

Bibliography

American Academy of Pediatrics (AAP) & American College of Obstetricians and Gynecologists (ACOG). (2002). *Guidelines for perinatal care* (5th ed.). Washington, DC: AAP & AGOG.

American Academy of Pediatrics (AAP) Section on Breastfeeding. (2005). Breastfeeding and the use of human milk. *Pediatrics, 115* (2), 496-506.

American Academy of Pediatrics, Committee on Genetics. (1996). Newborn screening fact sheets. *Pediatrics, 98* (3), 473-481.

American Academy of Pediatrics, Committee on Infectious Diseases. (2003). *Red book: 2003 report of the committee on infectious diseases* (26th ed.). Elk Grove Village, IL: The Academy.

American Academy of Pediatrics, Subcommittee on hyperbilirubinemia. (2004). Clinical Practice Guideline: Management of hyperbilirubinemia in the newborn infant 35 or more weeks of gestation. *Pediatrics, 114* (1), 297-316.

American Cancer Society (ACS). (2004). *Breast cancer.* Internet document available at http://www.cancer.org (accessed April 12, 2006).

American Cancer Society (ACS). (2006). *Cancer facts and figures 2006.* New York: ACS.

American College of Nurse-Midwives (ACNM). (2002). Abnormal and dysfunctional uterine bleeding. ACNM clinical bulletin No. 6. *Journal of Midwifery & Women's Health, 47* (3), 207-213.

American College of Obstetricians and Gynecologists (ACOG). (2003). Immunization during pregnancy. ACOG Committee Opinion No. 282. *Obstetrics and Gynecology, 101* (1), 207-212.

American College of Obstetricians and Gynecologists (ACOG). (2004). *Nausea and vomiting of pregnancy. ACOG practice bulletin No. 52.* Washington, DC: ACOG.

American College of Obstetricians and Gynecologists (ACOG). (2002). *Diagnosis and management of preclampsia and eclampsia. ACOG practice bulletin No. 33.* Washington, DC: ACOG.

American College of Obstetricians and Gynecologists (ACOG). (1998). *Postpartum hemorrhage. ACOG educational bulletin No. 243.* Washington, DC: ACOG.

American College of Obstetricians and Gynecologists (ACOG). (2000). *Scheduled cesarean delivery and prevention of vertical transmission of HIV infection. ACOG committee opinion No. 234*. Washington, DC: ACOG.

American College of Obstetricians and Gynecologists (ACOG). (2001). *Gestational diabetes. ACOG practice bulletin No. 30*. Washington, DC: ACOG.

American Dietetic Association (ADA). (2002). Position of the American Dietetic Association: Nutrition and lifestyle for a healthy pregnancy. *Journal of the American Dietetic Association, 102* (10), 1479-1490.

American Diabetes Association (ADA). (2004a). Gestational diabetes mellitus. *Diabetes Care, 27* (Suppl 1), S88-S90.

American Diabetes Association (ADA). (2003). Preconception care of women with diabetes. *Diabetes Care, 26* (Suppl 1), S91-S93.

American Diabetes Association (ADA). (2004b). Nutrition principles and recommendations in diabetes. *Diabetes Care, 27* (Suppl 1), S36-S46.

American Heart Association. (2005). American Heart Association guidelines for cardiopulmonary resuscitation and emergency cardiovascular care, Part 10.8: Cardiac arrest associated with pregnancy. *Circulation, 112* (24 Suppl), IV150-IV153.

American Heart Association Science Advisory. (2000). Assessment of functional capacity in clinical and research applications. *Circulation, 102* (13), 1591-1597.

American Psychiatric Association. (2000). *Diagnostic and statistical manual of mental disorders* (DSM-IV-TR) (4th ed., text revision). Washington, DC: American Psychiatric Association Press.

Aminoff, M. (2004). Neurologic disorders. In R. Creasy, R. Resnik, & J. Iams (Eds.), *Maternal-fetal medicine: Principles and practice* (5th ed.). Philadelphia: Saunders.

Ananth, C., Demissie, K., Smulian, J., & Vintzileos, A. (2001). Relationship among placenta previa, fetal growth restriction, and preterm delivery: A population-based study. *Obstetrics & Gynecology, 98* (2), 299-306.

Andres, R. (2004). Effects of therapeutic, diagnostic, and environmental agents and exposure to social and illicit drugs. In R. Creasy, R. Resnik, & J. Iams (Eds.), *Maternal-fetal medicine: Principles and practice* (5th ed.). Philadelphia: Saunders.

Anotayanonth, S., Subhedar, N., Garner, P., Neilson, J., & Harigopal, S. (2004). Betamimetics for inhibiting preterm labour. *Cochrane Database Systematic Reviews*, Issue 4, CD004352.

Association of Women's Health, Obstetric, and Neonatal Nurses (AWHONN). (2001). *Evidence-based clinical practice guideline: Neonatal skin care.* Washington, DC: The Association.

Association of Women's Health, Obstetric and Neonatal Nurses (AWHONN). (2003). *Fetal heart monitoring principles and practice* (3rd ed.). Dubuque, IA: Kendall/Hunt.

Ballard, J., Novak, K., & Driver, M. (1979). A simplified score for assessment of fetal maturity of newly born infants. *Journal of Pediatrics, 95* (5 Part 1), 769-774.

Balsells, M., Corcoy, R., Adelantado, J., Garcia-Patterson, A., Altirriba, O., & de Leiva, A. (2000). Gestational diabetes mellitus: Metabolic control during labour. *Diabetes, Nutrition & Metabolism, 13* (5), 257-262.

Bascom, A. (2002). *Incorporating herbal medicine into clinical practice.* Philadelphia: FA Davis.

Baskett, T. (2002). Shoulder dystocia. *Best Practices Research in Clinical Obstetrics and Gynaecology, 16* (10), 57-68.

Baxley, E., & Gobbo, R. (2004). Shoulder dystocia. *American Family Physician, 69* (7), 1707-1714.

Beck, L., Johnson, C., Morrow, B., Lipscomb, L., Gaffield, M., Colley Gilbert, B., Rogers, M., & Whitehead, N. (2003). *PRAMS 1999 surveillance report.* Atlanta: Division of Reproductive Health, National Center for Chronic Disease Prevention and Health Promotion, Centers for Disease Control and Prevention.

Bell, S. (2004). Pointers in practical pharmacology: Highly active antiretroviral therapy in neonates and young infants. *Neonatal Network, 23* (2), 55-64.

Benedetti, T. (2002). Obstetric hemorrhage. In S. Gabbe, J. Niebyl, & J. Simpson (Eds.), *Obstetrics: Normal and problem pregnancies* (4th ed.). New York: Churchill Livingstone.

Berg, T., & Smith, C. (2002). Pharmacologic therapy for peripartum emergencies. *Clinical Obstetrics & Gynecology, 45* (1), 125-135.

Bernasko, J. (2004). Contemporary management of type 1 diabetes mellitus in pregnancy. *Obstetrical and Gynecological Survey, 59* (8), 628-636.

Bernhardt, J., & Dorman, K. (2004). Pre-term birth risk assessment tools. Exploring fetal fibronectin and cervical length for validating risk. *AWHONN Lifelines, 8* (1), 38-44.

Blanchard, D., & Shabetai, R. (2004). Cardiac diseases. In R. Creasy, R. Resnik, & J. Iams (Eds.), *Maternal-fetal medicine: Principles and practice* (5th ed.). Philadelphia: Saunders.

Bowes, W., & Thorp, J. (2004). Clinical aspects of normal and abnormal labor. In R. Creasy, R. Resnik, & J. Iams (eds.), *Maternal-fetal medicine: Principles and practice* (5th ed.). Philadephia: Saunders.

Boyer, S., & Boyer, K. (2004). Update on TORCH infections in the newborn infant. *Newborn and Infant Nursing Reviews, 4* (1), 70-80.

Bricker, L., & Lavender, T. (2002). Parenteral opioids for labor pain relief: A systematic review. *American Journal of Obstetrics and Gynecology, 186* (5), S94-S109.

Burton, J., & Reyes, M. (2001). Breathe in, breathe out. Controlling asthma during pregnancy. *AWHONN Lifelines, 5* (1), 24-30.

Bushy, A. (2003). Strategies to facilitate communication with clients of another culture. *Lippincott's Case Management, 8* (5), 214-223.

Cates, W., & Raymond, E. (2004). Vaginal spermicides. In R. Hatcher et al. (Eds.), *Contraceptive technology* (18th ed.). New York: Ardent Media.

Cates, W., & Stewart, F. (2004). Vaginal barriers: The female condom, diaphragm, contraceptive sponge, cervical cap, Lea's Shield and FemCap. In R. Hatcher et al. (Eds.), *Contraceptive technology* (18th ed.). New York: Ardent Media.

Centers for Disease Control and Prevention (CDC). (2004). *Rapid HIV-1 antibody testing during labor and delivery for women of unknown HIV status: A practical guide and model protocol.* Internet document available at www.cdc.gov/hiv/rapid_testing (accessed November 7, 2005).

Centers for Disease Control and Prevention (CDC). (2002). Sexually transmitted diseases treatment guidelines. *MMWR Morbidity & Mortality Weekly Report, 51* (RR-6), 1-115.

Chervenak, F., & Gabbe, S. (2002). Obstetric ultrasound: Assessment of fetal growth and anatomy. In S. Gabbe, J. Niebyl, & J. Simpson (Eds.), *Obstetrics: Normal and problem pregnancies* (4th ed.). New York: Churchill Livingstone.

Clark, S. (2004). Placenta previa and abruptio placentae. In R. Creasy, R. Resnik, & J. Iams (Eds.), *Maternal-fetal medicine: Principles and practice* (5th ed.). Philadelphia: Saunders.

Contraception Online. (2003). Facts about injectable contraception. *The Contraception Report, 14* (3). Internet document available at http://www.contraceptiononline.org/contrareport/article01.cfm?art=256 (accessed October 27, 2004).

Cooper, E. et al. (2002). Combination antiretroviral strategies for the treatment of pregnant HIV-1 infected women and prevention of perinatal HIV-1 transmission. *Journal of Acquired Immune Deficiency Syndrome, 29* (5), 484-494.

Cowles, T., & Gonik, B. (2002). Perinatal infections. In A. Fanaroff & R. Martin, *Neonatal-perinatal medicine: Diseases of the fetus and infant* (7th ed.). St. Louis: Mosby.

Cunningham, F., Leveno, K., Bloom, S., Hauth, J., Gilstrap, L., & Wenstrom, K. (2005). *Williams obstetrics* (22nd ed.). New York: McGraw-Hill.

Curran, C. (2003). Intrapartum emergencies. *Journal of Obstetric, Gynecologic, and Neonatal Nursing, 32* (6), 802-813.

Davis, M. (2004). Nausea and vomiting of pregnancy: An evidence-based review. *Journal of Perinatal & Neonatal Nursing, 18* (4), 312-328.

Dialani, V., & Levine, D. (2004). Ectopic pregnancy: A review. *Ultrasound Quarterly, 20* (3), 105-117.

DiSaia, P., & Creasman, W. (2002). *Clinical gynecologic oncology* (6th ed.). St. Louis: Mosby.

Druzin, M., Gabbe, S., & Reed, K. (2002). Antepartum fetal evaluation. In S. Gabbe, J. Niebyl, & J. Simpson (Eds.), *Obstetrics: Normal and problem pregnancies* (4th ed.). New York: Churchill Livingstone.

Duckitt, R., & Harrington, D. (2005). Risk factors for pre-eclampsia at antenatal booking: Systematic review of controlled studies. *BMJ, 330* (7491), 565.

Duff, P. (2002). Maternal and perinatal infection. In S. Gabbe, J. Niebyl, & J. Simpson (Eds.), *Obstetrics: Normal and problem pregnancies* (4th ed.). New York: Churchill Livingstone.

Easterling, T., & Otto, C. (2002). Heart disease. In S. Gabbe, J. Niebyl, & J. Simpson (Eds.), *Obstetrics: Normal and problem pregnancies* (4th ed.). New York: Churchill Livingstone.

Ellertson, C., Evans, M., Ferden, S., Leadbetter, C., Spears, A., Johnstone, K., & Trusell, J. (2003). Extending the time limit for starting the Yuzpe regimen of emergency contraception to 120 hours. *Obstetrics & Gynecology, 101* (6), 1168-1171.

Expert Committee on the Diagnosis and Classification of Diabetes Mellitus. (2003). Follow-up report on the diagnosis of diabetes mellitus. *Diabetes Care, 26*, 3160-3167.

Florence, D., & Palmer, D. (2003). Therapeutic choices for the discomforts of labor. *Journal of Perinatal & Neonatal Nursing, 17* (4), 238-249.

Flores, M. (2003). Ibuprofen: Alternative treatment for patent ductus arteriosus. *Neonatal Network, 22* (2), 26-31.

Gibbs, R., Sweet, R., & Duff, W. (2004). Maternal and fetal infectious disorders. In R. Creasy, R. Resnik, & J. Iams, *Maternal-fetal medicine: Principles and practice* (5th ed.). Philadelphia: Saunders.

Gilbert, E., & Harmon, J. (2003). *Manual of high risk pregnancy & delivery* (3rd ed.). St. Louis: Mosby.

Gluck, J., & Gluck, P. (2005). Asthma controller therapy during pregnancy. *American Journal of Obstetrics and Gynecology, 192* (2), 369-380.

Hankins, G., & Suarez, V. (2004). Rheumatologic and connective tissue disorders. In R. Creasy, R. Resnik, & J. Iams (Eds.), *Maternal-fetal medicine: Principles and practice* (5th ed.). Philadelphia: Saunders.

Harman, C. (2004). Assessment of fetal health. In R. Creasy, R. Resnik, & J. Iams (Eds.), *Maternal-fetal medicine: Principles and practice* (5th ed.). Philadelphia: Saunders.

Hatcher, R. (2004). Depo-Provera injections, implants, and progestin-only pills (minipills). In R. Hatcher et al. (Eds.), *Contraceptive technology* (18th ed.). New York: Ardent Media.

Hatcher, R., & Nelson, A. (2004). Combined hormonal contraceptive methods. In R. Hatcher et al. (Eds.), *Contraceptive technology* (18th ed.). New York: Ardent Media.

Hawkins, J., Chestnut, D., & Gibbs, C. (2002). Obstetric anesthesia. In S. Gabbe, J. Niebyl, & J. Simpson (Eds.), *Obstetrics: Normal and problem pregnancies* (4th ed.). Philadelphia: Churchill Livingstone.

Hill, J. (2004). Recurrent pregnancy loss. In R. Creasy, R. Resnik, & J. Iams (Eds.), *Maternal-fetal medicine: Principles and practice* (5th ed.). Philadelphia: Saunders.

Hodnett, E., Gates, S., Hofmeyr, G., & Sakala, C. (2003). Continuous support for women during childbirth. *Cochrane Database Systematic Reviews,* Issue 3, art, CD 003766.

Hofmeyr, G. (2005). Evidence-based intrapartum care. *Best Practices Research in Clinical Obstetrics and Gynaecology, 19* (1), 103-115.

Iams, J., & Creasy, R. (2004). Preterm labor and delivery. In R. Creasy, R. Resnik, & J. Iams (Eds.), *Maternal-fetal medicine: Principles and practice* (5th ed.). Philadelphia: Saunders.

Jenkins, T.M., & Wapner, R.J. (2004). Prenatal diagnosis of congenital disorders. In R. Creasy, R. Resnik, & J. Iams (Eds.), *Maternal-fetal medicine: Principles and practice* (5th ed.). Philadelphia: Saunders.

Jennings, V., Arevalo, M., & Kowal, D. (2004). Fertility awareness-based methods. In R. Hatcher et al. (Eds.), *Contraceptive technology* (18th ed.). New York: Ardent Media.

Kilpatrick, S., & Laros, R. (2004). Maternal hematologic disorders. In R. Creasy, R. Resnik, & J. Iams (Eds.), *Maternal-fetal medicine: Principles and practice* (5th ed.). Philadelphia: Saunders.

Kowal, D. (2004). Coitus interruptus (withdrawal). In R. Hatcher et al. (Eds.), *Contraceptive technology* (18th ed.). New York: Ardent Media.

Kriebs, J. (2002). The global reach of HIV: Preventing mother-to-child transmission. *Journal of Perinatal & Neonatal Nursing, 16* (3), 1-10.

Kuczkowski, K. (2004). Nonobstetric surgery during pregnancy: What are the risks of anesthesia? *Obstetrical and Gynecological Survey, 59* (1), 52-56.

Landon, M., Catalano, P., & Gabbe, S. (2002). Diabetes mellitus. In S. Gabbe, J. Niebyl, & J. Simpson (Eds.), *Obstetrics: Normal and problem pregnancies* (4th ed.). New York: Churchill Livingstone.

Laros, R. (2004). Thromboembolic disease. In R. Creasy & R., & J. Iams (Eds*.), Maternal-fetal medicine: Principles and practice* (5th ed.). Philadelphia: Saunders.

Lawrence, R., & Lawrence, R. (2005). *Breastfeeding: A guide for the medical profession* (6th ed.). St. Louis: Mosby.

Lieberman, E., Ernst, E., Rooks, J., Stapleton, S., & Flamm, B. (2004). Results of the national study of vaginal birth after cesarean in birth centers. *Obstetrics & Gynecology, 104* (5 Part 1), 933-942.

Ludlow, J., Evans, S., & Hulse, G. (2004). Obstetric and perinatal outcomes in pregnancies associated with illicit substance abuse. *Australian and New Zealand Journal of Obstetrics and Gynaecology, (4) 44,* 302-306.

Ludmir, J., & Stubblefield, P. (2002). Surgical procedures in pregnancy. In S. Gabbe, J. Niebyl, & J. Simpson (Eds.). *Obstetrics: Normal and problem pregnancies* (4th ed.). New York: Churchill Livingstone.

Mahlmeister, L. (2003). Nursing responsibilities in preventing, preparing for, and managing epidural emergencies. *Journal of Perinatal & Neonatal Nursing, 17* (1), 19-32.

Maloni, J. (2002). Astronauts & pregnancy bed rest: What NASA is teaching us about inactivity. *AWHONN Lifelines, 6* (4), 318-323.

Maloni, J., & Kutil, R. (2000). Antepartum support group for women hospitalized on bed rest. *MCN American Journal of Maternal/Child Nursing, 25* (4), 204-210.

Mangurten, H. (2002). Birth injuries. In A. Fanaroff & R. Martin (Eds.), *Neonatal-perinatal medicine: Diseases of the fetus and infant* (7th ed.). St. Louis: Mosby.

Martin, J.A., Hamilton, B.E., Sutton, P.D., Ventura, S.J., Menacker, F., & Munson, M.L. (2005). Births: Final data for 2003, *National Vital Statistics Report 54* (2), 1-116.

Mayberry, L., Clemmens, D., & De, A. (2002). Epidural analgesia side effects, co-interventions, and care of women during childbirth: A systematic review. *American Journal of Obstetrics and Gynecology, 186* (5), S81-S93.

Mayberry, L., Strange, L., Suplee, P., & Gennaro, S. (2003). Use of upright positioning with epidural analgesia: Findings from an observational study. *MCN American Journal of Maternal/Child Nursing, 28* (3), 152-159.

McPhaul, K. (2004). Home care security: Nurses can take simple precautions to ensure safety during home visits. *American Journal of Nursing, 104* (9), 96.

Merenstein, G., Adams, K., & Weisman, L. (2002). Infection in the neonate. In G. Merenstein & S. Gardner (Eds.), *Handbook of neonatal intensive care* (5th ed.). St. Louis: Mosby.

Moore, T. (2004). Diabetes in pregnancy. In R. Creasy, R. Resnik, & J. Iams (Eds.), *Maternal-fetal medicine: Principles and practice* (5th ed.). Philadelphia: Saunders.

Mourad, J., Elliott, J., Erickson, L., & Lisboa, L. (2000). Appendicitis in pregnancy: New information that contradicts long-held beliefs. *American Journal of Obstetrics and Gynecology, 182* (5), 1027-1029.

Myers, M., Stanberry, L., & Seward, J. (2004). Varicella-zoster virus. In R. Behrman, R. Kliegman, & H. Jenson (Eds.), *Nelson textbook of pediatrics* (17th ed.). St. Louis: Mosby.

Nader, S. (2004a). Other endocrine disorders of pregnancy. In R. Creasy, R. Resnik, & J. Iams (Eds.), *Maternal-fetal medicine: Principles and practice* (5th ed.). Philadelphia: Saunders.

Nader, S. (2004b). Thyroid disease and pregnancy. In R. Creasy, R. Resnik, & J. Iams (Eds.), *Maternal-fetal medicine: Principles and practice* (5th ed.). Philadelphia: Saunders.

National High Blood Pressure Education Program Working Group on High Blood Pressure in Pregnancy. (2000). Report of the National High blood pressure education program working group on high blood pressure in pregnancy. *American Journal of Obstetrics and Gynecology, 183* (1), S1-S22.

National Institute of Child Health and Human Development (NICHD) Research Planning Workshop. (1997). Electronic fetal heart rate monitoring: Research guidelines for interpretation. *American Journal of Obstetrics and Gynecology, 177* (6), 1385-1390.

National Institutes of Health. (2000). *Antenatal corticosteroids revisited. Consensus Development Conference Statement.* Bethesda, MD: NIH. Internet document available at www.consensus.nih.gov (accessed August 1, 2005).

Nelson, N. (1990). *Current therapy in neonatal-perinatal medicine* (2nd ed.). St. Louis: Mosby.

Nick, J. (2004). Deep tendon reflexes, magnesium, and calcium: Assessments and implications. *Journal of Obstetric, Gynecologic, and Neonatal Nursing, 22,* 221-230.

Pagana, K., & Pagana, T. (2003). *Mosby's diagnostic and laboratory test reference* (6th ed.). St. Louis: Mosby.

Parilla, B. (2002). Estimation of fetal well-being. In A. Fanaroff & R. Martin (Eds.), *Neonatal-perinatal medicine: Diseases of the fetus and infant* (7th ed.). St. Louis: Mosby.

Perinatal HIV Guidelines Working Group. (2001). *Public Health Service Task Force recommendations: Use of antiretroviral drugs in pregnant HIV-1-infected women for maternal health and interventions to reduce perinatal HIV-1 transmission in the United States.* Internet document available at www.hivatis.org (accessed July 24, 2005).

Planned Parenthood. (2004). *Diaphragms* (updated July, 2004). Internet document available at http://www.plannedparenthood.org/bc/diaphragms.htm (accessed November 27, 2004).

Pollack, A., Carignan, C., & Jacobstein, R. (2004). Female and male sterilization. In R. Hatcher et al. (Eds.), *Contraceptive technology* (18th ed.). New York: Ardent Media.

Popovich, D., & McAlhany, A. (2004). Practitioner care and screening guidelines for infants born to *Chlamydia*-positive mothers. *Newborn and Infant Nursing Reviews, 4* (1), 51-55.

Resnik, J., & Resnik, R. (2004). Post-term pregnancy. In R. Creasy, R. Resnik, & J. Iams (eds.), *Maternal-fetal medicine: Principles and practice* (5th ed.). Philadelphia: Saunders.

Roberts, J. (2004). Pregnancy-related hypertension. In R. Creasy, R. Resnik, & J. Iams (Eds.), *Maternal-fetal medicine: Principles and practice* (5th ed.). Philadelphia: Saunders.

Samuels, P. (2002). Hepatic disease. In S. Gabbe, J. Niebyl, & J. Simpson (Eds.), *Obstetrics: Normal and problem pregnancies* (4th ed.). New York: Churchill Livingstone.

Scott, L., & Abu-Hamda, E. (2004). Gastrointestinal disease in pregnancy. In R. Creasy, R. Resnik, & J. Iams (Eds.), *Maternal-fetal medicine: Principles and practice* (5th ed.). Philadelphia: Saunders.

Seidel, H., Ball, J., Dains, J., & Benedict, G. (2006). *Mosby's guide to physical examination* (6th ed.). St. Louis: Mosby.

Sepilian, V., & Wood, E. (2004). *Ectopic pregnancy.* Emedicine at www.emedicine.com/med/topic3212.htm (accessed May 2, 2005).

Shehata, H., & Okosun, H. (2004). Neurologic disorders in pregnancy. *Current Opinion in Obstetrics and Gynecology, 16* (2), 117-122.

Shevell, T., & Malone, F. (2003). Management of obstetric hemorrhage. *Seminars in Perinatology, 27* (1), 86-104.

Sibai, B. (2002). Hypertension. In S. Gabbe, J. Niebyl, & J. Simpson (Eds.), *Obstetrics: Normal and problem pregnancies* (4th ed.) New York: Churchill Livingstone.

Sibai, B. (2004). Diagnosis, controversies, and management of the syndrome of hemolysis, elevated liver enzymes, and low platelet count. *Obstetrics & Gynecology, 103* (5 Part 1), 981-991.

Sibai, B., Dekker, G., & Kupferminc, M. (2005). Pre-eclampsia. *Lancet, 365* (9461), 785-799.

Simkin, P., & Ancheta, R. (2000). *The labor progress handbook.* Malden, MA: Blackwell Science.

Simpson, J. (2002). Genetic counseling and prenatal diagnosis. In S. Gabbe, J. Niebyl, & J. Simpson (Eds.), *Obstetrics: Normal and problem pregnancies* (4th ed.). New York: Churchill Livingstone.

Simpson, K. (2002). *Cervical ripening and induction and augmentation of labor* (2nd ed.). Washington, DC: AWHONN.

Simpson, K., & Atterbury, J. (2003). Trends and issues in labor induction in the United States: Implications for clinical practice. *Journal of Obstetric, Gynecologic, and Neonatal Nursing, 32* (6), 767-779.

Simpson, K., & Knox, G. (2001). Fundal pressure during the second stage of labor: Clinical perspectives and risk management issues. *MCN American Journal of Maternal/Child Nursing, 26* (2), 64-71.

Stenchever, M., Droegemueller, W., Herbst, A., & Mishell, D. (2001). *Comprehensive gynecology* (4th ed.). St. Louis: Mosby.

Stephenson, J. (2005). Reducing HIV vertical transmission scrutinized. *Journal of the American Medical Association, 293* (17), 2079-2081.

Stevinson, C., & Ernst, E. (2001). Complementary/alternative therapies for premenstrual syndrome: A systematic review of randomized controlled trials. *American Journal of Obstetrics and Gynecology, 185* (1), 227-235.

Stewart, F., Trussell, J., & Van Look, P. (2004). Emergency contraception. In R. Hatcher et al. (Eds.), *Contraceptive technology* (18th ed.). New York: Ardent Media.

Tiran, D., & Mack, S. (2000). *Complementary therapies for pregnancy and childbirth* (2nd ed.). Edinburgh: Baillière-Tindall.

Trussell, J. (2004). Contraceptive efficacy. In R. Hatcher et al. (Eds.), *Contraceptive technology* (18th ed.). New York: Ardent Media.

Tucker, S. (2004). *Pocket guide to fetal monitoring and assessment* (5th ed.). St. Louis: Mosby.

U.S. Department of Health & Human Services & U.S. Department of Agriculture. (2005). *Dietary guidelines for Americans 2005.* Hyattsville, MD: U.S. Department of Agriculture.

Warner, L., Hatcher, R., & Steiner M. (2004). Male condoms. In R. Hatcher et al. (Eds.), *Contraceptive technology* (18th ed.). New York: Ardent Media.

Weinberg, G. (2000). The dilemma of postnatal mother-to-child transmission of HIV: To breastfeed or not? *Birth, 27* (3), 199-205.

Weiner, C., & Buhimschi, C. (2004). *Drugs for pregnant and lactating women.* New York: Churchill Livingstone.

Weiss, N., & Bernstein, P. (2000). Risk factor scoring for predicting venous thromboembolism in obstetric patients. *American Journal of Obstetrics and Gynecology, 182* (5), 1073-1075.

Whitty, J., & Dombrowski, M. (2004). Respiratory diseases in pregnancy. In R. Creasy, R. Resnik, & J. Iams (Eds.), *Maternal-fetal medicine: Principles and practice* (5th ed.). Philadelphia: Saunders.

Wilson, R. (2000). Amniocentesis and chorionic villus sampling. *Current Opinion in Obstetrics and Gynecology, 12* (2), 81-86.

World Health Organization (WHO) Department of Reproductive Health and Research. (2004). *Medical criteria for contraceptive use* (3rd ed.). Geneva: WHO.

Index

Note: Page numbers followed by f indicate figures; those followed by t indicate tables; and those followed by b indicate boxed material.